JA + BM BAKER

BIOMEDICAL ETHICS
In A Canadian Context

BIOMEDICAL ETHICS
In A Canadian Context

Eike-Henner W. Kluge

Prentice-Hall Canada, Inc., Scarborough, Ontario

To
Aara, Graeme and Hagen

Canadian Cataloguing in Publication Data
Kluge, Eike-Henner W.
Biomedical ethics in Canadian context
Includes bibliographical references and index.
ISBN 0-13-085333-X
I. Medical ethics - Canada. I. Title.
R724.K58 1992   174'.2   C91-094064-9

© 1992 Prentice-Hall Canada, Inc., Scarborough, Ontario

All rights reserved. No part of this book may be reproduced in any form without permission in writing from the publisher.

Prentice-Hall, Inc., Englewood Cliffs, New Jersey
Prentice-Hall International, Inc., London
Prentice-Hall of Australia, Pty., Ltd., Sydney
Prentice-Hall of India Pvt., Ltd., New Delhi
Prentice-Hall of Japan, Inc., Tokyo
Prentice-Hall of Southeast Asia (Pte.) Ltd., Singapore
Editora Prentice-Hall do Brasil Ltda., Rio de Janeiro
Prentice-Hall Hispanoamericana, S.S., Mexico

ISBN 0-13-085333-X

Senior Project Editor: Maurice Esses
Manufacturing Coordinator: Anna Orodi
Copy Editor: Dick Hemingway
Book Design: Keith Thompson

1 2 3 4 5   RRD   96 95 94 93 92

Printed and bound in the U.S.A. by R.R. Donnelly & Sons

Table of Contents

Preface — xi

1. Meta-Ethics: The Nature of Ethics as a Discipline — 1
Meta-Ethical Theories — 2
   Ethical Emotivism — 4
   Ethical Relativism — 6
   Ethical Objectivism — 10
   Implications — 11
Conclusion — 12

2. Ethical Systems — 16
Introduction — 16
   An Example — 18
Teleological or Consequentialistic Systems — 20
   Ethical Egoism — 20
   Utilitarianism — 21
Deontological Theories — 25
Religiously Oriented Ethical Approaches — 29
Agapistic Approaches — 30
Utilitarian versus Deontological Approaches: A Comparison — 31
The Structure of Ethical Justification — 35
   The Pre-Conventional Level — 36
   The Conventional Level — 36
   The Post-Conventional, Autonomous or Principled Level — 36
A Sample Case — 39
Conclusion — 41

3. Codes of Ethics — 45
Introduction — 46
Codes of Professional Ethics — 47
   (1) Codes as Statements of Ethos — 48
   (2) Codes as Quasi-Legal Documents — 49

(3) Codes as Statements of Role-Specific Rules Unique to a Profession but Ethically Sui Generis	50
(4) Codes as Statements of Role-Specific Rules Derived from the General Framework that Govern Personal Interaction	52
A Model Code of Ethics for Physicians	53
Conclusion	71

4. The Physician-Patient Relationship — 77

Introduction	77
Models of Physician-Patient Relationships	78
The Paternalistic or Priestly Model	78
The Agency or Engineering Model	79
The Collegial Model	80
The Contractual Model	80
The Friendship Model	81
The Fiduciary Model	81
Analysis	83
Physicians as Decision-Makers	85
Argument from the Nature of the Profession	85
Analysis and Evaluation	87
The Argument from Patient Incompetence	91
Competence	92
Conceptual Competence	92
Volitional Competence	93
Emotional Competence	94
Valuational Competence	96
Extent of (In)Competence	97
Analysis and Evaluation	98
The Argument from Practice	99
The Argument from Emergency	100
Conclusion	102

5. Informed Consent — 111

Informed Consent: Duty versus Right	114
Informed Consent: Some Considerations of Practice	114
Standards of Disclosure	114
Full Disclosure	115
Professional Disclosure	115
Subjective Disclosure	117
Objective Reasonable Person Standard	117
Standards of Understanding	118
Obtaining Consent	120
Factors Affecting Freedom of Consent	122
Cultural Parameters	122

    Non-Cultural Parameters   124
        Freedom-Limiting Parameters—External   124
        Freedom-Limiting Parameters—Internal   126
    Truth-Telling and Therapeutic Privilege   128
    Reasons for Withholding Information   129
    Harm Caused   129
    Inadvisable Choice   130
    Reduced Effectiveness   131
    Placebos   132
    Conclusion   136

6. Proxy Decision-Making   141
    Introduction   141
    Possible Proxy Decision-Makers   144
    Criteria for Proxy Decision-Making   149
    The Permanently Incompetent Patient   151
    Conclusion   155

7. Experimenting with Human Subjects   160
    Introduction   160
    Experimentation and Consent   161
    The Nature of Experimentation   162
    Why Experiment?   164
    Experimentation versus Research   165
    Therapeutic and Non-Therapeutic Experimentation   166
    Guidelines for Disclosure   167
    Discussion   169
    Freedom and Autonomy   171
    Coercion   172
    Harm   173
    Reward and Enticement   174
    Boards and the Health Care Professional   175
    Conclusion   178

8. Health Care and Health   184
    Introduction   184
    The Definition of Health   186
    Health and Values   186
    Judging and Evaluating   188
    Health as an Evaluative Concept   190
    Right to Health versus Right to Health Care   194
    Origin and Nature of the Right to Health Care   195
    Duty versus Right   197
    The Rights of the Incompetent   198
    Conclusion   200

9. Health Policy and the Allocation of Resources: The Ethics of Discrimination — 205
Introduction — 206
Global Issues — 208
  Health Care Budgets — 208
    The Socio-Economic Capabilities of Society — 208
    The Prevailing State of Medical Sophistication — 208
    Average Health Profile of Members of Society — 209
    Competing Areas of Social Endeavour — 209
    Values of Society — 209
  Orientation — 210
Limitation — 211
Macro-Allocation — 212
  Primary Macro-Allocation — 212
    Possible versus Available — 213
    Statistical Needs — 213
    Equality versus Equity — 214
  Secondary Macro-Allocation — 215
Meso-Allocation — 217
  Merit — 217
  First-Come, First-Served — 218
  Ability to Pay — 219
  General Considerations — 219
Micro-Allocation — 220
  Possibility — 223
  Need — 223
  Priority: Life-Saving versus Quality-Enhancing — 224
  Status: Child versus Adult — 224
  Origin: Auto- versus Hetero-Induced — 225
  Lots — 226
Success — 227
Extent — 229
Non-Validated and Experimental Therapies — 230
Conclusion — 230

10. The Ethics of Deliberate Death: Euthanasia — 237
Introduction — 238
Some Considerations — 239
Euthanasia — 243
Ordinary versus Extraordinary — 243
Active versus Passive Euthanasia — 246
  Causality — 249
  Ethical Responsibility — 252

Direct versus Indirect Euthanasia	253
The Morality of Euthanasia	255
Life-Centred Arguments	255
Self-Realization	257
Professional Obligation	258
Pragmatic Arguments	259
Arguments in Favour	262
Living Wills	265
Voluntary versus Non-Voluntary	267
Conclusion	268

11. Abortion and the Status of the Fetus — 275

Introduction	275
Some Initial Considerations	279
The Ethical Status of the Human Fetus	279
Is the Fetus Ever a Person?	281
Does the Fetus Have Rights?	284
What Is the Relationship between the Right to Life of the Fetal Person and the Competing Rights of Others?	286
Abortion	288
Arguments in Favour of Induced Abortion	289
Arguments against Induced Abortions	291
Conclusion	291

12. The Right to Have Children — 302

Introduction	302
Historical-Legal Considerations	304
Some Ethical Issues	305
Some Arguments for the Right to Have Children	306
Argument from Biology	306
Argument from Desire	307
Realization of Personal Potential	307
Argument from Social Expectation	309
Interim Considerations	312
Argument from the Right of Personal Integrity	314
Control of Reproduction	315
Birth Control	316
Birth Control as Such	316
Methods of Birth Control	317
Type of Control	317
Abstention	317
Contraception	317
Sterilization	318
Relationship to People's Rights	319

Sterilization of the Mentally Handicapped 321
The Incompetent's Right to Have Children 323
Conclusion 325

13. Genetic and Pre-Natal Screening 330
Introduction 330
Some Historical Considerations 332
Some Arguments Against 335
Arguments Against Screening for Carrier Status 335
Arguments Against Pre-Natal Screening 336
Some Considerations About Genetic Screening 337
Carrier Status 338
Pre-Natal Genetic Screening 339
Fetal Diagnosis: Non-Genetic Prenatal Screening 341
Sex-Determination 345
Conclusion 347

14. New Techniques of Reproductive Technology 353
Introduction 353
In Vitro Fertilization and Associated Techniques 354
General Comments 354
Analysis and Replies 357
Gene Therapy and Genetic Engineering 361
Thesis 363
Antithesis 364
Analysis 366
Somatic versus Germ Line Therapy 367
General Considerations 368
Cloning 372
Surrogate Motherhood 374
Conclusion 376

Glossary 385
Bibliography 396

Appendix 1 414
Guide To The Ethical Behaviour Of Physicians 414

Appendix 2 419
Code of Ethics: Canadian Nurses Association 419

Index 428

Preface

In the past few decades, developments in medicine, nursing and associated professions have expanded the scope of health care beyond anything that could have been imagined in the past. The speed of these developments has been breathtaking, and in many instances it has left traditional perspectives on the delivery of health care struggling to adjust.

These developments have presented contemporary society with a challenge. The challenge is not technical in nature. It is how to proceed ethically—and in what direction. This challenge has not been ignored. Our society has come to recognize that health decisions are not simply medical decisions of technology but also moral decisions that involve the relationship between health care consumers, health care professionals and society at large. As well, Canadian society has started to re-appraise its understanding of the role of the individual in the social context and has moved the patient as person to centre-stage. As a result, the delivery of public health care is increasingly coming under scrutiny; and while society continues to expect technical competence from its health care professionals, it is also coming to expect ethical competence.

But this expectation of ethical competence no longer centres in standards developed by the health care professions themselves. There is a growing conviction that ethical standards are not like the rules of a game that depend on the whim of the players and that can be changed at will. Our society is becoming more and more persuaded that if ethical rules are truly ethical in nature—that is to say, if they truly deal with rights and obligations in a moral sense and cannot be reduced to expressions of custom and standards of etiquette—then they have a fundamental basis: a basis that is the same for all members of society, the health care professions included.

In this book I have attempted to build on these developments and on that conviction. It strikes me as important that health care professionals should be properly equipped to function in an ethically sensitized environment. While in the past, learning-by-doing and following the example of revered teachers may have been sufficient to prepare health care professionals for their task, the accelerated pace of contemporary society and a climate of heightened sensitivity no longer allow for the luxury of slowly developing an appropriate ethical perspective. Contemporary society expects that its health care professional will be able to deal with the ethical issues that arise in the delivery of health care the moment they enter professional life. We may regret this; nevertheless, it is a fact.

It is therefore crucial that contemporary health care professionals have some understanding of the ethical principles that govern society in general; and more specifically, of how these principles apply to the delivery of health care itself. At the same time, I think that it is important that health care consumers also have some understanding of the ethical challenges that face the health care professions, and of their own position in all of this. They should have some feel for the complexity of ethical decision-making in the arena of health care, and should be familiar with the principles that are appealed to when health care decisions are justified in ethical terms. To assist, an extensive Glossary of medical and philosophical terms is provided at the end of the book, beginning on page 385. This extensive Glossary, as well as the Index, will be especially valuable to laypersons who are trying to come to terms with these issues and the underlying ethical principles.

The number of issues that are encompassed by the notion of ethical decision-making in health care is of course quite daunting. It includes topics such as the nature of the health care professions, their relationship to one another as well as to government, to individual health care consumers and to society at large; it involves the concepts of personhood and disease, life and death; issues such as the allocation of resources, research and experimentation, population control, genetic intervention, mental health and its relation to law—to mention but a few.

Clearly no book can touch on, let alone deal adequately with all of these topics—or with the myriad of others that stand in the wings. Nor do I intend to do so here. The purpose of this book is to set out in a systematic fashion some of the ethical considerations that health care professionals should keep in mind in the conduct of their professional lives. To this end, I try to delineate some fundamental principles and relate them to several areas that currently are under public scrutiny.

I make no claim that these principles are generally followed—or even that they are explicitly recognized in the form in which I shall discuss them. On the contrary, part of the motivation for writing this book was the conviction that frequently this is not the case; that in many instances the ethical problems that arise in the delivery of health care could have been avoided by greater familiarity with (and appropriate attention to) the ethical principles involved in a given case.

The purpose of this book is therefore quite limited. It is to provide the readers with some conceptual tools that will allow them to evaluate the actions of health care professionals from an ethical perspective.

However, even to proceed on this basis would be a blueprint for failure. The delivery of health-care in the contemporary setting involves the participation of various professions. While these professions interact with each other more or less closely, each of them has its own professional mandate and each of them has its own area of expertise. It would be impossible to do justice to these distinct perspectives in the context of a single book. The issues are far too complex, and the perspectives far too varied. A focus is needed.

Therefore, while I have tried to discuss the various issues from a diversity of viewpoints, I have placed the major focus on one profession: the profession of medicine. There are several reasons for this—over and above the need for focus itself. The first is that many of the ethical issues that arise in the practice of medicine find analogues in the conduct of the other health care professions. Informed consent, the allocation of resources and codes of professional ethics are but three of a series of examples. (The *Guide to the Ethical Behaviour of Physicians* and *Code of Ethics: Canadian Nurses Association* are reproduced in the Appendices to this volume, beginning on page 414.) In these cases, what is said with respect to the practice of medicine can easily be transferred, with due alteration of detail, to the conduct of the other health care professions.

The second reason is that whether we like it or not, physicians are the major players in the arena of health care. They exercise tremendous control over who has access to health care, over the direction that health care takes, and how health care decisions are made at the level of the individual person. Therefore, it strikes me as appropriate that the ethics of medical practice should receive special consideration. By this I do not mean that the ethics of medical practice is somehow special in itself. I mean only that it should be considered carefully by all who become involved in health care, whether as suppliers of that care or as consumers.

Third, it seems to me that as a matter of general policy, the process of health care decision-making should be an open one. It should be based on ethical principles that apply to all people and that all people can understand. Focusing on ethical considerations as they apply to physicians, is to take one step closer to that goal. It is to lay open to non-physicians some of the ethical considerations that physicians should take into account in the ethics of their practice.

At the same time it is to assist physicians themselves. Because in all fairness, it is important to recognize that being a physician can sometimes be a very isolating experience. The majority of Canadians look to their physicians for more than merely technical help. They also look to them for personal guidance when they make their own health care decisions. That imposes a tremendous burden on the average physician: a burden whose nature the budding physician may not have realized at the outset of his or her career, but a burden that can take its toll in terms of addiction, broken marriages, suicide and other personal problems later on.[1] If physicians are familiar with the principles of medical ethics and how they apply to the various cases, and if patients are familiar with the ethical parameters that should guide physicians in their daily practice, then perhaps the two may mutually assist each other in the development of a less stressful and a more ethically oriented system of health care delivery. And if the other health care professions can be alive to some of the considerations that will be raised in the discussion of medicine, and if they can transfer some of the considerations to their own areas of practice, this effort may then foster a process of integration that will benefit the delivery of health care as a whole.

Finally, proceeding in this way also has a pragmatic purpose. The ethics of nursing has already received some discussion in the Canadian context. There is no such book on the ethics of the medical profession in the Canadian setting. This book, therefore, will fill a gap.

However, not all of the examples that will be used or issues that will be discussed will be drawn from the medical profession. There is a host of issues that concern other health care professionals as much as they do physicians. I have already identified some of them. They include informed consent, allocation of resources, competence, and so on. Furthermore, and perhaps much more importantly, most of these issues also concern the health care consumer, both on the individual level as patient, as well as in an aggregate sense, as society. The discussion that follows will attempt to indicate where and why the relevant issues arise, why they are issues, and the considerations that should guide the various players if they are to interact in an ethical fashion. The underlying principle will always be this: All participants, whether they be professionals or patients, are part of society. They are embedded in a social context that not only defines what they can do in a material sense, but also what they should (or should not) do in an ethical one. While the roles that the various individuals play may be different, the ethical principles that should guide how they engage in these roles are the same for all.

As I said, this book covers a host of issues. They range from codes of professional ethics to allocation of resources to reproductive technology. However, just as one cannot hope to deal with these issues from all possible perspectives, neither can one deal with all of them or to any great depth. I have therefore been selective in what I have included; and even topics that I have selected I have considered only as far as is necessary to allow some insight into the ethical principles that apply. My primary concern has been to provide some feel for how these principles function when trying to develop an ethically defensible solution to a particular issue. Readers who wish to pursue prticular topics in greater depth should consult the annotated list of Suggested Readings at the end of each chapter.

In other words, the overall purpose of this book is to provide an introductory schematic for how an ethically sophisticated physician might proceed in practice. The details of its application will depend on the will of the physician, the position of the patient and of the other health care professionals, and on the material facts of each case. Since it is intended primarily for the Canadian context, I have tried to use Canadian courts cases and have relied on Canadian authors whenever possible.

I owe thanks to the many persons who, over the years, have assisted me in developing and refining my views on ethics: Special thanks are due to the physicians and hospitals who, over the years, entrusted me with the responsibility of giving ethical advice—and for making sure that I experienced at first hand what the implications of that advice would look like; and to my legal colleagues, whose unfailing counsel has always been a source of joy. Of course paramount thanks are due to the patients who had faith in the process of ethical practice. Special thanks are due to the people who taught me: to Richard Brandt who originally taught me what a utilitarian approach to ethics looked like—and who so candidly admitted the shortcomings of such an approach; to William K. Frankena who, as my graduate advisor, taught me the nature and basis of a deontological perspective—and who was equally as candid in admitting its limitations; to Abe Melden, whose discussions during the years that he was my colleague deepened the understanding that I had gained; and to J.O. Urmson and H.D. Aiken who took me further down that road. Thanks also to John Burns, who made me examine my commitment to the patient as person. Finally, I owe special thanks to the students on whom I tried out many of the ideas that are contained in this book, and who challenged me with their comments and criticisms.

ENDNOTE

[1] See W.E. McAuliffe, M. Rohman, S. Santagelo, B. Feldman, E. Magnuson, A. Sobol and J. Weisman, "Psychoactive Drug Use Among Practising Physicians and Medical Students," *New England Medical Journal* 315: 13 (Sept. 25, 1986): 805–810; H.D. Kleber, "The Impaired Physician: Changes from the Traditional View," *Journal of Substance Abuse Treatment* 1: 2 (1984): 137–140; D. Hilfiker, *Healing the Wounds* (New York: Pantheon Books, 1985).

1
Meta-Ethics: The Nature of Ethics as a Discipline

> The new problem emerging for the 1990's shifts to the level of meta-ethics. It has to do with the nature of moral authority and what kinds of questions medical experts legitimately can answer ... The notion of a standard treatment, medically indicated treatment, or treatment of choice will be essentially seen from an evaluative stance—and an evaluation about which physicians have no particular expertise.
>
> Robert M. Veatch, *Medical Ethics Advisor* 6: 1(1990) p. 2.

This chapter introduces the reader to ethics as a discipline. It will also try to give the reader some reasons for accepting ethical objectivism rather than ethical relativism and ethical emotivism. At the end of this chapter, the reader should have some understanding of the difference between meta-ethics and ethics; be familiar with the difference between ethical emotivism, relativism, absolutism; and have some grasp of why ethical objectivism is the preferred meta-ethical approach in Canadian society. In order to achieve this end, it may help the reader to focus on the following questions:

1. What is a meta-ethical theory?
2. What is the point of a meta-ethical theory?
3. What is the difference between ethical relativism, ethical objectivism and ethical emotivism?
4. What meta-ethical theories are most commonly used in social practice in our society?

Meta-Ethical Theories

The *Code of Ethics* of the Canadian Medical Association starts with the following heading:

> Principles of Ethical Behaviour for all physicians, including those who may not be engaged directly in clinical practice.

It then lists seven principles that are supposed to guide the behaviour of "individual physicians and provincial authorities."[1]

The *Code of Ethics for Nursing* of the Canadian Nurses Association includes the following statements in the preamble to the *Code* itself:

> This Code expresses and seeks to clarify those ethical principles that are definitive of ethical nursing activity. For those entering the profession, this Code identifies the basic moral commitments of nursing and may serve as a source for education and reflection. For those within the profession, the Code also serves as a basis for self-evaluation and for peer review. For those outside the profession, this Code may serve to establish the expectations regarding ethical conduct of nurses.[2]

The passages that we have just quoted indicate that so far as the two major Canadian professional health care associations are concerned, there are certain types of behaviour that are ethically acceptable for their members in the delivery of health care and other types of behaviour that are not.

This perspective is not a uniquely Canadian phenomenon. It is shared by other professional health care associations all over the world. *The Code of Ethics of the American Medical Association, The International Council of Nurses Code of Ethics, The Royal College of Nursing Code of Professional Conduct, The Code of Ethics of the British Medical Association*—to mention but a few—all bear witness to this fact.

The question is, of course, whether all these associations are right. Are there things that are ethically acceptable or unacceptable in some absolute sense? Things that are ethically mandatory, forbidden or allowed? The short answer is—it all depends on how we understand the notion of ethics.

There are several ways in which the notion of ethics can be understood. One way is to see ethical statements merely as reflections or expressions of people's emotions. Therefore, according to this approach, if a particular code says that health care professionals should not kill patients who have an incurable disease it is not saying something that is true or false. It is merely expressing the feelings of the authors of the code. Similarly, if a code says that abandoning patients is prohibited it is not asserting some fundamental principle. It is merely expressing the feelings of the professionals who subscribe to the code. The code simply reflects their aversion to such behaviour.

A second approach to ethics says that the sorts of statements mentioned above and indeed statements of right and wrong in general, deal with more than merely emotions. According to this interpretation, ethical statements say something meaningful and cognitively significant, and make certain claims about the world. Therefore, according to this perspective, when a code says that killing incurable patients is wrong, it is doing more than merely expressing the feelings of the profession. It is saying, in fact, that the profession takes such killing to be wrong in some cognitive sense.

Moreover, according to this second approach, the validity of ethical claims is not absolute. It is relative. It may be relative to a given culture, to a given profession, or even to a specific person. According to this perspective there is no such thing as an absolute right or an absolute wrong. Different people, different professions, different groups and different cultures may have different points of view. For example, in Canada it is considered wrong to euthanatize defective newborns but it is considered acceptable in China. Muslim countries generally regard abortion as ethically indefensible, whereas those countries who do not subscribe to fundamental Islamic teachings—countries such as Canada and the U.S.—view it in an entirely different light.[3] Therefore according to this perspective all ethical principles and all ethical assertions are relative to the point of view of those who subscribe to them. Consequently the code of ethics of a health care profession would also have merely relative validity—relative to the profession that enunciates or promulgates it.

A third approach disagrees with both of these perspectives. It holds that there is an ethical right and an ethical wrong, and that being ethically right or wrong is neither something relative nor a reflection of how we feel about the matter. In this view, right and wrong are objective phenomena. It is up to us, as ethical people, to find out what they are and to act accordingly.

The first approach is called ethical emotivism; the second, ethical relativism; and the third, ethical objectivism. The difference between them is fundamental. It is also important because which one we accept determines what relevance we attach to ethical principles and, through them, to ethical judgements.

If we accept ethical emotivism, then the principles of any code of ethics—for example, of the *Code of Ethics* of the Canadian Medical Association or the *Code of Ethics For Nursing* of the Canadian Nurses Association—are merely more or less sophisticated expressions of a particular emotive stance. According to this, statements such as "Murder is wrong!"—or perhaps more to the point, "A nurse is obliged to treat clients with respect for their individual needs and values,"[4] or "An ethical physician will recognize that the patient has the right to accept or reject any physician and any medical care recommended to him,"[5]—have no greater binding force than exhortatory exclamations or disapproving grunts. Disagreement between people who hold different ethical positions have no more significance than a difference in emotional perspective.

On the other hand, if we accept ethical relativism our ethical statements will at least have cognitive significance. However, all of them will carry the implicit rider, "From our point of view!" For example, the statement "It is unethical to allow an incurable patient to die!" would be qualified by the tacit rider "so far as we are concerned." This would leave open the possibility that others might disagree with us, and that from their perspective allowing incurable patients to die would be perfectly acceptable.

However, if we did accept ethical relativism, ethical disagreement would still be impossible with people who did not share our basic principles. What was accepted by the one individual or group of individuals or even culture as being right (or wrong) would not be the same as what was accepted as being right (or wrong) by another individual, group of individuals or culture in the same setting. Therefore even though at first glance all of them would be talking about the same thing and making mutually opposed judgements, in actuality there would be no disagreement. After all, in this approach all ethical claims would carry the implicit rider "from my (our) point of view." Therefore, what at first glance looked like a disagreement would in fact be crossed monologues. Any arguments about basic ethical principles would be ruled out because to have a genuine disagreement there would have to be a prior agreement on the principles—which by definition is not the case.

Both ethical emotivism and ethical relativism have their points. Ethical claims do tend to be emotionally highly charged, and in many cases ethical disagreements merely become sophisticated yelling. It is fairly obvious there is no one set of ethical standards or imperatives accepted by all people. Different cultures have what look to be quite distinct stances and what is right in one setting may not be what is right in another.[6] For that matter, it may not even be right in the same culture at different times in its history. Capital punishment, slavery, and sexual discrimination are but three of many examples of attitudes and values in a culture changing over time. Such changes also occur even for different individuals within the same culture.

Considerations like these present a formidable challenge to systematic and reasoned health care ethics. Unless they can be met the very point of reasoning and of discussion is lost and the solution to ethical disagreement would then lie not in discussion and understanding but in political manoeuvring or even the use of force. This would be extremely troublesome in the Canadian context, with its deliberate and conscious acceptance of cultural diversity.

Of course, from a purely pragmatic standpoint it does not really matter whether we accept ethical objectivism as a matter of personal conviction. The main body of current medical ethics is based on the assumption that it is correct, and the ethics of medical decision-making is evaluated in that light. However, it is always easier to operate according to certain rules if they at have least a semblance of reasonableness about them. We shall therefore try to give some reasons for accepting ethical objectivism; and we shall do so by examining ethical emotivism and ethical relativism in terms of their own logic and in terms of how they agree with actual social practice.

Ethical Emotivism

The practical basis of ethical emotivism is the fact that ethical disagreement can be a highly emotional affair. All of us have found on occasion that disagreement over what we consider unethical can easily turn into a highly charged confrontation of attitudes where no amount of reasoning is likely to convince the other party. Even when our—or, for that matter the other person's—logic is shown to be faulty, we still tend to insist on our position because it just "feels" right. "I just know I'm right" or "I can't argue with you—you just don't see!" are expressions that capture our attitude very well.

It is this fact of unshakeable emotional commitment that has led some ethical emotivists to conclude that it is the emotional commitment itself that is really the focus of ethical judgements: that ethical judgements are nothing more than sophisticated verbal expression of an emotional conviction. According to them, "Murder is wrong!" really amounts to "Murder: Booh!"; "Kindness is ethically laudatory" into "Kindness, Yeah!", etc.[7]

Of course, not all emotivists have been so radical in their position. Some have admitted that ethical statements do have cognitive components. They have said that while ethical judgements are essentially nothing more than sophisticated emotional exclamations, they also involve an attempt to evoke similar attitudes in others.[8] More recently, some ethical emotivists have gone further still and have presented ethical judgements as convoluted attempts to recommend a certain kind of behaviour to others—linguistic expressions of our willingness to generalize or universalize the attitudes contained in and expressed by the relevant expressions.[9]

However, no matter how one approaches ethical emotivism the fact remains that it faces some serious objections. First, we do genuinely disagree over ethical matters—and this disagreement is more than merely a disagreement in our attitudes. Second, while our ethical positions—what we take to be ethically right or wrong, etc.,—have strong emotional overtones, for all that they are not identical with these emotions themselves.

An example may illustrate the first of these points. Suppose someone were to say, "Euthanasia is wrong!" or "Physicians have a duty treat AIDS patients without discrimination!" and suppose that someone were to reply, "So that is how you feel about the matter." Suppose further that the first person were to respond, "No, it's not merely how I feel about it—although, of course, I do—it's also true!" We would not feel that such a response was inappropriate.

In other words, the fact that the first person's response distinguished between the emotive aspect of these ethical assertions and the claim that they are true would not strike us as confused, but simply as setting the record straight. We would agree that while these claims may involve or evoke emotional reactions, we would not feel that it was these emotive parameters that were at issue but rather that the real issue was which one of these positions is correct. However, with this we would in fact be accepting the claim that there is a distinction between the emotive and the cognitive parameters of ethical assertions.

As to the distinction between the emotive stance adopted by people and what they are is saying in ethical terms, the following may serve to illustrate this distinction:

> Dr. B. is a physician in a community in southern Saskatchewan. One of Dr. B's patients, who suffers from impaired kidney function, comes to Dr. B. and announces that she is pregnant. Dr. B. examines the young woman, performs the appropriate

tests, verifies the fact of pregnancy but discovers that the young woman's kidney function is increasingly compromised by the pregnancy. In Dr. B's estimation, if the young woman goes ahead with the pregnancy, her health may well be seriously compromised. Dr. B. consults with some experts, who confirm her diagnosis and prognosis. Dr. B. counsels the young woman and explains to her that there are medical indications for performing an abortion. The young woman decides to have an abortion. However, in all of this Dr. B. has not let the young woman know that her own private morality is opposed to abortions. Dr. B. accepts intellectually that the choice belongs to the young woman: that she has the right to decide whether she wants an abortion; but at the same time Dr. B. has tremendous emotional difficulties with what this entails.

If ethical emotivism were correct—that is to say, if ethical judgements were simply more or less sophisticated expressions and/or reflections of a particular emotive stance—Dr. B. could not have done what she did. She could not have accepted that *ethically* the young woman had a right to have an abortion, while emotionally rejecting her choice on a private level.[10]

Ethical Relativism

While emotivist meta-ethical theories are essentially non-cognitivistic in nature—that is to say, while emotivist theorists say that ethical theories really have no cognitive meaning but only emotive content—both ethical objectivism and ethical relativism stand at the other conceptual extreme. Both maintain that ethical statements are cognitively significant; and while they accept that ethical statements may evoke emotional associations, their significance does not lie in the associations themselves.

However, at this point the two part company. Ethical relativism maintains that the ethical assertions are not absolutely valid. It contends that each ethical judgement carries the tacit rider that it is a judgement from-a-certain-point-of-view, and that it holds only for the particular person who makes it or for the conceptual or cultural framework within which it is made.[11] In this approach, statements like "It is unethical for nurses to withhold medicines from their patients!" "To participate in an abortion is to participate in murder!" are really short for something like "From the perspective of the Canadian Nurses Association it is unethical for nurses to withhold medicines from their patients!" and "From our perspective to participate in abortion is to participate in murder!"

Persons who share the same conceptual framework—as for instance members of the same culture, sub-culture, or even group—will probably share the same ethical tenets.[12] Others, however, whose values differ, probably will not. Therefore, they need not and perhaps will not agree with these ethical judgements even if they are able to understand them.

Ethical relativism therefore maintains that there are no absolute ethical truths and no universal ethical tenets binding on all people. As an ethical theory, it has a fairly ancient lineage. Already in ancient Greece certain well-travelled individuals[13] noted that the customs and laws of different states frequently differed; sometimes even fundamentally so. What was considered right or wrong in one society did not necessarily have the same status in another, and vice versa, and standards and injunctions could not be generalized. In fact, they found that the only safe generalization they could make was that conceptions of right and wrong were state-relative. From this they concluded that therefore there are no universal ethical standards, and that ethical judgements are relative to their particular social dimensions.

In more recent times social scientist have adduced a similar line of reasoning. For instance, they have argued that because some cultures practise infanticide, therefore infanticide cannot be wrong absolutely speaking but only from our perspective;[14] that because public execution for marital infidelity is practised in some cultures, it cannot be ethically objectionable in an absolute sense but only from our particular point of view, and so on. The bottom line is always the same: there are no universal ethical laws, no universal ethical standards, because as a matter of fact none are universally shared.

There is something very comforting and convenient about ethical relativism. If ethical judgements are framework-relative, and if different cultures operate with different valuational concepts, then no matter how heinous the practices of a given culture may seem to others, so long as they are justifiable in terms of the ethical concepts of the culture in which they are practised, they are above reproach. The other society's condemnation might be anthropologically interesting, but it can go no further. At least not in any ethically relevant sense. Therefore, all other things being equal, ethical relativism leaves the actions of individuals and groups immune from outside attack.

Criticism of Relativism

However, despite its appeal, it strikes us that there are several points on which this line of approach can be criticized. The first was already pointed over two thousand years ago by Socrates: ethical relativism confuses the question of what is the case—of what as a matter of fact is believed, legislated, or otherwise promulgated as correct by a group of individuals—with the question whether people who believe this are correct in doing so. Believing that one is right does not necessarily make one right—in ethics any more than in mathematics or in embryology. (1)

begs Q

A second point is that this approach involves a version of what could be called (2) a consensus theory of truth. This theory of truth would assume that something is true if and only if everybody agrees with it. Conversely, the theory would hold that if someone disagrees with a proposition, then it is not true. The reasoning that underlies the argument in favour of ethical relativism seems to be that if there were universal agreement on ethical propositions, then they would be binding on everybody.[15] However, since there is no such agreement, it follows that no ethical injunction is universally binding.

However, a moment's reflection shows that this consensus approach would be rather silly. Universal agreement does not make statements true. We merely have to recall the history of witchcraft, of chemistry and physics, and even medicine itself. All sorts of propositions were universally accepted—like the claim that witches could change into cats, that combustion is due to phlogiston, that nature abhors a vacuum and that melancholy is due to an imbalance of the four humors. However, that did not make these propositions true.

Furthermore, strictly logically speaking, it does not follow from the fact that there is no universal agreement on matters of ethics that therefore there are no universally valid ethical propositions. Logically, there could be all sorts of reasons for the fact that people don't agree on such propositions—including the possibility that people are just not sufficiently sophisticated to appreciate and understand the nature of ethical statements themselves. The work of Kohlberg and Piaget should be remembered in this regard.[16]

On the other hand, even if there were universal agreement, this would not establish the validity of ethical claims. Racial discrimination could not be ethically justified in this fashion—and neither could the claim that we ought to kill socially useless people, the thesis that one sex is superior to the other, and so on. We could (and probably would) still ask, "But is that really ethically defensible?"[17] If agreement guaranteed truth, that question could be meaningless. But it is not. Therefore, there is a difference between being accepted, universally or otherwise, and being ethically true.

It is also possible to question ethical relativism from a more pragmatic viewpoint: If it was correct, then social practice would be fundamentally at variance with it. For instance, those who sat in judgement and who prosecuted Nazi war criminals during the Nuremberg trials did not justify their judgements by saying, "We are the stronger, therefore we will judge according to our own ethical standards. Your actions are ethically above reproach when considered from the viewpoint of your own system; but since we have prevailed over you by force of arms and can enforce our standards, we will judge you according to them." Rather, they believed that no matter what was accepted or legitimate according to the standards of the accused, what the accused did was ethically wrong in some absolute sense that transcended individual ethical frameworks. The accused knew or should have known this. The fact that Nazi society at the time accepted their behaviour was not accepted as exculpation.

We submit that the prosecution at Nuremberg was quite correct in adopting this approach. Nothing else would have given their judgements ethical legitimacy. The reason war criminals were condemned by the Nuremberg tribunal was not that the killing of millions in concentration camps was wrong according to the standards of the victors. Unless there are universal and non-relative ethical principles, the prosecutors would have had to say that the criminals were ethically every bit as good as their judges; that it was merely the fact that the prosecutors were on the winning side that gave their judgements validity. After all, the actions of the accused were justified according to their own personal perspectives.

We can generalize this beyond the context of Nuremberg. We frequently make ethical claims about practices in other societies and the principles that supposedly motivate them. We condemn the torture and repression in countries like Peru and Chile; we object to the deliberate killing of female infants in countries like China;

and we maintain that drug trafficking is ethically reprehensible no matter what. Our critique of these things is not blunted by the realization that these practices may well be defensible within the framework of the other society or from the perspective of the other point of view. On the contrary: We decry the very fact of such ethical divergence as being fundamentally misguided.

An ethical relativists could of course attempt to explain this away as a logical aberration of social practice, and as illegitimate in itself. However, by doing so, the relativist would be overstepping the limits of our credulity. We generally do not think that we are engaged in an enterprise of crossed monologues when we debate with someone who does not share our ethical principles; nor do we think the application of our ethical standards to war criminals, murderers, drug traffickers and the like reduces to a question of force. Or on a more positive note: We usually do not think that the obligation to help the less fortunate in other countries—the starving and dispossessed, the diseased and otherwise needy— is merely a relative matter that disappears when we adopt a different perspective. We think that there is an absolute ethical obligation to help these people, irrespective of what our personal beliefs or cultural context may be. We would condemn the adoption of principles that did away with such an obligation as a deliberate and callous perversion of the true ethical state of affairs.

When it comes to actual practice, therefore, ethical relativism ceases to be fashionable and goes by the board.

There is a reason for this. It lies in the realization that ethical judgements are not moves within conceptual games, where different players may operate with different premises and play according to different rules. We generally believe that in some way or other, ethical judgements are statements about the world. We tend to believe that opposing ethical judgements about people are genuinely in conflict with each other. We also tend to accept that they cannot both be true; that at least one of them must be unacceptable. And here it is no good replying that ethical judgements always carry the rider, "according to my point of view," "according to system x," or some such. We still want to ask, "But does your point of view (system x, etc.) correctly characterize the ethical state of affairs? " That question lies at the very heart of ethical disagreement. It is not answered by pointing to the fact of disagreement itself.

We can put the point differently. When people disagree in their ethical assessments of a given situation—say, of the acceptability of abortion—we cannot convince them that they are wrong by showing them that the position of the people with whom they disagree follows from the other people's moral premises. It is these very premises that are being rejected. Disagreements in ethics cannot be solved by establishing the internal consistency of the ethical claims that are made. To assume that is to confuse derivation with ethical validity. That is to say, it is to confuse the question of whether certain judgements follow from the basic concepts of a particular ethical framework, with the question of whether these concepts and the judgements based on them capture the ethical aspects of the world.

Ethical Objectivism

In actual practise, then, what is ethically right and wrong, obligatory or permissible, forbidden or allowed, is not considered a relative matter. We take it to be a question about the ethical facts of the world.

However, if we assumed that there are objective ethical facts, what would they be like?

It is difficult to answer this question. However, it may help to think of them as emergent in nature. The notion of emergence can be illustrated from the context of everyday life by considering such things as the taste of a cookie. The taste we experience is a result of the chemical properties of the flour, the sugar, the spices, their interaction with our tongue, the nerves in our tongue, our brain, and so on. However, the fact of the matter is that there is nothing like the taste we experience in the basic material constituents of the cookie we eat. A cookie is composed of atoms and molecules that have electromagnetic, nuclear, and other properties. The interrelationship and combination of these propeties gives rise to the properties of the cookie. At the same time, these new properties are not mere summations of the more basic properties. They are new and qualitatively distinct in nature with a logic all their own.

We find another example in the human brain. The individual neurons that make up the brain are not themselves conscious or aware in any sense. They are merely electrochemically active. However, the integrated firing of these neurons gives rise to a wholly new type of phenomenon: conscious awareness. The individual mind emerges as a totally different, totally new entity at the level of the brain functioning as a whole. It cannot be reduced to the activities, natures, and qualities of any neuron or group of neurons.[18]

We can find another illustration of this when we look at the behaviour of population groups. The behaviour of these groups is very real and predictable. However, it is not merely a summation of the behaviour of individual members of the group. The mutually affective interrelations between individual members give rise to social profiles whose qualitative nature is quite distinct from that of individual persons. Social psychology and sociology are based on this fact.

These examples illustrate the ubiquity of emergence-relations in ordinary life. However, they also allow us to make two observations that are very important to applied ethics.

First, to be aware of something that is emergent in nature, and to appreciate its nature as emergent, requires a perspective whose logic is more elevated than the logic of the more basic entities that give rise to the emergent thing. Since emergence is a function of relations among more basic entities, an awareness of an emergent property requires that we transcend that level. To use an example we gave before, a neuron cannot be aware of the awareness of the brain of which it is a part. Not all people are capable of an awareness that encompasses their social relations as a whole. This is important for applied ethics, because some people remain tied to the level of individual agents without ever being able to see them in the context of social interactions. Such individuals are ethically blind.[19]

Second, the relations that allow something to emerge in this sense can hold only between things that have a certain qualitative nature. For instance, no matter how cookies and marbles are combined, they will not give rise to something that is consciously aware. Emergent qualities, therefore, are not to be found in any and all contexts: only when certain preconditions are met.

What, then, are emergent entities? To give a proper philosophical account of them would transcend the scope of the present discussion. The most we can say here is that emergent entities are ontologically complex: they are, so to speak, their ontologically more primitive parts—but their parts-in-relation.

Implications

If this is correct, then several things follow. First, it follows that ethical properties and relations, in particular rights and obligations, are objective. They come into being as soon as people enter into interrelationships with each other in the appropriate way.

Second, the fact that these ethical properties and relations are objective does not entail that everyone will be aware of them—any more than the objective nature of numbers and number-relations, or of sociological and psychological facts, entails that everyone will know them. In each case, awareness of them requires a certain level of conceptual sophistication. We should therefore not be surprised that people disagree on matters of ethics.[20] If developmental psychologists and social psychologists are right, people mature and develop in different ways and at different rates. The nature and direction of their cognitive development is also influenced by the culture in which they live, the challenges they face and so on. Therefore it would be surprising if all people did in fact agree in their ethical perspectives.

Third, it follows that ethical rights and obligations, etc., cannot be discussed in the same way and on the same level as other things, like hot-dogs, cats or paper airplanes, nor be treated like contractual arrangements. Their logic is different and we should not expect ethical terms to yield non-ethical analysis.

Fourth, we would expect ethical facts and relations to be situation dependent. Since they depend on the natures of individuals that give rise to them through their interrelationship and on the natures of these relationships themselves, we would expect that variations in any one these will yield different ethical facts.

However, we must be careful here. This does not mean that ethics is relative after all. We can use the analogy of sociology to illustrate the point. Sociology deals with patterns of interrelationship among groups of people. It tries to express these in terms of sociological laws. However, the fact that are such general law-like patterns does not mean that they will manifest themselves in the same way all the time. How they manifest themselves on a given occasion is a function of the specific nature of the groups of people involved and the material facts of the case. However—and this is the point of the analogy—this does not mean that therefore these sociological laws or general patterns are relativistic.

If ethical objectivism is correct, then a similar thing is true of ethics. The fact, if it is a fact, that there are objective ethical patterns or laws does not mean that they must express themselves in the same way all the time. On the contrary. What it means is that how they manifest themselves is a function of the particular nature of the context. And this has one further consequence that is very important: It means that ethical judgements require careful attention to the particulars of the specific cases.[21]

For the rest of this book we shall adopt an objectivist approach to ethics; and when we use the term "ethics" we mean it in this objectivist sense.

Conclusion

What, then is ethics? That is to say, what is ethics in the objectivist sense?

As a discipline, it is a branch of philosophy. It deals with questions of right and of wrong conduct; with what we ought to do and what ought to refrain from doing, and what we may do if we please. It considers issues of rights and obligations, and tries to determine what this means for individual people and how such rights and obligations are related to the social context in which people are embedded.

Ethics is not the only discipline that deals with such issues. Law and theology, psychology and sociology as well as other disciplines deal with them as well. However, what distinguishes ethics from these disciplines is its methodology, its basic operating assumption, and the nature of its claims.

Ethics differs from psychology and sociology in that it is prescriptive in nature and not descriptive. What this means is that ethics is not concerned with how individuals or groups of people feel—or even the reasons why they feel in a certain way. Nor does it focus on the customs that groups of people follow and have adopted as a matter of historical fact. Such data are of interest to ethics only insofar as they are the basis of a quite different question: whether people *ought* to follow these customs or whether they *ought* behave in these ways.

Furthermore, ethics does not try to answer these questions by looking at what people have decided to do as a matter of social rules or convention, or by considering the nature and origin of the psychological make-up that characterizes a certain point of view. Instead, ethics tries to deduce its claims from basic ethical principles, or by looking at the nature of what it is to be a person and from the nature of human social interaction itself.

In a sense, then, ethics is much more like law and religion. Law and religion are also prescriptive. They also lay out what people ought to do and how they ought to behave. However, both law and religion differ from ethics in the source and nature of their pronouncements. Law is largely concerned with the rules that a particular society has chosen to govern the behaviour of its members. These rules may be rooted in tradition, as in the common law tradition of the English-speaking world; or they may be the outcome of conscious decisions by a legislative body, as in statute-law of countries like France and Germany; or they may be the result of a combination of both—as in Canada, with its civil tradition in Quebec and its common-law tradition in the other provinces.

However, no matter how these rules or laws are derived, they are not the result of an analysis of ethical principles or based on what it is to be a person. Furthermore, laws have binding power only within in the political boundaries that define a nation. If they have applicability beyond that—as for example with some so-called international laws like those that prohibit slavery—then it is rooted in an agreement among the nations themselves.[22]

As to religion, it also tells people what they ought to do or what they ought to refrain from doing. If the injunctions are peripheral to the religion, then they are sometimes justified in terms of a process of reasoning that involves other injunctions and beliefs. However, the central and basic injunctions of a religion are not open to such a discussion. They find their basis in some belief or series of beliefs whose acceptability is not open to debate. The believer must either accept this belief or cease to be a member of that religion. An example would be the belief of a Christian Scientists that disease is the result of insufficient faith and therefore can be cured by restoring faith to an appropriate level and in an appropriate fashion; or the belief of Jehovah's Witnesses that the use of blood contravenes a fundamental law of God; or, finally, the belief of some traditional Christian sects that contraception is against God's dictates. While religion allows reasoning about rules and prescriptions of behaviour, it allows this only within the framework of beliefs that are fundamental to be religion itself. This does not man that religions may not contain ethical rules and principles. Most religions do. It just means that the way these principles function, and their ultimate justification, is fundamentally different.

Objectivist ethics claims universal validity, rationality and objectivity. It claims that the rules, principles or injunctions with which it deals are not pronouncements that are discovered by some special gift or insight. Nor are they mere reflections of some tradition. Instead, it maintains that they are objective statements that describe certain kinds of relationships that hold between persons within a social context. These relationships are best expressed by using terms like "ought," "right," and "duty," and by considerations that deal with autonomy, beneficence, and the like.

By laying claim to universal validity, ethics does not maintain that therefore everyone will behave ethically or that therefore everyone will accept the same ethical standards. That would be like saying that since the structure of social dynamics follows certain principles studied in sociology, therefore every member of society was aware of them. Such awareness presupposes a certain level of conceptual sophistication and insight. Not everyone has that. And so it is with ethics.

ENDNOTES

[1] *Code of Ethics*, The Canadian Medical Association (Ottawa, December 1986), reproduced in Appendix 1.

[2] *Code of Ethics for Nursing*, Canadian Nurses Association (Ottawa: 1990) 7, reproduced in Appendix 2.

[3] For a good presentation of different cultural values and their impact on the ethics of health care decisions-making, see proceedings of the *Conference on Transcultural Dimensions* (Washington: Fidia Research Group, 1990)

[4] CNA *Code*, Value I, 13.

[5] The Royal College of Physicians and Surgeons of Canada, clause 5.

[6] See note 3, above.

[7] See A.J. Ayer, *Language, Truth and Logic* (Gollanz: London 1948) Ch.6.

[8] See C.L. Stevenson, *Ethics and Language* (New Haven: Yale University Press, 1944).

[9] See R.M. Hare, *The Language of Morals* (Oxford: Oxford University Press, 1952) for a critical discussion of ethical emotivism. For a more detailed analysis, see R.B. Brandt, *Ethical Theory* (Englewood Cliffs, N.J.: Prentice Hall, 1959).

[10] Someone might attempt to explain such a stance in terms of self-deception. However, it is not at all clear that such an attempt would be successful, since it would have to deny the reality of the overt emotional stance. For an interesting recent discussion of emotion, see Robert M. Gordon, *The Structure of Emotions: Investigations in Cognitive Philosophy* (New York: Cambridge University Press, 1987).

[11] See R.B. Perry, *Realms of Value* (Cambridge, Mass.: Harvard University Press, 1954) and E. Westermarck, *The Evolution and Development of the Moral Ideal* (New York: MacMillan, 1906).

[12] There is no guarantee that this will be the case. For an historical version see E. Westermarck, *Ethical Relativity* (New York: Harcourt Brace, 1932). For a critique see G.E. Moore, *Ethics* (London: Cambridge University Press, 1912) and Brandt, *Ethical Theory*, (ref. note 9).

[13] The so-called Sophists.

[14] See note 3, above.

[15] Actually, not everyone; only everyone who counts. That in itself presents a problem for the theory. The sort of critique that we have run here is sometimes called the "open question" attack.

[16] See Lawrence Kohlberg, *The Philosophy of Moral Development* (Chicago: Harper and Row, 1971). See also Chapter 2 for a more extended discussion of this issue.

[17] This, again, is a variant of the "open question" argument.

[18] The precise nature of the relationship between neural processes and consciousness is still a matter of philosophical controversy.

[19] It is here that we find the conceptual basis for the claim that children—and schizophrenics—are ethically incompetent.

[20] For a variant of this point, see Brandt, *Ethical Theory*, (full ref. note 9) 241–269.

[21] For more on this, see Chapter 2 on the Principle of Relevant Difference.

[22] Strictly speaking, this is not quite true. The so-called natural law tradition maintains that there are certain laws—the *ius gentium*—which apply to all people and are grounded in the nature of humanity itself. This finds its earliest expression in the writings of the Stoics, and entered Roman jurisprudence through Cicero and Seneca. In the Middle Ages it was combined with a Christian perspective by St. Thomas Aquinas for example. In the 16th and 17th centuries it was modified and rationalized by Grotius, Montesquieu, Rousseau, Spinoza, Pufendorf and Wolff on the continent, and in the English-speaking world by thinkers like Locke, Adams, Paine and Jefferson. However, when this perspective is pursued to its ultimate foundation, it turns out to be based on the thesis that there are certain fundamental ethical principles that derive from and that apply to human nature.

SUGGESTED READINGS

- Frankena, W.K. "Morality and Moral Philosophy," from W.K. Frankena. *Ethics*. Englewood Cliffs, N.J.: Prentice-Hall, 1963, 1–10.

  This is the first chapter of a good introduction to ethical theory by one of the most prominent North-American ethical theorists of the last few decades. Although published some time ago it is a classic in its field.

- Harman, Gilbert. "Ethics and Observation," from *The Nature of Morality: An Introduction to Ethics*. Oxford: Oxford University Press, 1977.

  A somewhat more theoretical discussion of the relationship between ethics and the world of ordinary experience. A good companion piece to Frankena's discussion, although it takes a bit more work.

- Kohlberg, Lawrence. "Indoctrination versus Relativity in Value Education," from Lawrence Kohlberg, *The Philosophy of Moral Development*. Chicago: Harper and Row, 1971.

  A discussion of how ethical awareness is developed, and its place in the overall social context by a pioneer in the discipline of social ethics and ethics education. Kohlberg builds on some of the pioneering work of Piaget in the developmental theory of value perception.

- Stevenson, C.L. "Working Models," from C.L. Stevenson, *Ethics and Language*. New Haven: Yale University Press, 1944, 20–36.

  This is an excerpt from Stevenson's classic presentation of an emotivist approach to ethics. It should be read in conjunction with Frankena's and Taylor's expositions.

- Taylor, Paul. "Ethical Relativism," from Paul Taylor, *Principles of Ethics*. Belmont, Calif.: Wadsworth, 1975.

  A critical discussion of the notion of ethical relativism by one of the more balanced writers on the subject.

2
Ethical Systems

This chapter discusses the four major approaches to ethical decision-making current in the Canadian context. At its conclusion, the reader should be familiar with the two major types that are encountered most frequently in the health care context and should be able to discuss some of their advantages and disadvantages. The reader should also have some idea of the nature of ethical decision making.

The following questions may be useful as a focus while reading this chapter:

1. What are the fundamental features of teleological, deontological, religious and agapistic ethical approaches respectively?
2. What is the major teleological system? How does it work in practice?
3. What are some advantages of a utilitarian approach? Some disadvantages?
4. What is the basic thrust of a deontological system? How does it work?
5. What is meant by ethical justification? And how does it differ from the psychological account of levels of ethical decision-making?

Introduction

Scientific and academic disciplines often see bitter controversies between rival theories. Physics is a good example. The debate between quantum mechanics and relativistic physics is as long-standing as it is well-known. Both theories claim to be about the world; each has its own strengths and weaknesses; and yet, the two are mutually incompatible. Quantum mechanics provides a satisfactory description of the world at the sub-atomic level. However, it is essentially useless at the macro-level of stars and galaxies. Here relativistic physics comes into its own. Unfortunately, relativistic physics fails at the level of atoms. A great deal of current theorizing in physics is devoted to developing a theory that combines both quantum physics and relativistic physics into one overall scheme.

There are two points about this controversy that are important for ethics: First, the fact that the two theoretical approaches do not agree in certain areas does not mean that physics is bankrupt as a science. Second, the fact that the two theoretical approaches have their own strengths and weaknesses does not mean that they cannot agree in some of what they say.

In some ways the situation in ethics is very similar to that of physics. There are several competing theories that claim to describe the ethical nature of the world correctly. They disagree with each other in some of their conclusions while they agree in others, and they overlap in their claims from time to time. At a fundamental level, however, they are incompatible. And as in physics, there is as yet no generally accepted ethical theory that combines the insights of all of them into an overall and consistent system.

This does not mean that no such theory is possible. In the pages that follow, we shall try to show how the consistent development of one particular ethical approach—the deontological one—goes a long way towards fulfilling the aim of a unified global theory. We have chosen this approach because more than any other, it reflects what is beginning to emerge from current ethical discussions, legal judgements and public sentiment. However, in order to understand this approach, and to be able to see both its strengths and its weaknesses clearly, we have to be aware of the other major ethical approaches that have currency.

These fall into three major groups. They are either *teleological*, or goal directed; *deontological*, or rule or law centred; and *agapistic*, or love oriented.

In general terms, the difference between these types of systems comes out in the sorts of considerations they find relevant in reaching their conclusions. A teleological approach is consequentialistic. This means it focuses on the anticipated outcome of a given situation or action. For instance, a teleological approach would be more concerned about the overall consequences of prohibiting soliciting for the purposes of prostitution than with the rights of the individual prostitute in absolute terms independently of considerations of outcome.

On the other hand, a deontological approach concentrates on balancing rights and duties, and tends to reject purely outcome-oriented considerations as mistaken.[1] This is not to say that a deontological approach necessarily ignores outcomes. Instead, it maintains that there is more to the story: that questions of rights and duties can and indeed should be raised independently of such outcome-oriented considerations. To continue with our example, a deontological approach might ask whether, on balance, the rights of the prostitute to conduct her business and to free and unhindered expression are outweighed by the rights society to freedom from nuisance and from the things that are associated with prostitution, and by the prostitute's own duties towards other members of society. In other words, a deontological approach would not focus on the social importance of the consequences but would concentrate on balancing rights (and duties).

Finally, an agapistic approach evaluates ethical situation by asking what the ethics of brotherly love would dictate. While the conclusion it reaches may on occasion be the same as that decided by the other approaches, there is no guarantee that this would be the case. For instance, it might conclude that letting someone die would show more of love and concern than keeping the person alive by heroic means that involve an unacceptably low quality of life.

Of course, there are also religiously oriented approaches to what is right and wrong: to what is forbidden, permitted or allowed. As we indicated in the previous chapter, these do not have quite the same conceptual underpinnings as the three sorts of approaches we just identified; nor are they open to discussion and debate concerning the legitimacy of their fundamental premises. But for all that, religiously grounded considerations often do play a role in the debate about ethical issues. Therefore if we were to consider religiously oriented approaches from the same perspective as philosophically oriented ethical ones, we would have to say that they tend to ignore outcomes and considerations of duties and rights in and by themselves. These latter become important only when they have a bearing on the interpretation of the religious directives that form the moral basis of the religions themselves. It is these directives that are considered decisive. The directives may be entirely different from anything sanctioned by either utilitarian, agapistic or deontological approaches. Consequently the injunctions derived from them may also be fundamentally different. The example of transfusions in the case of Jehovah's Witnesses illustrates this rather well. They may also differ from religion to religion. For instance, no other religion commands abstention from blood in any form as a matter of ultimate law.

An Example

We can illustrate the difference between these ethical approaches by considering how they could line up on the issue of abortion. A teleological approach might focus solely on social outcome and argue that the acceptability of induced abortions varies depending on the circumstances. In some cases, for example overpopulation, induced abortions would be acceptable because they would ease socio-economic strain. In others, such as societies that suffer from under-population, the opposite would be true. In each case, the ultimate goal of social survival would entail a different evaluation.

On the other hand, from a deontological perspective there could only be one answer: It all depends on how the conflicting rights and duties of the relevant parties are balanced. While social considerations are not necessarily ruled out, they become relevant only insofar as they can be translated into the language of competing and conflicting duties and rights.

An agapistic ethics would reject induced abortions out of hand, because it would view the deliberate killing of one living being, certainly the deliberate killing of a human being, in order to benefit another, as a violation of the fundamental tenet of love. It would be inclined to see the tragedy inherent in the death of a woman for lack of abortion as a natural and unavoidable consequence of life itself. In that sense, agapistic ethical approaches tend to be much more accepting of unpleasant consequences than most other perspectives.

Finally, a religiously oriented position might well condemn induced abortions as a matter of fundamental belief. In fact, most religions have injunctions to that effect. With such an approach it does not matter what social considerations enter into the equation: a society that allows an infringement of these injunctions would be unethical. The only exception would be if the fundamental beliefs of the religion contained something that said that under certain circumstances abortion would be alright: for instance, when the life of the mother is at stake. But here again, this sort of exception would be limited only to the exceptive belief itself.

This example of induced abortion also highlights a point we made above. Different ethical systems may occasionally agree in the conclusions they reach. However, this does not mean that the systems are essentially the same. Nor does it mean that it does not matter which approach we adopt. All it shows is that different ethical approaches occasionally provide the same answer. We still have to decide which one is acceptable and should be followed.

This observation entrains another. The fundamental requirement for any ethical system is not simply that it should be internally consistent or pragmatically useful, that it agrees with what other people, our society, our culture or even our tradition finds acceptable. It is whether it provides a framework that can guide whoever follows it to ethically acceptable actions. And it should do this not simply as a matter of good fortune.

That is to say, it should lead to an ethically acceptable outcome not simply because it just so happens that the approach happens to provide an ethically acceptable answer in a particular case. If that were sufficient, then the hardened criminal whose perverse perspective enjoined him or her to do what a morally good person would also do under those circumstances, would be as good as the morally good person.[2] Instead, the ethical system must allow the person who follows it to arrive at an ethically acceptable answer as a matter of course. This is why a discussion and evaluation of competing ethical systems is not a matter of purely academic relevance. It impacts on the conduct of actual practice.

At the same time, such analysis and discussion can be carried to extremes. Each system we have mentioned has sub-systems, and each of these in turn has variations. A complete analysis of all this would get us bogged down in pure theory, and we would never reach the subject-matter of bioethics itself. We shall therefore refrain from such analysis. Fortunately it is not necessary to go to such lengths. While Canadian society does include groups who follow agapistic and religious approaches, it tends to stick almost exclusively to the teleological and the deontological ones in its social and legal practice.[3] We shall therefore focus most of our theoretical discussion on these two approaches.

But even here we shall be brief. In this we are guided by Aristotle's remarks in the *Nicomachean Ethics*:

> Our treatment will be adequate if we make it as precise as the subject matter allows. The same degree of accuracy should not be demanded in all enquiries any more

than in all the products of craftsmen ... The educated person looks for as much precision in each subject as the nature of the subject allows.[4]

Or—we would add—as the nature of the enterprise demands. Those who look for a more detailed examination of these purely theoretical matters are referred to the various works devoted to theoretical ethics.

Teleological or Consequentialistic Systems

Ethical Egoism

As we indicated a moment ago, teleological ethical approaches are con-sequentialistic in nature. This means that they focus on the expected outcomes of our actions. There are two very general kinds of approaches that share this characteristic: those that are *egoistic* and those that are *utilitarian.*

Egoistic approaches take individual persons as the focus of their ethical considerations. However, the term "egoistic" is somewhat misleading. Usually when we call someone egoistic we mean that this person thinks only about her- or himself. This is not what the term means when it is used in an ethical sense. In order for egoism to count as a genuine ethical approach, it must be based on ethical principles that can be stated in purely formal terms independently of reference to a specific person.[5]

In other words, the primary principle or injunction of ethical egoism cannot be something like "maximize the good for me," or "maximize the good for Jezebel Murchie!" Instead, it must go something like this: "For any person *a*, all and only those acts are obligatory if they advance or maximize the good for *a*; and all and only those are a matter of right if the right in question is a right for *a*."[6] In terms familiar to health care professionals, ethical egoism requires them to look out for their own good rather than that of their patients, of the hospital, of society or anything else.

So far, we have said nothing about what this "good" that is supposed to be aimed at is like. With good reason. There are several interpretations of what it actually is. Some say that it is *hedonistic*, which is means it consists in pleasure or well-being; others say that it is *ideal*, that it centres in things like honesty, justice, or beneficence.[7] Still others maintain that it is eudaemonistic or happiness-oriented; and some even maintain that it is a mixture of any or all of these.[8]

Ethical egoism can accept any of these definitions of the good. It is therefore a very useful theory. Furthermore, it allows health care professionals to avoid having to make judgements about the values of their patients. In that sense, it is very congenial to the multicultural Canadian setting.

However, ethical egoism has several features that should make it unacceptable as a guide for health care professionals. In the first place, it demands that when the good of a patient is in conflict with that of the health care professional, the good of the professional takes priority. This is hardly something that most health care professionals would accept.

Of course, this is not a logical argument against ethical egoism. But if health care professionals believed that they had a duty towards their patients, which overrode their own interests, then the professionals could certainly not accept this theory.

The other thing is that ethical egoism cannot provide any way of allowing health care professionals to rank the competing demands of different parties in an institutional and global fashion. The issue is important because health care delivery depends on such ranking. Without it, the planning of health care budgets is impossible. However, what is the good for the planner, for the physician or for the nurse, may conflict with what is the good for the patients. Furthermore, the same difference may exist among the goods of the patients themselves. For instance, one patient may require a transplant, where the only available organ belongs to another patient; or one patient may need a bed which is already occupied by another patient. One patient may require the physician's attention just when another patient needs her or his attention, and so on. Ethical egoism provides no way of resolving this sort of conflict. However, an ethical system that does not allow the resolution of such conflicts fails in practice.[9]

Utilitarianism

Utilitarianism is by far the most common consequentialistic or teleological ethical theory in our society.[10] It is frequently used by health care administrators in their decision-making. For instance, it underlies the cost/benefit and cost/effectiveness considerations that go into deciding whether to expand an emergency department or to add a psychiatric wing.

Utilitarian approaches focus on outcomes or goals. They differ on how the nature of these goals are to be determined. Some utilitarians claim a special sort of insight or intuition is involved.[11] This intuition is supposed to show that the good is an intrinsic value. That is to say, it is supposed to be something that has value in and by itself whether or not anyone actually values it or finds it valuable. Others focus on the nature of human beings as central and maintain that the good has to be determined in terms of that nature, perhaps in the full realization of its capabilities and potentials—whatever that may amount to.[12] Still others reject both of these positions and instead look to the current preferences of society and say that the nature of this good is a matter of socially accepted preference. While the first two allow for *a priori* reasoning independently of considerations of social practice, social preference utilitarianism is empirical in outlook and finds the basis for its claims in social attitudes. Furthermore, while the first two types of approaches would yield an absolutistic sort of answer as to the nature of the good to be aimed at, the preference-based approach has to admit that the good aimed at may change over time.

Finally, utilitarian theories may differ on how the test of utility is to be applied. Act-utilitarianism proceeds on a case-by-case basis. Its basic principle, which is sometimes called the *principle of utility*, may be expressed like this: "An act is right if, all other things being equal, it produces or is likely to produce the greatest amount of good for the greatest number of people." Therefore an act utilitarian approach requires that we examine each situation and reach a decision for it.[13] This means that health care professionals who face ethical decisions could not follow general rules or guidelines of ethical decision-making. Instead, they would have to calculate utility separately and anew for each individual case.

Rule utilitarianism, on the other hand, maintains that utility should be determined only for general rules of conduct. If we were to express its basic tenet in the form of a principle, we could put it like this: "Those rules of conduct are morally obligatory that produce or are likely to produce the greatest amount of good for the greatest number of people."[14] In other words, it is these rules that must be justified in terms of utility. This approach therefore allows physicians to develop and follow rules of conduct similar to those contained in the codes of ethics of the various health care professions. When it comes to actual decision-making, all that the professionals then have to do is see what the rule means when it is applied to the situation in question.[15]

It is important to note that both types of utilitarianism leave open the nature of what counts as the good. As in the case of ethical egoism, this good may be hedonistic, eudaemonistic, ideal or mixed in nature.[16]

The relationship between the consequentialistic approaches we have sketched are shown in Figure 2-1.

At first glance, the differences between these various types of consequentialistic or teleological theories may seem pragmatically irrelevant. However, this is not true. If we return for a moment to the question of abortion, consider the following case:

> A small-town hospital is deciding whether to perform induced abortions. Some of the physicians who have privileges at the hospital say that they are personally opposed to abortions and will not participate in any way. Two of the local physicians are willing to do them. The hospital board has to decide whether to brave the storm of protest that it thinks will come from the more outspoken members of the community when word gets out that it is doing induced abortions, or simply to continue with its previous policy of not doing abortions.

For the sake of discussion, let us ignore the impact that criminal legislation and the Code of Ethics of the medical profession would have on this case, and consider only the variations possible under the various utilitarian approaches.

Let us begin by assuming that the hospital board is *rule utilitarian*. Then if it were moved by *hedonistic* considerations it would try to balance the problems the community would face if the hospital did abortions, against the problems the community were to face if the hospital continued not to do them. Here it would take into account such factors as the demand on social resources necessary to raise unwanted children; the cost of taking care of failed abortion attempts by women

FIGURE 2-1
Teleological System

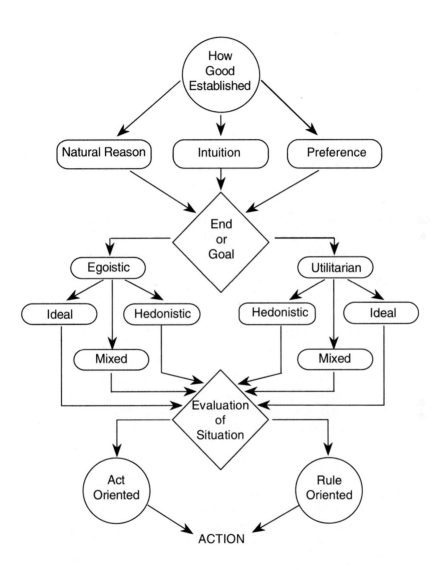

who try to induce their own abortions or who have had a non-medical person try and do them; the cost of the abortions themselves and the impact that they would have on health care within the community, and so on. On balance, the hospital would probably decide that the greatest amount of pleasure and/or material good for society would be achieved if it allowed abortions. The storm of protest would be more than outweighed by the long-term material considerations in health cost savings alone.

If the board decided to adopt an ideal utilitarian perspective, it might well reason differently. It would consider that ideal values like compassion and respect for life are fundamental in our society. It would balance these against the strong emphasis that our society places on self-determination and would try to arrive at a solution. It might then reason that the respect for life is just as fundamental a value in our society as self-determination. From this it might then decide that a balanced approach would be the most appropriate. In other words, it might decide to allow abortions but only under certain conditions, such as in cases of rape or incest, in cases where they were medically indicated, and only as long as the pregnancy was not far enough advanced to allow the foetus to survive. In other words, it might place something like a 20–24 week limit on induced abortions. It would therefore not allow abortion on demand. It would say that although autonomy is a fundamental value, it does not amount to licence, and that any rule of conduct that reflected this perception would have to take this into account. Autonomous persons must be accountable for their actions—even in things like pregnancy. The board might even go so far as to reason that this sort of approach would contribute to a responsible attitude in both men and women. That attitude would probably carry over into other areas of health care consumption.

If the board adopted a mixed utilitarian perspective, it would try to balance ideal and hedonistic considerations against each other. It would be impossible to say beforehand what the board might decide, because its decision would depend on the relative weight that it attached to the various parameters.

Finally, if the board decided to be *eudaemonistic* in its utilitarian outlook it would look for statistical data about the psychological sequelae of abortions as opposed to denial of abortions. It would compare these with data about societal mood when abortions are performed and when they are not. On this basis it would reach a decision. In the current social climate, this would probably mean that the board would opt for allowing abortions to be performed.

If the board were to approach the issue from an *act utilitarian* perspective, it would not try to decide what *policy* it should adopt. Instead, it would set up a committee to look at each case separately and without any hard and fast guidelines except the principle of utility. It is unlikely that any hospital board would operate for long in that fashion. An act utilitarian approach does not easily lend itself to making policy decisions.[17]

Deontological Theories

As we mentioned before, health care administrators frequently use a rule utilitarian approach when deciding what to do. It is not surprising that they should do that. The job of health care administrators is to develop and implement health care policies. By their very nature, these policies are intended to provide the greatest amount of quality health care for the greatest number of people. They therefore tend to fit the mixed rule utilitarian pattern.

At the level of practice, however, the situation is different. Here the individual patient is the focus of primary concern. This comes out very clearly in the codes of ethics of the various health care professions.[18] That is why the deontological perspective is considered ethically more appropriate in this setting.

Deontological perspectives are oriented around the conviction that in and by themselves, the consequences of an action do not determine whether the action is ethically acceptable. Instead, a deontological perspective maintains that whether an action is ethically acceptable depends on whether it is in accordance with, and is performed out of respect for, certain absolute and universal principles. The principles of autonomy, and equality and justice are several well-known examples of such principles.[19] For instance, the principle of autonomy would give a competent[20] patient the right to reject a particular form of treatment even if what the patient had chosen was not in the patient's best interest from a medical perspective. Likewise, equality and justice would entail that if it would be unjust to kill someone—for instance Ghengis Khan or Josef Stalin—then we could not ethically kill that person even if a greater number of people would suffer. The old Roman proverb captures this uncompromising outlook of a deontological approach: "Let justice be done though the heavens falls!"

Like utilitarian theories, deontological theories come in various versions. In fact, we can identify three major types. The first is monistic. It holds that there is only one basic principle from which all judgements and rules of right and wrong are ultimately derived. The position of Immanuel Kant is probably the best-known (and most influential) example. Kant called his basic principle the "categorical imperative," and gave several formulations of it—five, to be exact.[21] All of them, so he claimed, were equivalent to one another. Two of these formulations are of special interest for the health care context. The first, he simply called "categorical imperative" as such. It goes like this:

> Act only according to that maxim by which you can at the same time will that it should become a universal law.[22]

The second, which he called the "practical imperative," he expressed as follows:

> Act so that you treat humanity, whether in your own person or in that of another, always as an end and never as a means only.[23]

Perhaps we can clarify the meaning of these imperatives by means of an example. Suppose that a physician has a patient with metasticized cancer of the lungs. The cancer is inoperable; it is inaccessible to chemotherapy and radiation treatment, and most likely it will be fatal within a year, a year-and-a-half at most. Let us suppose further that the physician knows that the patient is psychologically labile. If the patient were to be told of her condition, she would react extremely emotionally and might even suffer psychological harm. Let us also suppose that the physician wants to spare her patient the psychological trauma that she is convinced will result if this information were to be disclosed to the patient before the disease had progressed to the point of seriously incapacitating her. The physician therefore lies to the patient about the diagnosis and prognosis.

While this sort of action may be defended from a humanitarian perspective, Kant would argue that it is unethical because it fails the first test. The maxim of the act—the general rule according to which the physician would here be acting— would be something like this: Lie when motivated by humanitarian considerations. However—so Kant would say—if this maxim were to be elevated to the level of a universal law, it would become the precept that anyone, on any occasion involving humanitarian motives, should lie. However, what counts as a humanitarian motive is very much an idiosyncratic matter that depends on the perception and the private values of the individual who has the motive. There are not, and there cannot be, general, universal and absolute standards in this regard. Consequently if the maxim became a law, no-one could ever be sure that in fact he or she was not being lied to by other people on all sorts of occasions. Not only would that completely erode our confidence in what we are told by other,[24] it would also mean that for all practical purposes the distinction between lying and telling the truth would disappear. The maxim would thus fail the universalizability test and defeat itself.

Not only that, Kant would argue, in keeping with his second formulation, that to lie to a patient, even under circumstances such as these, is to withhold from her the information that she should have if she is to be able to make reasonable, rational and appropriate decisions about how to conduct the rest of her life. In other words, it would be to treat her not as what she really is—namely an autonomous rational being who is an end-in-herself—but as an object, something to manipulated.[25]

The question whether these two formulations of the categorical imperative really are equivalent has been the subject of some theoretical debate.[26] We shall not enter into it here. Instead, let us turn to another type of deontological approach: deontological pluralism. The best-known example of this sort of approach is that of W.D. Ross.

Ross argued[27] that there is a whole series of fundamental ethical principles. He said that the list should include the principles of fidelity, of making reparation for harm caused, of rendering service for service rendered, of assisting the distribution of happiness according to merit, of doing whatever one can to promote the good for others (beneficence), of not injuring others (non-malfeasance), and of improving "our own condition in respect of virtue and intelligence."[28]

Ross also maintained that these principles—and indeed ethical principles in general—hold only *prima facie*. That is to say, they are only abstract and general approximations which serve as guides. They do not hold absolutely. Instead, they license or enjoin expectations and obligations whose actual force or effectiveness must be examined by considering their relative strengths with respect to one another on a given occasion.

In other words, according to Ross the actual force of a *prima facie* principle is functionally determined by the context in which the actual situation is embedded. This context would include not only the nature of the relevant acts themselves, but the ethical weight of the personal, social and material factors, for instance, that characterize the situation as a whole.[29] Only when all of this is taken into account can we say what is an actual right/duty rather than a *prima facie* one.

Another pluralist deontological theory of note has recently been proposed by John Rawls, particularly in his book *A Theory of Justice*.[30] It is an attempt to construct a theory of justice on the basis of several general principles that are absolutely ordered with respect to one another as to precedence or priority. For instance, Rawls suggests that justice in human interactions takes priority over equity of distribution of economic goods.

Rawls maintains that the theory he has constructed is only a partial theory. It deals only with justice, and it does not attempt to explain all ethical concerns. However, in spite of this, it is an improvement over the theory proposed by Ross in that the air of extreme vagueness that surrounded the latter is attenuated to a considerable degree.

However, what we have outlined so far captures only one aspect of the diversity of the deontological approaches. Deontological theories also differ in the orientation of the principles that form their basis. Some are quality oriented, others are person-oriented. *Quality-oriented* approaches maintain that certain moral qualities have intrinsic value. The justice oriented perspective of Rawls is a good example. *Person-oriented* approaches, as their name suggests, find their focus in the concept of a person. The Kantian system is here representative. Its governing assumption is that ethical laws necessarily will have persons as their focus. Persons are beings of ultimate and incommensurable value. That fact, so Kant claimed, will be reflected in the natures of the laws themselves. It is therefore not surprising that this sort of approach places a strong emphasis on personal autonomy. It prohibits lying to patients under any and all circumstances—a position that may be somewhat too uncompromising for medical practice.

The deontological systems are shown in Figure 2-2.

Unfortunately, situations in real life do not fall neatly into any one of the ethical rubrics that we have just sketched. Our social, legal and medical practices combine all of them together into a mélange that[31] sometimes leads to severe problems in planning and delivery. For example, proponents of emergency health care sometimes advance deontological arguments that focus on the need of particular individuals and direct these considerations against proponents of increased preventive health care measures who use a utilitarian perspective to point to the common good. Both sides claim justice and equality as underwriting their positions, and both sides

FIGURE 2-2
Teleological System

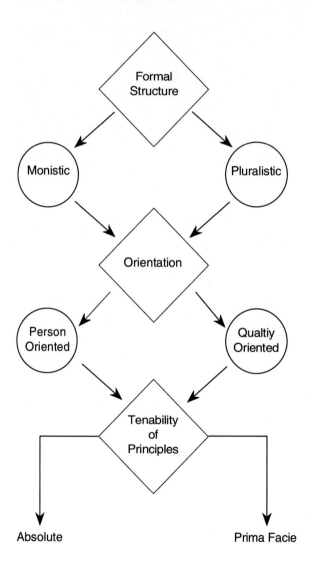

talk about rights and obligations. Both sides employ similar language—although they mean different things.[32] The situation sometimes has the appearance of crossed monologues. A proper understanding of the ethical theories that underlie these distinct perspectives may go a considerable way towards facilitating a solution.

Religiously Oriented Ethical Approaches

Before leaving our discussion of ethical theories, we should briefly consider religiously oriented approaches. Of course the Charter of Rights and Freedoms prevents policy planners from giving precedence to any religious persuasion, and it does prevent people in the public sector from acting on their personal religious beliefs in a way that discriminates against the rights and liberties of others. Therefore, in Canada at least, religious orientation cannot form the basis of any policy planning in the health care sector, and cannot constitute a reliable guide to professional actions by physicians engaged in the delivery of health care.

Still, it is a fact that the actions of many physicians are guided by their personal religious beliefs. This has come out very clearly in the intra-professional debate that surrounds induced abortions, DNR orders and similar issues. It is therefore important to have at least some understanding of the logic of religious approaches to ethics per se, and to see why even though they may provide personally satisfying guides to moral living, they are not acceptable as a professional ethical basis.

Canadians subscribe to a wide variety of religious beliefs. They include the various Christian, Muslim, Jewish, Sikh and Native Indian perspectives—to mention but a few. However, if we were to try and classify them in purely ethical terms, we would have to say that most of them are like deontological theories. They postulate fundamental principles to guide ethical conduct.

However, they differ from the deontological theories in how they arrive at these principles and in their implications. For instance, these principles find their ultimate basis not in independent or "unaided" reasoning, like the principles of other ethical approaches, but in some fundamental belief or experience.

Furthermore, unlike philosophical ethical approaches, religious approaches do not countenance the possibility that a particular principle may in fact be wrong (e.g. when it conflicts with others), or that the belief-system *as a whole* may have to be re-examined and changed for the sake of consistency. Instead, the fundamental principles and tenets of these approaches are essentially immune from question or revision because they define the belief systems themselves, and because they have a basis in belief that raises them above rationalistic critiques. What has to change is not the beliefs themselves but how they are interpreted. The current controversy surrounding abortion provides a good example of how religiously oriented ethical perspectives work. While they allow for discussion up to a certain point, when a fundamental tenet of belief is threatened all discussion ceases.

As we have said, we shall not discuss religious approaches further because it would be pointless. The Charter of Rights prevents policy makers from basing their decisions and recommendations on religious convictions. Therefore, any formulation of health care policy has to be made independently of them. This does not mean that the decisions that are made or the policies that are enacted will necessarily be at variance with religious beliefs. In many cases, the two will probably overlap. However, the religious belief cannot be the reason for the policy. Therefore, when we are trying to understand the ethical reason that is supposed to justify a particular decision, the consideration of religious views will not help.

The same thing is true for individual health care professionals. Like everyone else, they are entitled to hold their own values and perspectives. They are also entitled to act on them. However, and this is very important, they are entitled to act on them only so long this does not infringe on their duties as professionals and only as long as it does not infringe on rights of the health care consumers. Furthermore, they are entitled to act on them only if the decisions that they reach can also be defended in terms of independent ethical considerations. We shall explore some of the implications of this later, when we deal with such issues as the physician/patient relationship, abortion and reproductive technology.

Agapistic Approaches

As to agapistic approaches, they are perhaps most appropriately characterized as ethics of love. This is often interpreted as meaning love for all living beings. Within the recent past Albert Schweitzer[33] was its most famous Western proponent. In the Canadian setting this perspective has started to gain increasing adherence from ecology-minded persons and from those concerned with animal rights. In general terms, then, an agapistic approach, when it is interpreted in this fashion, demands that we consider all living things as ethically equivalent. To use the term coined by Peter Singer, who is one of the best-known current exponents in bioethics, we should avoid "speciesm."[34]

If this is what agapism amounts to, it faces serious problems in the health care setting. The problem is not that it is internally inconsistent as an ethical theory, but that it is difficult to apply it in practice and remain a health care professional. If we take it in the form we have just indicated it does not allow us to make any distinction between different types of living things. Therefore, if we followed it, we could not institute public health measures to control disease vectors, or take any steps to save the life of human beings in preference to other living things.

On the other hand, if agapism is interpreted in a more species-oriented way, by distinguishing between different kinds of living things, then we have ask ourselves what the basis of that distinction would be and why we should draw the line here rather than there. For instance, why should we think that birds occupy a more privileged ethical niche than filarial worms or tripanosomes? Why should we be more concerned over groundhogs than, say, micro-phages or viruses? Any attempt to give an answer would immediately involve us in a slide down a slippery slope which, once begun, is difficult if not impossible to stop without adopting an arbitrary position that would be open to the "speciesm" criticism raised by Singer.[35]

This is not to say that the agapistic approach has no relevance to the Canadian health care scene. Canadian society accepts the principle of respect for life as an important value. It even enshrines it in certain laws and regulations. However, Canadian society does not commit the logical mistake of confusing love and respect with obligation. Life, all life, merits special consideration and must be treated with respect. It might even be an appropriate object of love. But the fact that we respect or love something does not mean that therefore we have an obligation towards it. Of course, we may voluntarily accord certain rights to something because we love or respect it. But that is an entirely different matter. Agapistic perspectives do have something valuable to say for biomedical ethics. However, what they have to say can be accommodated by accepting the premise that consistent ethical behaviour is governed not only by respect for ethical rights and obligations, but also by respect for personal and subjective values.

Utilitarian versus Deontological Approaches: A Comparison

It should be clear by now that it is not entirely irrelevant what kind of ethical system or approach someone adopts. Each type of approach has its characteristic strengths and weaknesses. For instance, the essentially calculative outlook of the utilitarian approach has much to recommend it. It allows for the introduction of cost-benefit and cost-effectiveness considerations. This counts for a great deal because, at least in principle, it allows us to construct a calculative framework of weighted parameters which is independent of subjective variables while at the same time being capable of implementation in an objective fashion.

Furthermore, it facilitates the use of social and family-based considerations that allow the physician to place treatment of the individual patient in the social context in which the patient is embedded. This is a powerful argument in our increasingly socially conscious setting.

Nevertheless, it seems to us that utilitarianism suffers from a severe shortcoming. Surprisingly enough, this shortcoming lies in this very calculative feature that is touted as its advantage. By focusing on the social good—the greatest amount of good for the greatest number of people—utilitarianism seems to allow, at least in principle, the sacrifice of individual right and justice in the name of the common good. It therefore appears to operate on the principles that the end justifies the means, and that the end at which we must always aim is the aggregate total of the greater good. This stands opposed to the basic value that our society seems to place on the individual person, and on the fundamental rights and duties that it accords to individuals.

Furthermore, Canadian court cases seem to have a deontological thrust. Decisions like *Mulloy vs. HopSang*, *Reibl vs. Hughes*, and *Hopp vs. Lepp* as well as *Morgentaler vs. The Queen*, *re Eve* and *Malette vs. Shulman* illustrate this rather well. These decisions, and others like them, focus on the individual person as an autonomous decision-maker. They portray the individual patient as a centre of rights and obligations, and they evaluate the acceptability of a given course of action not in terms of utility but, as we shall see later, with reference to the interplay of existing duties and rights. They also bespeak a perception of the principles of equality and justice that is entirely deontological in nature.

This must not be misunderstood. It does not mean that Canadian law as it stands—whether with respect to statutes, the Charter, or its various cases and interpretations—is a perfect reflection of a deontological approach. It is not. Neither the law nor social norms are of pristine ethical purity. Considerations of a utilitarian nature that focus on the common good obtrude themselves. The not-withstanding clause of the Charter is itself a case in point, and legal health test requirements for entry into Canada as an immigrant is another.

Our laws therefore evince admixtures of utilitarian, religious or even agapistic considerations. But these are exceptions. By and large the deontological perspective is dominant. We tend to place a fundamental emphasis on the individual person as a being of ultimate and incommensurable value, and in theory at least, we tend to believe that questions of right and wrong should be decided with reference to universal and absolute principles that preserve, as far as possible, the autonomy of the person.

This still leaves us with a fundamentally important question: Are there any reasons for preferring one ethical system or approach to ethical issues over another? In our estimation there are. The most important reason is that we think that the deontological approach is ethically correct.[36] As to practical reasons, we have already indicated why we think that neither a religiously oriented approach nor an agapistically grounded ethical stance is very useful as a generally acceptable professional guide. But that leaves deontological and utilitarian approaches. Are there ethical reasons for preferring one over the other?

We think that there are, and that they favour a deontological approach. These reasons are both theoretical and practical in nature. The theoretical ones centre around the concepts of justice and fairness, and the notion of a right.

To put it in a nutshell, we believe that in the end, neither the concepts of justice and fairness nor the notion of a right can find proper expression in a utilitarian system. Justice and fairness lose their usual meaning entirely. Instead of dealing with the condition of the individual in relation to others, they have to be redefined in terms of the common good. As one group of authors put it, from a utilitarian perspective "What may be required is that individuals and individuality be sacrificed on rare occasions to prevent even greater sacrifice of or *harm* to numbers of others."[37] It seems that to us that such a perspective loses the meaning of justice and fairness, and replaces it with the notion of—well—utility.

In our estimation, the notion of a right fares no better. A right is claim had by an individual on others, where these others have a corresponding obligation.[38] The binding force of the right/obligation lies in the interrelationship between the individuals concerned. On a utilitarian approach, however, these interrelations lack binding force. It is only the greater good that is of interest. Unfortunately, there is no accepted account of what constitutes that good.[39]

An inveterate utilitarian might reply that such a critique is short-sighted; that it applies only to the approaches we have identified as act- and preference-utilitarianism. It leaves rule utilitarianism untouched. Rule-utilitarianism believes that fairness and justice are fundamental rules by which to evaluate the acceptability of a given action precisely because only by accepting fairness and justice as fundamental principles will overall utility be served.[40]

Those taking a utilitarian approach might even try to put this defense in terms of a concrete example. For instance, by agreeing that act-utilitarianism could require the active termination of health-care efforts for those suffering from haemophilia because the expenditure involved would have a much greater overall effect when reallocated to community health projects. From a standpoint such as this, therefore, what would ordinarily be considered an obligation to provide the haemophiliacs with medical services on the basis of fairness and justice, would go by the board. Furthermore, preference utilitarianism, which bases itself on societal preference, might or might not agree. It all depends. However, so the rule utilitarian might argue, these are not weaknesses. Fairness and justice in themselves have an overall social utility because when they are consistently aimed at, they tend produce a socio-psychological climate which is more effective in promoting overall aggregate welfare than any other maxim.[41]

However, such a rule-utilitarian response would be deceptive. No matter how the rule-utilitarian may attempt to explain it away, the fact remains that neither the rule of fairness nor the rule of justice can play the role of fundamental principles in a rule-utilitarian setting. Both are merely very general pragmatic guidelines. Their purpose is to maximize utility. That is why they are instituted as rules and whence they derive their binding force. In other words, if it should turn out that following them leads to social fragmentation or similar results, or that a greater likelihood of social survival would be guaranteed by following other rules, both justice and fairness would have to be rejected. Rule utilitarians tend to argue that when the consequences of dropping these rules are completely analyzed, it will emerge that abandoning them can never be justified from a utilitarian perspective. However, that is merely a claim. It has never been substantiated. The issue becomes particularly important when we approach the question of how to allocate health care resources justly and fairly in light of changing demographic circumstances. With due alteration of detail, a similar point can be made for the principle of autonomy.

Finally, we should always keep in mind that the reason utilitarianism is so attractive is that it promises to set ethical decision-making on an objective footing by providing a calculative basis. However, that promise is illusory. In order to calculate utility, we have to be able to assign numbers to degrees of goodness, we have to be able to calculate the extent of its distribution, weigh the significance of its qualitative variations, and so on.

However, none of these parameters are clear. The greatest good: Of what sort and of what intensity? As defined how, or by whom? On what basis? For the greatest number of people where? At what point in history? For what duration? Questions could be multiplied, but this will give us some idea of what is at stake. For all of the time that utilitarianism has existed, it has never succeeded in specifying the calculative parameters necessary for its implementation in a precise, let alone usable, fashion. Promises have been held out but never fulfilled.

The recent introduction of Quality Adjusted Life Years and similar measures, which hold out the promise of quality-of-life considerations in a collective fashion into resource allocation considerations, are but further examples along that line. As the proponents of these measures themselves admit,[42] these measures have to balance economic values with personal values. The answer is not provided by the calculative parameters, which assume that an appropriate non-calculative evaluation has already taken place. While this in itself does not suffice to rule out utilitarianism as a viable ethical theory, it certainly throws doubt on its attractiveness.

A theory that promises an advantage but does not deliver, and moreover, whose delivery requires the ability to forecast the future, fails the test of possibility. The more recent attempts by preference utilitarians to settle the issue fare even less well. Given the constantly shifting nature of social opinions, guidelines would exist for the moment only, to be overturned by the next poll.

We therefore favour a deontological approach. While it may lack the calculative promise of utilitarianism, it focuses on the most fundamental aspect of medical ethics: the interplay of obligations and rights in the fiduciary setting between the physician and the patient. However, it also seems to us that the approach of Kant or Ross and even that of Rawls is not entirely satisfactory for the medical setting. We think that instead a combination of their respective insights provides a more usable deontological perspective. Such a combined approach can be represented by six basic principles:[43]

1. The Principle of Autonomy and Respect for Persons:

    All persons have a fundamental right to self-determination that is limited only by unjust infringement on the rights of others.

2. The Principle of Priority:

    Rights can be ranked according to logical, natural, and voluntary priority.

    a) *Logical:* If a right can be exercised if and only if a particular condition is satisfied, then the existence of the first right entails a right to bring about that condition, and the latter is logically prior to and more fundamental than the former, for example, health and life.

    b) *Natural:* Rights that arise out of the nature of a certain situation take precedence over rights established by agreement or convention, for example justice over education.

c) *Voluntary:* Every competent person may voluntarily subordinate an otherwise prior or more basic right to a lower one.

3. Principle of Impossibility

    A right that cannot be fulfilled under the circumstances is ineffective as a right, and an obligation that cannot be met under the circumstances ceases to be effective as an obligation; for example, the obligation to save life is ineffective in the context of a moribund patient.

4. Principle of Best Action:

    Whoever has an obligation also has the ethical duty to discharge it in the best manner possible under the circumstances; for example, if there is a duty to respond to a code, the duty is to do so as quickly as possible.

5. Principle of Relevant Difference:

    A right is effective to the degree that nothing in the relevant circumstances contravenes the conditions under which it arose; for example, the presumption of a right to health care is prudence and responsibility. Therefore, a deliberately imprudent and irresponsible life style affects the priority of an otherwise equal claim.

6. Principle of Equality and Justice:

    A right is effective to the degree that it preserves or promotes justice; for example, a right to preferential health resource allocation is based on this as a matter of justice and equity.

We shall use these principles in the discussions that follow. We believe that they allow not only theoretical neatness in the analysis of bioethical problems but also permit the practical resolution of conflicts. The deontological perspective and the requirements of practice need not be incompatible.

The Structure of Ethical Justification

Before we conclude this chapter on ethical theory, a brief word is necessary about the structure of ethical justification. All of us are concerned that our ethical decisions be above reproach. Unfortunately, there is no way to guarantee that they are. The best we can do is to think clearly and to try to make sure that we do not confuse legal considerations with ethical ones, and keep psychological convictions and personal values distinct from ethical principles. Here it is useful to keep two points in mind:

> What people take to be true is not necessarily the same as what is true; nor is the depth of a conviction a reliable guide to the truth of what is believed.

What leads a person to accept a certain statement or adopt a particular decision is not necessarily the same as what justifies his position in the first place.

These facts are trivial and commonplace. However, they are frequently overlooked. When this is done, it leads to a confusion of the *psychology of ethical decision-making* with the *ethical justification or acceptability of a given decision.*

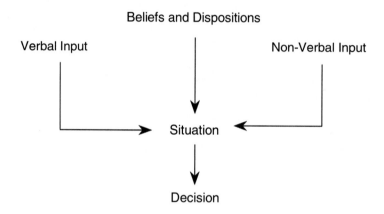

FIGURE 2-3
Psychological Parameters of Decision-Making

That is to say, ethical decision-making can be analyzed psychologically as well as ethically. Psychologically it can be analyzed by focusing on the generality of concepts that the individual uses and the level of his or her social integration. Jean Piaget has done this for children[44] and Lawrence Kohlberg for children but also adults.[45] Kohlberg's schema is something of a classic in this regard.[46] It divides moral decision-making into six stages of increasing generality and degrees of acceptability and justification. These are as follows:

The Pre-Conventional Level

This is the level at which a small child operates before it has become a acculturated into the society in which it lives. Kohlberg identifies two stages within this level.

Stage 1 is the level of punishment and obedience orientation. The person who operates at this level adjusts his or her behaviour essentially in response to reward or punishment alone. There is no reflection about the meaning of these. Obedience is central.

Stage 2 is more reflective. Kohlberg describes it as the level of instrumental relativistic orientation: a kind of *quid-pro-quo* orientation modified by awareness of rules of punishment and obedience.

FIGURE 2-4
Rule-Oriented Ethical Decision-Making

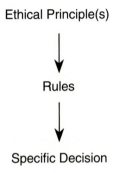

The Conventional Level

At this level the person has become acculturated, and has acquired the conventions of the society in which he or she lives. Again, Kohlberg distinguishes two stages. *Stage 3* he describes as the stage of interpersonal concordance or "good boy-nice girl" orientation. In other words, it is the stage at which people orient themselves according to the conventions of their society, and tend to conform to or fulfill descriptions applied to themselves.

Stage 4, what Kohlberg calls the law and order orientation, is self-explanatory. It is a convention-oriented perspective that is legalistic in outlook, and tends to evaluate all actions in legalistic terms.

The Post-Conventional, Autonomous or Principled Level

This is the level at which Kohlberg thinks we find truly ethical or moral behaviour. Again he distinguishes two stages. *Stage 5*, the social contract legalistic orientation stage, is similar to stage 4, except the perspective is wider and conceptually deeper than mere attention to the rules of law and order. The reason for these rules enter into the considerations of the person who operates at this level. *Stage 6*, the level of universal ethical principle orientation, is the level of a truly autonomous moral person who determines what is ethically appropriate on the basis of general principles. The more general the level at which the individual is operating, and the more universal the principles that form the basis of the actions, the more appropriate are the actions of that person in an ethical sense.

However, as other commentators have already pointed out,[47] this is not a schema of ethical justification. There is no guarantee that there is any concordance between the generality (universality) of a principle and its ethical correctness. Nor are conceptual breadth and social integration guarantees of moral correctness. At best, what it shows is levels of psycho-social integration—a different thing entirely.

What Kohlberg, Piaget and others like them have done is produce an analysis of the psychology of ethical decision-making from the perspective of levels of sophistication. However, the justification structure for ethical decision-making looks quite different. Figure 2-4 (on page 37) gives some indication of how it looks for rule-oriented ethical systems.

The structure in Figure 2-4 can itself be broken down into parts:

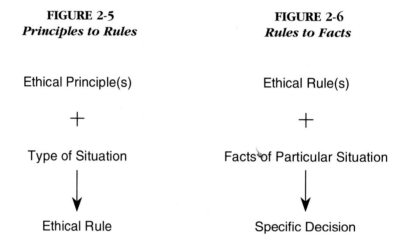

FIGURE 2-5
Principles to Rules

Ethical Principle(s)
+
Type of Situation
↓
Ethical Rule

FIGURE 2-6
Rules to Facts

Ethical Rule(s)
+
Facts of Particular Situation
↓
Specific Decision

All rule oriented ethical systems require this sort of justification structure of their decisions.

As to act oriented systems, their justification structure is similar. The only difference is that the specific decision will be reached directly on the basis of an ethical principle or several principles without reference to intervening and more particular rules:

Finally, a word of warning. While it is true that the schemata we have sketched represent the justification structure of ethically acceptable decision-making, this does not mean that they also represent the actual process of ethical decision-making. That process *is* a matter of psychology. It involves individual as well as cultural

FIGURE 2-7
Act-Oriented Ethical Decision-Making

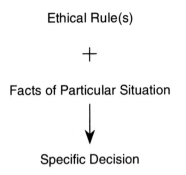

variables. Here the work of Piaget, Kohlberg and others is useful in illuminating what actually occurs.

On the other hand, what we have said about the ethical justification structure concerns not the psychology but the acceptability of an ethical decision. If such a specific decision cannot be analyzed in this fashion it will not be ethically defensible. The ethical relations must be there, even though the individual decision-maker neither employs nor is aware of them.

A Sample Case

To illustrate some of the differences between the utilitarian and deontological approaches that we have sketched so far, let us consider the following rather simple case.

> A young woman consults her physician for a condition that turns out to be genital herpes. What ought the young woman to do? What ought the physician to do?

If we assume a hedonistic egoistic system, then the physician should be concerned only for her welfare, and the patient should be concerned only about hers. The physician would therefore be unlikely to counsel her patient to inform her sex partner(s) of her condition, and the patient is unlikely to volunteer such information because it will probably be contrary to advancing her interests. The physician would probably take whatever action might be in her best interest—which probably means that she would simply follow the laws of reporting as they apply in this case. Furthermore, the physician would probably provide the young woman with whatever relief she is able to give simply because it is likely to advance the professional interest of the physician herself.

If the physician was an ideal egoist, then her actions would be different. She would be guided by values such as of honesty and compassion. She might therefore decide that the young woman cannot ethically hide her condition from her sex-partners because that would not foster ideal values like truthfulness, justice and so on in the woman. She would probably counsel the woman to reveal that she has genital herpes to her partners, and she would take appropriate steps to make sure that the young woman does in fact do so. (Something like this underlies a great deal of the virtue-through-suffering approach to life.)

A mixed egoistic approach would involve a combination of these different sorts of actions.

On the other hand, if the physician has a utilitarian outlook, she will operate on the basis of the principle of utility. The welfare of the young woman (however the term "welfare" may be understood) then recedes into the background except insofar as it has a bearing on the total good for the greatest number of people. The right course of action will then be determined on a balancing and calculative basis. But that is not all. The distinctions between ideal, mixed, and hedonistic goods would now apply with even greater force. For, as John Stuart Mill already pointed out, the mere quantity of the good is not the only parameter in a utilitarian calculation. Neither is its distribution. Its quality is also important.

But the difference does not stop here. The variations in method of determination now enter in. As an act utilitarian, for instance, she would evaluate the situation on its own merits. Should would take into account the various factors of the case, such as the general health status of the young woman, the threat the illness represents to others, the socio-economic, psychological and political implications of the situation. She would then attempt to arrive at some calculation of what action would produce the greatest amount of good for the greatest number of people under the circumstances. If this mean that the wishes of the young women had to be overruled—e.g. by tracing contacts—the physician would still go ahead.

If the physician were a rule utilitarian, she would consider the particular facts of the case only insofar as they related to the general rules of conduct which she, as a physician, believed would advance the greatest good for the greatest number of people. She would therefore counsel according to a set of rules that she believed advanced overall utility. In this case, these rules would probably require that the young woman disclose that she has herpes to her partner(s) because in this estimation, these rules would tend to maximize the public good.

Finally, if the physician were a preference utilitarian, she would follow current social standards on the issue. Obviously, there can be no a *priori* answer here as to how the judgement would go. We would have to look and see.

If the physician followed a deontological perspective, the results would again be different. As a person oriented deontological physician she might focus on the principles of equality and justice as they apply to persons. Her counsel would then be the result of a balancing of the rights of the young women against the right of others in society. She would therefore recommend disclosure—and would let the young women know that unless she gave her some reliable indication that her recommendation had been followed, she (the physician) would take the appropriate actions herself.[48] On the other hand, if the physician was a quality oriented deontologist, she might define justice not simply in human terms but view it as something that is not partisan to any particular life form. Living beings other than people would enter the equation. Under these circumstances it might well be similar to an agapistic approach.

Conclusion

We began our discussion by saying that there are four major kinds of approaches to ethical decision-making. After giving a brief sketch of each, we suggested that really only two of them, the utilitarian and the deontological, find much representation in the Canadian setting. Of course, in light of what we said in the first chapter, this does not count for much. Ethics cannot be done by consensus—nor should it be influenced by what a particular country or region finds or does not find acceptable. That is why we went further. We suggested that so far as we could determine, only the deontological approach really captures what to us is central to ethics: the interrelationship of rights and duties between person and person.

Perhaps we should end on this note. Health care is concerned with the delivery of a certain kind of service to persons. Whether we are dealing with public health measures or intensive care treatment, ultimately it is the individual person who is central, and it is the individual person's rights that have to be balanced against the competing rights of others—and whose obligations have to be evaluated in a similar manner. Therefore it seems to us that there is a congenial fit between the person-oriented perspective of a deontological approach and the raison d'être of health care itself. In the chapters that follow, we shall draw out some of the implications of this conviction.

ENDNOTES

[1] See W.K. Frankena, "Morality and Moral Philosophy," from W.K. Frankena, *Ethics* (Englewood Cliffs, N.J.: Prentice-Hall, 1973), and Brandt, R.B. *Ethical Theory* (Englewood Cliffs, N.J.: Prentice-Hall, 1959), for analogous discussions.

[2] Immanuel Kant focuses on this fact in his discussion of the notion of a good will in his *Foundations of the Metaphysics of Morals*, I.

[3] Some evidence for this is found in Canadian court cases dealing with medical malpractice, negligence and similar issues; as well as in the Charter of Rights and Freedoms, which effectively rules out the use of a particular religious or valuational perspective as guiding public policy. Sections 2 and 15 are here particularly implicated. For more detailed discussion of the various individual cases that illustrate the point, see the chapters that follow.

[4] *Nicomachean Ethics* I: 3.

[5] Compare Brandt, *Ethical Theory*, 369 and elsewhere.

[6] Brandt, *Ethical Theory*. It will therefore be apparently that ethical egoism is not quite what is usually understood by the term "egoism" in ordinary discourse.

[7] See Brandt, *Ethical Theory*, 395. See also A.C. Ewing, *The Definition of Good* (New York: Macmillan, 1947) Chapter 6.

[8] We shall encounter this again in our discussion of utilitarianism. Teleological theories generally lack agreement about what constitutes the Good.

[9] See Brandt, *Ethical Theory*.

[10] Aside, that is, from religiously oriented ethical approaches. Some of these also contain consequentialistic reasoning.

[11] See G.E. Moore, *Principia Ethica* (Cambridge: Cambridge University Press, 1903).

[12] W.R. Ross, *The Right and the Good* (Oxford: Clarendon Press, 1938).

[13] See Brandt, *Ethical Theory*, 380–391.

[14] Strictly speaking, this is an oversimplification. A complete formulation would require that we introduce qualifiers that allow for the resolution of conflict among rules, where that set of rules is correct which, when followed conscientiously by all members of society, would maximize the welfare or good for all. See Brandt, *Ethical Theory*, 253f.

[15] Brandt, *Ethical Theory* 253–258 and 396–405.

[16] For some interesting discussion on this issue, see Henry Sidgewick, *The Methods of Ethics* II: 3; J. Bentham, *The Principles of Morals and Legislation* 1–4; J.S. Mill, *Utilitarianism* 2, 4, etc. See also Brandt, *Ethical Theory* and G.E. Moore, *Principia Ethica*.

[17] Mill, *Utilitarianism*, calls the principle of utility "the greatest happiness principle." This is somewhat misleading because it seems to assume a eudaemonistic interpretation of the good.

[18] See *Code of Ethics for Nursing*, value II; *Code of Ethics* of the CMA, clause 5, etc.

[19] For a discussion of the Principle of Beneficence and also of Malfeasance see pp. 88 to 91 below.

[20] For the significance of this condition, see Chapter 5.

[21] Compare A.J. Paton, *The Categorical Imperative* (London: Hutcheson, 1947).

[22] Kant, *Foundations of the Metaphysics of Morals*, 422.

[23] Kant, *Foundations*, 429.

[24] For a similar point see S. Bok, *Lying* (New York: Random House, 1978), Chapter 4.

[25] We shall discuss this more thoroughly when we discuss therapeutic privilege. See Chapter 5.

[26] See Paton, (ref. note 21).

[27] Ross, (ref. note 12), Chapter 2.

[28] Ross, Chapter 2.

[29] Ross, Chapter 2.

[30] John Rawls, *A Theory of Justice* (Cambridge: Harvard University Press, 1971).

[31] This emerges clearly in such cases as *Mulloy vs. HopSang, Reibl vs. Hughes* and other cases. We shall have more to say on this when we come to discuss informed consent.

[32] This is particularly apparent in recent discussions surrounding the issue of resource allocation. For more on this, see Chapter 9.

[33] Albert Schweitzer, *Civilization and Ethics*, 3rd ed. (London: Black, 1949).

[34] Peter Singer, *Animal Liberation* (New York: Avon Books, 1975).

[35] For other critiques of the sanctity-of-life doctrine that is central to the agapistic approach, see W.K. Frankena, "The Ethics of Respect for Life", in Stephen F. Barker, ed., *Respect for Life in Medicine, Philosophy, and the Law*, (Baltimore: Johns Hopkins U.Press, 1977), 24–62; Edward W. Keyserlingk, *Sanctity of Life or Quality of Life in the Context of Ethics, Medicine, and the Law*, Study Paper for the Law Reform Commission of Canada (Ottawa: Law Reform Commission, 1979), 9–47; Marvin Kohl, "The Sanctity-of-Life Principle," in Marvin Kohl, ed., *The Morality of Killing: Sanctity-of-Life, Abortion and Euthanasia* (London: Peter Owen, 1974), 3–23; Helga Kuhse, *The Sanctity-of-Life Doctrine in Medicine: A Critique* (Oxford: Clarendon Press, 1987), Chapter I and elsewhere.

[36] In this we adopt a perspective similar to that of Tristam Engelhardt, Jr., Paul Ramsay, Robert Veatch and others.

[37] R.B. Edwards and G.C. Graber, *Bio-Ethics* (Harcourt, Brace Jovanovich: San Diego and New York, 1988) 17.

[38] Compare R.R. Faden and T.L. Beauchamp, *A History and Theory of Informed Consent* (New York and Oxford: Oxford University Press, 1986) 6ff.; Brandt, *Ethical Theory*, 336ff.; Frankena, *Ethics*, Feinberg, *Social Philosophy* (Prentice-Hall: Englewood Cliffs, N.J.: 1973) For a somewhat different analysis, but one which still portrays rights as claims, see Ronald Dworkin, *Taking Rights Seriously* (Cambridge: Harvard University Press, 1977) 9ff., 188–192ff. and elewhere.

[39] See T.A. Mappes and J.S. Zembaty, *Biomedical Ethics* (McGraw-Hill: New York and St. Louis, 1986) 16 and elsewhere.

[40] Compare Brandt, *Ethical Theory*, 306–326.

[41] See R.B. Brandt *A Theory of the Good and the Right* (Oxford: Clarenden Press, 1979), 164-182.

[42] Michael Drummond, "Guidelines for Health Technology Assessment: Economic Evaluation," in D. Feeny, Gordon Guyatt and Peter Tugwell, *Health Care Technology: Effectiveness, Efficiency and Public Policy* (Montreal: Canadian Medical Association &The Institute for Research on Pubic Policy, 1986) esp. 122 f.

[43] What follows is based in part on J.E. Magnet and E.W. Kluge, *Withholding Treatment from Defective Newborn Children* (Cowansville: Brown Legal Publ.,1985).

[44] J. Piaget, *The Moral Judgement of the Child* (Geneva: 1926). M.R. Harrover, in "Social Status and the Moral Development of the Child, *British Journal of Educational Psychology* 4(1934) 75–95 casts doubt on the universality of the stages identified by Piaget. However, he does not impugn the fact of such development.

[45] Lawrence Kohlberg, *The Philosophy of Moral Development* (Chicago: Harper and Row, 1971). For a relatively recent restatement of his position by the author, see "The Future

of Liberalism as the Dominant Ideology of the West," in R.W. Wilson and G.J. Shoichet, eds., *Moral Development and Politics* (New York: Praeger, 1980).

[46] See F.L. Kohlberg, "Development of Children's Orientation towards A Moral Order: First Sequences in the Development of Moral Thought," *Vita Humana* 6 (1963), and "Stage and Consequence: The Cognitive Developmental Approach to Socialization," in D.A. Goslin, ed., *Handbook of Socialization Theory and Research* (Chicago: Rand McNally, 1969) Ch.6.

[47] Compare M.L. Hoffman, "Moral Development," in P.H. Mussner, 3rd. ed., *Carmichael's Mantel of Psychology* (New York: John Wiley and Sons, 1970) vol.2, 276–281; and F.H. Cohen, "Stages and Stability: The Moral Developmental Approach to Political Order."

[48] For more on physicians' obligations to third parties, see Chapter 3.

SUGGESTED READINGS

- Bowie, Norman E. ed. *Ethical Theory in the Last Quarter of the Twentieth Century.* Indianapolis: Hackett Publishing, 1983.

  This is a collection of essays by Stevenson, Frankena, Brandt and Melden on value-judgements, moral-point-of-view theories, utilitarianism and rights-based approach. It can serve as a useful way of focusing some of the perspectives in the other readings mentioned.

- Frankena, William K. "Deontological Theories," from W.K. Frankena, *Ethics*. Englewood Cliffs, N.J.: Prentice-Hall, 1963.

  This selection from Frankena's classic introductory text on ethical theory discusses various types of deontological theories and attempts to relate them to one another.

- Haering, Bernard. "Ethos, Ethical Code and the Morality of the Physician," from Bernard Haering, *Medical Ethics*. Notre Dame, Ind.: Fides, 1973. Chapter 4.

  Bernard Haering is a Catholic theologian who writes on medical ethics. This excerpt is from his text, which for years has served as a standard and middle-of-the-road guide to Catholic physicians.

- Pellegrino, E.D., and J.P. Langan, J.C. Harvey, eds. *Catholic Perspectives on Medical Morals*. Dordrecht: Kluwer Academic, 1989.

  A good collection of essays on the interrelationship between catholicism and ethics in the context of health care. It addresses foundational issues within the pluralistic perspective that characterizes contemporary catholic thought. The points raised in these discussions can be applied to other religious perspectives.

- Taylor, Paul. "Utilitarianism," from Paul Taylor, *Principles of Ethics: An Introduction*. Belmont, Calif.: Wadsworth, 1975.

  A classic exposition of utilitarian theory for those who do not want to go to the full-length work of Richard Brandt and others.

3
Codes of Ethics

> While throughout antiquity merely technical skill and empirical proficiency constituted the equipment of the average physician who as a craftsman was trained through apprenticeship with another physician-craftsman, the medical "scientist" studied philosophy. The ethics of these physicians became identical with that of the philosophical school to which they professed allegiance as scientists.
>
> L. Edelstein, "The Professional Ethics of the Greek Physicians" Bulletin of the History of Medicine 1956, Vol. 30 reprinted in L. Edelstein, *Ancient Medicine* (Baltimore: Johns Hopkins Univ. Press, 1967) pp. 332–333.

> A moral code, if it is to be a code, must be formulable, and if it is to be a code to be observed it must be formulable in rules of manageable complexity.
>
> J.O. Urmson, "Saints and Heroes," reprinted in Joel Feinberg, ed., *Moral Concepts* (Oxford: Oxford University Press, 1979) p. 70.

This chapter examines the notion of a code of ethics for physicians using the theoretical concepts developed in the preceding chapter. At the end of this chapter the reader should have an analytical understanding of the various codes that govern the conduct of professional medicine in Canada at the present time.

Questions to keep in mind while reading this chapter include:

1. What is the difference between professional medical ethos, professional medical protocol and professional medical ethics?
2. What is the basis of a code of professional medical ethics, and from what does it derive its binding power?
3. What are the limits of a code of professional medical ethics?
4. What are the implications of medicine as a professional service monopoly?
5. Why should a code of ethics for the profession of medicine include statements of rights as well as statements of duties?

Introduction[1]

In 1978 the Canadian Medical Association adopted a Code of Ethics with the following words:

> A physician should be aware of the traditional standards established by his forebears and act within the general principles which have governed their conduct.
>
> The Oath of Hippocrates represented the desire of members of that day to establish for themselves standards of conduct in living and in the practice of their art. Since then the principals established have been retained as our basic guidelines for ethical living with the profession of medicine.
>
> The *International Code of Ethics* and the *Declaration of Geneva* (1948), developed and approved by The World Medical Association, have modernized the ancient codes. They have been endorsed by each member organization, including The Canadian Medical Association, as a general guide having worldwide application.
>
> The Canadian Medical Association accepts the responsibility of delineating the standards of ethical behaviour expected of Canadian physicians.

The Association then identified the following as the principles that should govern the behaviour of ethical physicians:

1. Consider first the well-being of the patient.
2. Honour your profession and its traditions.
3. Recognize your limitations and the special skills of others in the prevention and treatment of disease.
4. Protect the patient's secrets.
5. Teach and be taught.
6. Remember that integrity and professional ability should be your best advertisement.
7. Be responsible in setting a value on your services.

It went on to interpret these principles under three general headings: Responsibilities to the Patient, Responsibilities to the Profession, and Responsibilities to Society. In October of 1987, the Association reaffirmed the *Code* and its interpretation without change. Similarly in 1985, after several years of discussion, analysis and consultation, the Canadian Nurses Association promulgated a new *Code of Ethics for Nursing*. Other health care professions in Canada, both before and since, have considered and adopted similar codes as binding on their members.[2]

The development and promulgation of such codes would be a matter of purely historical interest if it were not for one very important fact: Although in and by themselves these codes are not legally binding on the members of the various professions, all Canadian Provinces and Territories have enacted legislation that identifies these codes as delineating the ethical standards of conduct which society may reasonably expect of physicians. This statutory recognition, in turn, is closely followed in case law.[3] Therefore, the development and promulgation of these codes in effect constitutes a legally sanctioned fixing of the ethics of the professions. The preamble of the recent CNA *Code of Ethics* puts the point rather well:[4]

> This Code expresses and seeks to clarify those ethical principles that are definitive of ethical nursing activity. For those entering the profession, the Code identifies the basic moral commitments of nursing and may serve as a source of education and reflection. For those within the profession, the Code also serves as a basis for self-evaluation and for peer review. For those outside the profession, this Code may serve to establish expectations regarding the ethical conduct of nurses.

With due alteration of detail, the *Code of Ethics* of the Canadian Medical Association has to be seen in a similar light.

The fact that codes of ethics are characterized in this way would hardly occasion unease if it were not for three things. First, these codes are generally developed by the professions themselves independently of the rest of society, essentially on the basis of the experiences and perspectives of the members of the respective professions. This suggests that in the eyes of these professions, the technical expertise required of individuals in order to become members of the profession, and the experiences of the respective professionals themselves in the conduct of their business, are sufficient to allow the profession alone to decide what does and what does not constitute ethically acceptable behaviour.

Second, it suggests that since the codes of the various health care professions are distinct from each other, the ethics of the various health care professions are also distinct from each other and somehow unique. More precisely, it suggests that the ethical principles mentioned by each profession apply only to those who are formally associated with the relevant professions and who earn their living in the exercise of the relevant vocation.

Third, since the codes of the various health care professions are not merely restatements of codes already adopted in other countries, it suggests that in the eyes of Canadian health care professions, the special ethical principles which supposedly govern the conduct of these professionals differ from country to country.

All three suggestions may be questioned. The first may be called the fallacy of expertise,[5] the second may be called the fallacy of uniqueness and the third the fallacy of nationality. However, to appreciate fully what this involves, and to connect it with our discussion in the preceding chapters, we shall approach the whole issue of codes somewhat more circuitously by beginning with the question: What is such a code supposed to be?

Codes of Professional Ethics

There are four common ways of responding to this question. A code of professional ethics can be seen either

1. as a statement of the ethos of the profession;
2. as a quasi-legal document outlining the judicial position of the profession;

3. as a statement of the unique role-specific rules that govern the conduct of the profession and that are not part of a universal ethical framework; or as

4. as a statement of the role-specific rules that govern the conduct of the profession but which derive from the general framework within which all ethical rules are embedded.

(1) Codes as Statements of Ethos

The word "ethos" may be defined as "the underlying sentiment that informs the beliefs, customs or practices of a group or society; the character or disposition of a community, group or person."[6] Therefore, if we understand the notion of a code of ethics in this sense, then the function of a code of professional ethics will be to reflect the way the majority (or perhaps more correctly, the way the most vociferous and/or influential part) of an association or profession feels about the issues that arise in the conduct of the profession.

Such an approach to codes of professional ethics is not uncommon.[7] However, there are several considerations that may be raised against it. For instance, it may be argued that if we really took this interpretation of the nature and role of these codes seriously, then any association which tried to develop a code of ethics really would be wasting its time if it engaged in analysis and deliberation. Especially if it deliberated about what is right and what is wrong, or about what ought and what ought not to be done, etc. All of this would be quite inappropriate because it would provide no real clue about the membership's opinion or position on these issues. Instead, if this interpretation was correct, the correct way to proceed would be to conduct an opinion poll among the members of the profession. The appropriately generalized and statistically analyzed results of that poll would then provide the clauses of the code itself.

It is unlikely that many people would take a code that was produced in this way seriously. But even if they did, a code that was developed in this way would be suffer from a tremendous disadvantage: It would lack ethical binding power. As Socrates has already pointed out, the fact that most people agree on a certain course of action or agree to be bound by certain rules does not show either that the people are correct or that the rules are ethically valid. To be sure, they may be; but that would be a matter of coincidence. Agreement itself is no guarantee of anything except agreement. Furthermore, history has many examples of agreements that in fact were ethically wrong. For example, once upon a time it was generally agreed (even among women) that women were not persons, that ethnic minorities could be discriminated against, and so on.

In effect, an association that developed a code of ethics in this manner would have to accept the possibility that what it promulgated as its code of ethics might actually be ethically unsound.

Of course, not all consequences of this sort of approach would be negative. An association that accepted it would find itself in the interesting (and possibly advantageous) position of never really having to worry about ethical problems at all. It could simply right an otherwise unacceptable practice by inducing its members to change their minds on how they thought about the particular matter. After all, on this interpretation the evaluative standards of the code would be mere reflections of the majority opinion—and that may change, or be changed. However, it is unlikely that many would accept this kind of group-centred ethical voluntarism.[8]

Furthermore, those in charge of preparing such a code would face a rather onerous task. They would have to update their Code continuously. Not, however, because the Association, its membership or its executive comes closer to the truth or to a correct answer, but because the opinion of the membership undergoes continual change. The vagaries of everyday existence, of personal and professional interaction, all take their toll and are reflected in changes in personal attitudes and perspectives. While such responsiveness may be considered a virtue in some contexts, in professional areas requiring guidelines the uncertainty that would result from this fluctuation would be disastrous.

(2) Codes as Quasi-Legal Documents [9]

On the other hand, if we were to take a code of ethics to be a quasi-legal document these difficulties would be avoided. A code would then be merely an attempt by the profession to outline its judicial position and that of its members, but without having recourse to the judicial machinery that exists in the context of the law itself. Adherence to the code then would become a matter of quasi-legal obligation. It would find its ultimate test in the courts.

This approach has much to recommend it. For instance, it would explain the use of codes of ethics by the disciplinary bodies within the professions when they sit in judgement on the conduct of their members in disciplinary hearings. It would also explain the courts' recognition of professional codes of ethics as guidelines when they attempt to decide whether a legal breach of professional obligation has occurred; and why the courts are usually reluctant to overturn the decisions that have been reached by professional disciplinary tribunals, and so on. After all, if this perception of codes of professional ethics is correct, then the two—that is to say, legal cases and codified professional guidelines—are functionally related to one another.

However, while this approach would be correct in focusing on the closeness of legal decisions and codified guidelines, the fact remains that two are not the same; nor should codes of professional ethics be construed in this fashion. Codes of professional ethics in general, and those of the health care professions in particular, do indeed have legal standing. However, the reason for this is not that the codes reflect any underlying judicial sentiments or state of affairs. Instead, they tend to have legal standing because the law assumes that professional codes of ethics are more likely than not to be ethically appropriate, and it is extremely reluctant to overturn what it takes to be ethically correct. The law attempts to follow the ethics, not ethics the law.[10]

Which brings us to a second consideration: There is nothing particularly ethical about a code of health care ethics that is construed in this way. If this interpretation were correct, then all that a code of ethics really amounted to would be a statement of ethos based on social sentiment with the added weight of legal sanctions. Sanctions, however, even when legally grounded, do not add ethical weight to anything. They merely add an element of coercion.

(3) Codes as Statements of Role-Specific Rules Unique to a Profession but Ethically Sui Generis

If we understood the code of ethics of a profession as a statement of the role-specific rules that are ethically unique to that profession, we would avoid the pitfalls that beset interpretations (1) and (2). The reason is that this interpretation would centre around two claims: First, on a very general level, the claim that the existence of a profession per se gives rise to ethical parameters that do not obtain outside of the professional context; and second, on the claim that the specific nature of a particular profession gives rise to special ethical parameters which, although they might find analogies in other professions or walks of life, nevertheless are never quite the same.

However, one can legitimately ask whether the first claim is really true. Does the existence of a profession really give rise to special ethical parameters? And more importantly, are these parameters unique to each distinct profession?

There are reasons for replying both in the negative and in the affirmative. On the negative side we could say that membership in a profession or in a professional organization is really nothing more than an artificial, conventional relationship. In and by itself it no more touches the ethical status of the individual than any other conventional affiliation. On the positive side we could argue that while this is true, the criteria on which such membership is based do have ethical import. Unlike clubs, unions and the like, professional associations have criteria of competence that individuals must meet in order to qualify for membership. These criteria, however, do entail special rights and obligations. Codes of professional ethics therefore are really more or less formal expressions of these particular ethical implications.

As to the second claim, which centres around the notion of responsibility, it is important to note that there are several requirements that anyone must meet before being held morally responsibility for a particular act.[11] These requirements include: *free will*: The act in question must be voluntary and originate with the actor; *awareness*: The actor or agent must aware of and understand the nature of what it is he or she is doing; *intention*: The individual must intend the particular thing or outcome that results.

However, the degree of responsibility that falls on a particular person increases as the person's awareness and understanding of the act in question increases. Everyone is presumed to have free will, and all other things being equal, everyone is presumed to be free to the same degree. Furthermore, everyone is deemed capable of forming intentions. However, not everyone is presumed to have equal understanding, technical competence, or skill. In fact we can say as a general maxim of ethics that the greater someone's degree of understanding and expertise, the more she or he is presumed capable of exercising judgement in those actions that involve her/his area of competence.

It is upon these grounds that the difference in ethical expectations between the health care professionals and lay persons is based; and it is here that there enters the connection between increased responsibility and membership in a professional association. Professional associations admit as members only those who have a certain degree of expertise in their respective areas. That is why someone who is formally identified as a health care professional is subject to greater ethical scrutiny, and why the fact of association indirectly licenses greater expectations. A difference in ethical status is created by the fact that the member meets the pre-conditions for membership itself.

A difference of this kind is heightened further by the fact that the profession also holds itself out to the public as having such a heightened expertise. As a profession it also holds out a promise. Therefore, both the professions as well as the individual professionals, by the very fact of identifying themselves in this way, invite more stringent ethical evaluation. Therefore, when someone enters into a contract with a member of a profession, he or she may legitimately expect a greater degree of proficiency from that member simply by virtue of his or her professional association.

However, if this is true, then a curious consequence follows. In that case it does not really matter how that expertise is acquired or whether it is exercised in the context of an institutionalized formal professional association. If the crux of the matter is the possession of expertise, then how it is acquired is irrelevant. (The surgeon in Chicago who, as it turned out, had never gone to medical school but had acquired his knowledge and expertise initially as a military medic and later, so to speak, "on the job," could not escape responsibility for his actions by pointing to his lack of formal education and training.)

In our society, at the present time, those who possess this expertise usually have undergone a period of institutionalized formal training and have a certificate or diploma to prove it. In some instances, membership in a professional association is a legal requirements for anyone who wishes to put his or her competence into practice. However, so far from being an absolute truth, this merely reflects the institutionalized way in which competence and expertise are usually acquired in our society. It also reflects the politics of professional practice. However, there is nothing illogical, contradictory, or otherwise wrong-headed about the suggestion that the necessary competence or expertise can be acquired outside of such a context; nor does it follow that an individual is exercising technical competence at an unacceptable level simply because he/she is practising outside of the pale of professional affiliation. All these are merely accidental and socially relative features that have to do with the politics of enforcing professional standards.

This consideration certainly has a point to make. Heightened ethical responsibility also falls on those who have the appropriate degree of technical expertise, whether they are formally associated with the rest of the profession or not. However, it would be foolhardy to ignore the fact that in our society expertise and formal association do generally go hand in hand; and that as professionals, those who have the increased expertise do hold themselves out as having such.

Therefore, interpretation (3) is correct when it insists that physicians are subject to special ethical constraints; and correct also when it suggests that the types of situations that they encounter (or are likely to encounter) because of the nature of what they do is distinct. It may also be appropriate to try to capture this in a special code, for heuristic and possibly pedagogical reasons.

However, it would be hasty to conclude from this that therefore the nature of the ethical rules and principles that bind the profession are unique. If anything, it suggests the fourth interpretation is correct.

(4) Codes as Statements of Role-Specific Rules Derived from the General Framework that Govern Personal Interaction

No matter how we look at it, physicians as professionals are different from other people. The fact of their professional status and of their qualifications increases the degree of their moral responsibility.

In and by itself, this does not require a special code of ethics to regulate or guide their behaviour. The ethical principles that are involved are not different from those that guide other members of society. On the contrary, the fact that physicians are members of society, and the fact that they operate in a social context, entails that they are subject to the same ethical principles that govern everyone else.[12]

However, it is true that there are certain more or less clearly identifiable issues that arise frequently in the practice of any profession: issues that have an ethical core and that require an ethical resolution. It is to these issues that the codes of ethics of the professions are directed. In other words, the function of such codes is to provide guidance for those situations that are likely to strike the professional as being ethically difficult. This means that in principle it is possible to dispense with such codes. After all, they are really nothing more than applications of the same general ethical principles that govern all social interactions. In practice, however, such codes are very useful because they spell out how the general ethical principles apply to certain types of difficult situations. Furthermore, they alert the professional to the type of conduct that the profession expects of its member in these circumstances, and serve as guides against which the actions of the members of the profession can be measured. For practical reasons, therefore, such codes are invaluable.

Therefore, a professional code of ethics should not be understood as containing something that is ethically peculiar and unique. It should be seen as nothing more than a particularized version of a universally applicable moral code, where the specifics of that particularization are a function of the nature of activities in question.

Professional codes of ethics do not indicate a conviction that different ethical principles apply. They indicate an acceptance of the fact that the distinct knowledge of the members of the relevant profession, and the fact that the members represent themselves as having a particular type of expertise, imply a commitment to and an acceptance of a higher-than-normal level of ethical responsibility.

From this it follows that if a profession wants to construct a code of ethics, it should determine what formal rules of action follow when the general ethical principles, that apply to society in general, are applied to the activities that are characteristic of the profession.

We mentioned that Canadian medicine has codes of ethics. The question we should therefore ask is whether the clauses of these codes follow from the general ethical principles that apply to society as a whole. However, to answer that question would involve us in an analysis of tremendous proportions. That might be useful. However, it strikes us that it would be more useful still—and certainly more constructive—to give a brief sketch of what a code of ethics for the medical profession might look like if it were to developed wholly on the basis of the nature of medicine itself and the fundamental principles of the deontological ethical perspective that we identified in the preceding chapters.

A Model Code of Ethics for Physicians

However, before proceeding with this task, we would like to clear up a possible misunderstanding. This involves what we previously called the fallacy of nationality. It consists in assuming that a code of ethics can be specific to a particular nation. The fact is that ethics and nationality have nothing to do with one another. Nationality has no ethical significance. It is an entirely legal notion. What does have ethical significance is the socio-economic milieu in which the profession of medicine may be exercised. Not, however, because it is tied to the ethics of a particular country in some peculiar, unique and nontransferable manner. The reason is that the socio-economic milieu constitutes the set of conditions that particularize the general ethical principles that apply to all people, to the particular context in question. Wherever and whenever conditions are similar, there the general principles must be applied in a similar way.[13] We must therefore ignore any nationalistic parameters that may be associated with a particular code of ethics except insofar as the conditions of practice are relevant to the foundation of appropriate rules.

We should also keep in mind that a code of ethics must walk a fine line between generality and specificity. To be practically useful, it must be sufficiently free of specifics to allow application to the whole array of situations that characterize the profession of medicine in general. At the same time, it must be specific enough to distinguish it from the ethics of other professions.

Finally, we should be careful to distinguish between two parameters that are liable to be confused: the nature of medicine on the one hand, and the conditions of contractual sale of the services by the physician on the other. The ethical parameters involved in these two and that follow from them are quite distinct. The ethical parameters that follow from the first derive only from the role that the individual plays as a physician. Therefore the rights and obligations that are here involved hold for all physicians as such, independently of their area of practice or specialization. The rights/obligations that might arise from their particular and specific conditions of employment or practice—e.g., length of duty, level of remuneration and the like—are irrelevant.

It is precisely these conditions of employment or practice however, that are central in the second case.[14] The conditions under which a physician or group of physicians agree to perform certain services may raise obligations that do not hold for others. An example here would be the service contract conditions that physicians at a given hospital might agree to as a matter of employment by that hospital; or the conditions that a provincial medical association might agree to in its bargaining with a particular provincial government.

It is the first sorts of considerations, the rights and obligations that derive from the nature of medicine, that are central for a code of ethics for physicians, not the second. They give rise to at least nine general themes. Four of them may be expressed as rights and five as obligations.

The obligations are:

1. advancement or realization of functional potential of the patient
2. respect for the autonomy of the patient
3. primacy of services to the patient
4. repayment of social debt
5. professional integrity

The rights are:

6. adequate information and decision-making authority
7. adequate working conditions
8. preservation of ethical integrity of his/her own personhood
9. fair and equitable treatment and remuneration

We shall consider these in turn.

1. Physicians have an obligation to promote their patients' health potential to the greatest degree possible under the circumstances.

This obligation is rooted in the function of medicine as a profession. That is to say, every human being has a unique nature or make-up. This nature, both psychological and physiological, determines the potentials of that individual. Sometimes the realization of these potentials is prevented because of some dysfunction or condition suffered by the individual. In other words, the individual may be unhealthy relative to the state of optimal functional excellence that is possible for him or her in virtue of his or her make-up or nature.[15]

Medicine is centred in the notion of health. That is to say, the essential role of medicine is to promote and maintain the greatest degree of health possible for a given individual under the circumstances. The nature of medicine as a profession and the concept of the health potential of an individual therefore coincide on this point. Anyone who becomes a physician therefore accepts the role of physician as defined by the nature of the profession. It follows that anyone who becomes a physician also accepts the obligation to promote each patient's health potential to the greatest degree possible.

However, no professional activity can take place in a socio-economic vacuum. For physicians this means that the competing obligations they have towards their various patients (as well as towards society), the lack of sufficient resources, and so on, put constraints on the range of actions open to them as physicians. This means that there are cases in which the attainment of the optimal state of health for a given patient—of a patient's full health potential—is not possible.[16]

However, this does not mean that therefore physicians have no duty whatsoever. Rather, it means that physicians must adjust their activities to the nature of the situation, and that they must strive for the greatest degree or level of health possible for their patients under the circumstances. Furthermore, since not all patients have the same health potential, physicians cannot expect to achieve the same level of functional performance for all of their patients. Nor should physicians aim at the same level in each case. That would be to deny the individual variations that characterize the patients themselves.

2. Physicians have an obligation to respect their patients as persons

This duty has three separate components: autonomy, confidentiality and equality of treatment.

Autonomy

In all but the most unusual of circumstances,[17] practising physicians deal with patients who are not mere bodies or biological organisms but are persons.[18] After all, practising physicians are not biological mechanics. The principle of autonomy requires that persons not be treated as mere objects. This means that patients may not simply be treated according to whatever will most easily, most effectively, or most expeditiously, produce the outcome that the physicians have in mind. Instead, patients must be treated as persons: as beings of incommensurable value who have a fundamental right to self-determination.

This in turn means that insofar as this is possible, physicians have an obligation to allow their patients to make the decisions about the direction that their medical care ought to take.[19] In contemporary jargon, physicians must allow their patients to give an informed consent or an informed refusal for the care that is planned.

This entails three things: first, patients must be given whatever information is necessary for informed consent on their part to be possible. Second, it means that this information must be presented to them in a way that is appropriate to their level of understanding. Third, it means that physicians have no right to impose their own values on their patients or to influence their patient's decision-making in an untoward manner.[20]

All of these points are important for actual practice. Physicians must constantly keep in mind that the ultimate right to decide whether to accept or reject a particular form of treatment belongs to the patient. This is true even though such a decision might conflict with the religious and/or ethical views of the physician.[21] Anything else would be a denial of the patient's moral autonomy.[22] Physicians must always remember that expertise in matters of health care is not the same as expertise in ethics, and that knowledge of facts is not knowledge of values. They must also remember that the professional status of physicians does not confer a superior authority that allows them to override the goals set by a patient through the autonomous exercise of informed consent.

Of course, there are situations where patients are incapable of giving informed consent because their autonomy is compromised. In such cases, physicians may have a duty to act as proxy decision makers. However, this duty arises only under certain conditions.[23] Specifically, it arises only in emergency contexts where it is not possible to contact or consult an appropriate proxy decision maker such as a next-of-kin, the relevant social agencies, or the courts, for example.

Furthermore, even when time is of the essence, if the incompetent patients are known to have indicated how they would wish to be treated under the sort of circumstances that obtain, or if there is some reasonably accessible indication to this effect, then physicians have a duty to determine and follow these indications.[24] Of course, if no such indications and/or values are known or are reasonably ascertainable under the circumstances that prevail, then physicians must decide on the basis of current social values. That is to say, they must employ the standards of the objective reasonable person.[25] It may be the case that these standards correspond to the position that the physicians themselves would adopt. However, they need not be. However that may be, under no circumstances may physicians point to their professional status and claim a right or a duty to make a decision solely on the basis of what they as professionals take to be correct. That would be to violate the principle of autonomy and commit the fallacy of expertise.

Confidentiality

Other more specific obligations follow from the duty to consider patients as autonomous moral agents: for instance, the duty of confidentiality and the duty of equality of treatment.[26]

The duty of confidentiality is grounded in the fact that, all other things being equal, patients do not seek physicians out in their capacity as private individuals. They seek them out in their capacity as health care professionals. Therefore, the access that physicians have to information about their patients is predicated on their functioning in a professional capacity, and the information that patients provide is given, disclosed, or otherwise made available on the assumption that physicians will use it only in a professional context. Therefore, physicians do have the right to use whatever information is relevant to and necessary for the conduct of their professional role towards their patients. However, they may not use or divulge this information in an identifiable form in any other fashion without express permission of the patient.[27] That would violate the autonomy of the patients and would contravene the conditions of the physicians' access to the information in the first place.

There are exceptions to this. However, they are very limited. They tend to involve situations where physicians become privy to information that leads them to believe that in their professional opinion the patients' condition and/or actions, etc. constitute a clear and present danger to other parties, or that they otherwise violate or threaten to violate the rights of others in an ethically unacceptable fashion. Here confidentiality must be breached.[28] However, such a breach would be justified by the principle of autonomy as well as the principle of equality and justice.

Another sort of situation involves epidemiological research and quality assurance studies. Here certain data about patients, suitably de-identified but retaining all the relevant health-care related data, must be revealed. Most provinces have laws that allow the disclosure of otherwise privileged information in this sort of case. The reason is that the development and planning of health services cannot proceed without such information. Therefore access to health-services is predicated on such information being made available by patients to appropriately qualified persons. However, the ethical requirement still remains that if the relevant information can be used in a de-identified fashion, then it should be revealed only in that way.

Furthermore, confidentiality in the strict sense of the term must also be breached by physicians when their patients are incompetent and a medical decision has to be made. Here the relevant information must be passed on to the appropriate proxy decision-maker(s).

Confidentiality may also be breached when other health care professionals are appropriately involved in the treatment of a patient[29] and require the relevant information. There are still other occasions when confidentiality may be breached. However, we shall leave further discussion of this topic to the chapter on informed consent.[30]

Equality

The principle of equality is one of the fundamental principles of deontological ethics. This principle should therefore govern all human interaction, professional or otherwise. However, it presents a special problem for the practice of medicine. It sometimes happens that different patients compete for the professional services of one and the same physician. Likewise, it sometimes happens that different patients compete for the same limited resources that a physician has at his or her disposal. The temptation here is to resolve the problem along utilitarian lines by trying to calculate the greatest good for the greatest number of people and then act on the basis of that calculation.[31]

However, that is unacceptable from a deontological perspective. It would reduce the patients from the status of autonomous moral agents to objective quantities who have merely calculative value. Instead, physicians should try to find a solution to the problem by balancing the competing rights of the patients relative to each other under the circumstances that prevail. In other words, physicians should try to apply the principle of equality and justice, and the principle of priority. Of course this may not always be easy to do. However, we shall postpone further discussion of this until Chapter 9.

3. Physicians owe a primary obligation of service to their identified patients

Since the Canadian context is essentially one of socialized medicine, physicians who are acting as a health care professional may be seen as the embodiment of society's attempt to fulfil its obligation of health care towards its various members.[32] Typically, therefore, although by no means exclusively, the exercise of professional medical activity involves patients. In our society this usually occurs within an institutionalized setting; which is to say, in a setting that recognizes the distinctive role of the physician as health care provider and that perceives this role as defined in historically sanctioned and legally circumscribed terms.[33]

Invariably, such settings include more or less clearly formalized criteria of practice. A patient may therefore be defined as someone who meets these criteria in an operant sense. It follows that physicians, in their capacity as health care professionals, stand in a special relation to their patients in a way they do not stand towards non-patients. This relationship is usually referred to as the physician/patient relationship.[34]

However, this is only half the story. In principle, the domain of persons towards whom the physician stands in a physician/patient relationship includes all persons who meets these criteria. However, it is impossible for any one physician to fulfil the right to health care for such a large number of people. The mere attempt to do so would guarantee that no-one's needs would be sufficiently served. A single physician can only fulfil the right to health care for a limited number of patients at any one point in time. Therefore, the class of patients for which a particular physician is responsible cannot be co-extensive with the class of patients in general. The question therefore is, how can the class of patients for which a physician is responsible be defined?

Two sorts of considerations are here relevant. One focuses on the institutional, the other on the non-institutional context. The physician in an institutional[35] setting has no say over who will be a member of the group of patients towards whom a duty of service is formally recognized. The more or less mechanically operating institutional determinants assign specific duties on the basis of ability and training, as well as on the basis of such criteria as urgency, temporal priority and likelihood of success and so on.

However, things are different in the non-institutional setting or private sphere. Here physicians have some choice about whom to take as a patient.[36] As long as reasons for refusing to accept someone as a patient are not unacceptably discriminatory in an ethical sense—e.g., on the basis of colour, creed, or ethnic extraction—and as long as the refusal itself does not contravene the conditions of service access tacitly contained in the establishment of medicine as a service provider monopoly, physicians have a right of refusal that is as firmly entrenched as that of any other profession in a similar position.

Furthermore, all other things being equal, the fact that physicians are persons guarantees them the right to terminate the physician/patient relationship if the conditions under which it was entered into[37] are not being met from the side of the patient.[38] This would be the case, for example, if a patient competently, knowingly and deliberately[39] ignored the advice of the physician or even went against it.

However, sometimes not all things are equal—and herewith we come to the exceptive clauses that we noted before. We mentioned emergency contexts. Here their expertise and training imposes a duty to act on physicians even when the individuals in question are not their patients.[40] We shall not detail the reasons any further. Among other things it would require on analysis of the ethical equivalence between bringing about an outcome by acting directly and positively, and bringing about the very outcome by deliberately refusing to act.[41] For now, suffice it to say that physicians who deliberately refrain from appropriate action in an emergency situation become responsible for the foreseeable outcome of that failure.[42] Therefore, even if the law does not as yet place what is sometimes called a good-Samaritan obligation on the physician, ethics—deontological ethics as we have described it—does.[43] Another sort of exception derives from geographic factors. Canadian physicians may find themselves in geographic locations where they are the only physicians within reasonable reach of the patients. In such a case the right of refusal and the right of termination are diminished to such a degree that unless the physicians have made appropriate arrangements to allow the patients equal opportunity of access to other physicians without undue hardship for the patients, they must act as though the physician/patient relationship was in place.

4. Physicians have a professional obligation towards society

This obligation has three roots: the social cost of the education of physicians, the social origin of the knowledge and skills that physicians acquire, and the fact of professional monopoly.

To begin with education: Professionals in general and physicians in particular do not fully pay the cost of their education. Tuition fees cover but a fraction of the total cost involved in educating them;[44] nor do the services provided by them while they are being educated and trained constitute anything like an adequate recompense to society. Equality and justice therefore entail that anyone who voluntarily accepts a medical education thereby accepts the obligation to render an appropriate return. That return may take several forms. For instance, providing a certain amount of free medical service for society, the way in which lawyers do for indigent clients; or adjusting fee schedules to reflect the fact of this social obligation; or restraining what otherwise would be an unfettered freedom to seek and serve clients of their own choice.[45]

Furthermore, the knowledge and skills that are acquired by physicians also have a social component. They are neither the property of the physicians who acquire them nor are they the property of the medical profession as a whole. They have been developed over generations and even millennia, through a process of mutually cooperative effort that involves physicians as well as other professionals such as biochemists, physicists, engineers, and many others. Furthermore, society as a whole has also been involved in this effort. For instance, it has made the development possible in a socio-economic sense. Furthermore, it has provided subjects for experimentation, and it has given physicians the opportunity to practise. Without all of this, medicine would not exist nor have come into being as a scientific discipline.

These factors license an expectation of appropriate social return. Given the nature of this indebtedness, one of the most appropriate forms of repayment would be for the physician and for the profession to serve in an educative capacity both to individuals and to the public. This is sometimes expressed by saying that the physician has an obligation to educate.[46]

The third root of social obligation lies in the fact that by law, medicine is a professional service monopoly. No-one who does not meet certain standards, set and controlled by the medical profession itself, may practise medicine in Canada.[47] This does not mean that no-one except a physician may provide health care services. Nurses, physiotherapists, chiropractors and other professionals also provide health care. What it means is that non-one except a duly recognized physician may perform operations, prescribe medications and so on. This situation is not a necessary or inevitable social development. Other societies and other times—even our own society in the past—have handled things differently. Rather, the fact of this professional service provider monopoly is the result of a conscious and deliberate decision on part of our society and of the profession of medicine itself.[48]

Society has several reasons for acting in this fashion. One, of course, is to control the number of physicians and to make it economically attractive to enter the profession.[49] This reason played considerable role in the early Canadian setting[50] as well as in other countries.[51]

Another reason is to try to guarantee standardization and control of quality of service. Historically, this was the consideration that figured most prominently in the health care acts and legislations in Canada since the Act of 1818 in Upper Canada, and that was re-emphasized in the Flexner Report of 1910. All other things being equal, this has remained the strongest reason why society has persisted in retaining the monopolistic status of the profession in this way.

However, the fact of monopoly entails three consequences for the delivery of medical services by the profession: quality, ubiquity and universality.

Quality

Monopoly means that for all practical purposes, the profession has control over medical education, licensing and the setting of standards. It thereby acquires the duty of making sure that these standards are the best possible under the circumstances, and that they are policed effectively.[52] However, this does not mean that quality control becomes a purely in-house matter to be handled entirely by the profession, as it were in the bosom of the profession itself.[53] Rather it means that whatever policing body society ultimately might see fit to institute, the profession has an obligation to assist it to the best of its ability; and that as professional capabilities change, these changes should be incorporated into the qualitative standards suggested by the profession itself.

Ubiquity

The obligation of ubiquity of service arises from the fact that the existence of the monopoly prevents anyone who is not a member of the profession from practising medicine. However, this means that unless the profession undertakes to ensure that all areas of the country (provinces) that require medical services are in fact supplied with them, these affected areas will be denied reasonable access to health care.

This in turn would mean two things: First, the people who live in those areas would thereby be treated differently from people in other areas; i.e. they would be the subjects of discriminatory deprivation. Second, if there is a right to health care—and we shall later agree with the Lalonde Report[54] and argue that there is—then that right would be violated.

On both counts, if the profession allowed this to occur, it would be acting unethically. By not supplying the needs in these instances, it would be creating a service vacuum which could not be filled by anyone else because of the fact of its monopoly. Ethically speaking, the profession may not allow this to happen. The fact of monopoly creates the obligation of ubiquity of service. It is a nice question how that obligation could be met in geographically remote areas or in otherwise disadvantaged locations. Perhaps the suggestion of a B.C. and of an Ontario task-force on the subject which suggests "compulsory medical service in areas of need"[55] is the most feasible method. But whatever the solution, the onus of discharging it rests squarely on the shoulders of the profession itself.

Universality[56]

Universality of service is closely related to ubiquity. It is the obligation to ensure that the number of appropriately trained physicians in a given area is adequate to permit equitable access to health care. Over and above this, however, it is also the obligation to ensure that no type of medical condition is ignored by the profession—even if the condition should be a dangerous one such as Hepatitis B, bubonic plague, or

AIDS.[57] In support of this, we again return to the notion of service provider monopoly itself. The existence of this monopoly entails that no-one except a physician may act in a medical capacity. Therefore the profession's failure to act in such contexts—or its refusal to do so—would ensure that those who suffer from the relevant conditions will be cut off from medical aid. If the profession were to allow this to occur, it would not be living up to the condition of its monopoly.

Of course this does not mean that it falls to each individual physician to fulfil this particular obligation. Nor does it fall to group of physicians identified in an a priori and discriminatory fashion. That would be to confuse an obligation that falls to the profession with an obligation that falls to the professional.[58] It simply means that the profession has the duty to find some equitable means of distributing the discharge of this obligation among its members.

5. Physicians have an obligation of professional integrity[59]

This duty is perhaps best understood by beginning with disciplinary proceedings by professional associations against their members.

Professions usually have boards, bodies, or committees that deal with any problem that might arise in the conduct of their members.[60] These are usually referred as disciplinary committees. Moral charges, accusations of technical incompetence, or allegations of contravention of guidelines set by the association, etc. are here implicated. Transgressions of these regulations, standards or guidelines are usually referred to as breaches of professional integrity and standards of practice. They are considered violations of the code of ethics of the profession, and are dealt with by more or less draconian measures, depending on the nature of the infraction. The profession of medicine also has such bodies. They are under the jurisdiction of the Colleges of the various provinces.

However, a code of professional ethics is different from a code of personal ethics. That is to say, all members of society engage in a variety of roles. In and by themselves, none of these roles exhaust the nature of the individual. A physician may be a father or mother, an alderman, a member of a hospital board, a husband or wife, a son or daughter, and so on. Although all of these roles may be united in the same individual, they are logically distinct.

Each of the roles that an individual fulfils is governed by the general system of ethical principles that hold for all members of society. However, given the distinct nature of these roles, it follows that how well or ill a particular physician fulfils one role may be quite independent of, and irrelevant for, how well or ill he or she fulfils another. Therefore, it would be irresponsible and illogical to assume as a matter of course that simply because it is one and the same person who fulfils these various roles, therefore if he or she fulfils one role badly then by that very token he or she fulfils other roles badly as well.

In other words the fact of malfeasance in one role in and by itself does not amount to, nor does it imply, malfeasance in another. The same may be said, of course, for excellence. We need merely consider the fact that excellence as spouse or daughter has no implications whatever with respect to excellence as an alderman or a physician.

A code of professional ethics deals with individuals only in their capacity as professionals. That is to say, such a code deals with the professionals as individuals exercising their technical skills and fulfilling their professional duties. Consequently such a code is different from a code of personal ethics. It does not deal with, nor does it contain, ethical maxims that govern the behaviour of the individual as a private person. The fact that the professional also happens to be a private person and vice versa does not change the situation. The situation is different if and only if the act of the individual as a private person is also and at the same time an act of the individual as professional, or when such an act has direct bearing on how well he or she can fulfil the relevant professional role.

It therefore follows that a code of professional ethics is not the place for injunctions that deal with the personal conduct of professionals outside of their professional capacity; nor are considerations of moral turpitude, inefficiency and the like as practised in a private sphere relevant when considering the professional integrity of a person. The only exception, again, is when such acts or situations impinge on the conduct of the individual as a professional or when they have an effect on the ability of the profession as a whole to fulfil its mandate.

For instance, trust is an important element of the physician-patient relationship. Therefore if a physician as private person behaves in such a way that prospective patients will feel unable to trust him or her, then the capability of the physician to act in a professionally appropriate way will be seriously undermined. And if the offending behaviour is so flagrant that it brings the profession as a whole into disrepute, then this would clearly impair the ability of the profession to fulfil its mandate. Therefore in cases like these, there is a cross-over between private and public life. However, in all such cases it is very important to establish a causal link between the activity of the professional as a private person and the professional as a public person.

Likewise, professional integrity should not be confused with loyalty to the profession as an association. Except for the purely ethical aspects that we have tried to detail, the rules and precepts laid down by an association of professionals for their own internal governance, for the advancement of the fortunes of a majority of its members, or for an increase in the respect in which the profession is held by individuals who are not members of the group,[61] have no inherent ethical value. They are on a par with the rules of clubs, corporations, and the like. While adherence to them may be a condition of membership in the association, it is not and cannot be an ethical requirement in the sense of an ethical rule of conduct that grows out of the nature of the profession itself.

In other words, if the notion of professional integrity is understood in an ethically relevant sense, it focuses only on those obligations that arise for the individual professional insofar as he or she is a professional. Here we can identify three parameters: competence, confidentiality, and policing of professional standards.

Competence[62]

When physicians become physicians in the full-fledged formalized sense of that term, they become members of a monopolistic service profession. By seeking and gaining entry into the profession, they incur an obligation to have, maintain and update their technical competence with respect to the skills normally expected of someone in their position.

However, this obligation extends further than merely the actual possession of these skills. It also includes the obligation to realize the limits of their professional practice. Consequently, it entails the further duty of consultation when the limits are reached, and of withdrawal from cases when these limits are overstepped.

Furthermore, competence is governed by more than merely the possession of certain skills or the realization of their extent and limits.[63] It is also affected by the conditions under which these skills are employed, both with respect to the work environment—the actual working context—as well as with respect to the conditions of the workers: the professionals themselves. If either of these is deficient the result is incompetence, and except under emergency conditions, the decision to act as a professional in such contexts is a decision to compromise professional integrity.

It follows that except in emergency contexts, physicians have an obligation to employ their skills only under material conditions that do not compromise their professional activity and under personal conditions that do not interfere with their professional functioning. In more specific terms, this means that except in emergency situations when any professional help is better than none, physicians should not venture to perform medical acts that do not lie in their area of practice. Furthermore, it means that when physicians are too tired or otherwise personally incapable of working in a proper professional manner at a level that society has come to expect as a standard of normal practice, they should refrain from acting as physicians.[64]

It will be obvious that physicians also have the further duty to try to make sure that conditions which impair their capacity to act in an appropriate fashion as professionals do not obtain in the first place.[65] In other words, they cannot just accept unreasonably long hours or other conditions of practice if they impair their ability to function properly. Of course it may not always be possible to do something about this immediately. However, physicians owe it both to themselves and to their patients to try to make sure that they can function as we have indicated.

Confidentiality[66]

We have already touched on confidentiality in a different context. Consequently it requires little comment. As we noted then, the nature of medical practice is such that physicians have access to information about patients to which others are not privy except by explicit admission on part of the patients themselves. Since physicians have access to it only in the context of their professional activity—which is to say, as a professionals and not as private persons—they have a right to use that knowledge only insofar as their professional association with the patient is concerned. Furthermore, physicians have a right to do this only insofar as it does not compromise the moral autonomy of their patients. Anything else would constitute a breach of trust.

However, as we had occasion to observe under (2), there will be exceptions to this. There will be situations in which maintaining patient confidentiality would violate the autonomy and welfare of others.[67] For instance, if a patient had tested positive for AIDS, was married and it turned out that her spouse did not know that she was sero-positive. Here the physician would have to balance the conflicting concerns. Since the life and welfare of a third party is predictably at risk, the physician must breach confidentiality.[68] This does not mean that the physician should divulge the relevant information without further ado. The more appropriate thing to do for the physician would be to suggest to the patient that the patient divulge the particular information to the spouse. It is only when the patient refuses or fails to do that, that the physician has the duty to take the appropriate action.

It should also be clear that situations that involve incompetent patients also require a breach of confidentiality. However, there is no way around that. The appropriate proxy decision-maker must have access to the relevant information, otherwise he or she cannot make a decision. Furthermore, since the proxy decision-maker is here taking the place of the incompetent person, divulging the relevant information to the appropriate proxy decision-maker is like divulging it to the individual him- or herself.

Policing of Professional Standards[69]

As we said above, physicians have knowledge and skills not shared by the remainder of society. Furthermore, they also enjoy a monopolistic position. These facts entail an obligation to ensure that physicians live up to the standards of competence that can reasonably be expected of someone in their position. This point was already covered under the rubrics of technical competence and of social obligation.

However, the obligation extends further. The position in which physicians find themselves by virtue of their specialized knowledge and skills give them a special advantage when it comes to evaluating both their own performance as well as the performance of their colleagues. It also allows them an informed opinion about the standards of some other professionals who are not physicians but nevertheless are legitimately engaged in the delivery of health care—nurses and technicians for example. In these contexts, physicians have an obligation to take appropriate action when the relevant standards of the other profession are not met. Not to do so would be to deliberately allow an unacceptable situation to continue as though, in fact, it were acceptable. It would be to live a lie. No more blatant an example of compromise of professional integrity could be imagined.

At the same time, the ethical position of medicine as a profession must be kept in mind. As we have said repeatedly, the profession is not a private organization set up for the benefit of its members. As a profession, it is the formalized expression of the public trust placed in a certain group of individuals to fulfil the obligation of health care.[70] Its duties and powers derive from this trust and this delegation of obligations. The institution and maintenance of professional standards therefore is not a private in-house affair of relevance only to the profession. It is of social importance.

Society is the ultimate ground of the profession's privileged status. Therefore society has the right of unhindered access to information about the implementation and policing of professional standards. The implementation of these standards, therefore, and of disciplinary procedures, must be open to public scrutiny at all stages.[71]

It follows that the traditional notion that the profession of medicine should be self-policing is only a partial truth. It extends only as far as the contents of competence judgements and professional standards are concerned. It does not extend to the manner in which these standards are examined. Any attempt to ignore this amounts to an arrogation of ethical independence that does not in fact exist. Therefore, if a physician has followed the appropriate in-house procedures but has good reasons to be convinced that these procedures are inadequate in bringing the true facts to light, then that physician has a duty to go beyond and outside the boundaries of the professional apparatus itself. Not to do so would amount to placing loyalty to an association before a professional obligation to society. That would also be a breach of professional integrity.

RIGHTS

No obligation is without a corresponding right. Minimally, an obligation entails a right to the fulfilment of those conditions that make the execution of the obligation possible.[72] This is also the case in medicine.

6. Physicians have a right to adequate information and power (authority) to allow them to fulfil their professional duties

This right needs little discussion. It is merely a particularized version of the ethical principle of impossibility: One cannot have an obligation to do the impossible. If physicians have to have certain information to fulfil their role and duty as physicians—for instance, whether a particular patient is an IV drug user—then they also have a right to that information. Otherwise they cannot make a proper diagnoses or prescribe appropriate treatment.

Similarly, once a patient has accepted a particular course of treatment, then the physician must have the authority to manage the details of that course of treatment. Unless there is such authority within their delegated realm of responsibility, physicians cannot practise. Of course the situation is different when the details change radically from what was understood by the patient when he or she accepted the treatment. For instance, when a patient has agreed to a particular form of chemotherapy, but the physicians decides that it should include a certain type of surgery that was not part of the original agreement. However, when that happens the physician is really proposing a new form of treatment that is importantly different from what was agreed to, so a new consent is necessary. The sort of thing that we are considered is the power to order the details that are necessary to carry out an agreed-to therapy itself.

7. Physicians have the right to working conditions that are sufficiently adequate to allow them to fulfil their professional duties[73]

The same ethical principle that underlies (6) also underlies (7). However, this must not be misunderstood. It does not mean that physicians have the right to working conditions that are personally pleasant to them. Nor does it mean that physicians have a right to conditions which would make their work easier than would normally be expected, and so on. The only thing it means is that when conditions are such that physicians cannot fulfil their professional duties even with the best of intentions without becoming morally guilty, then the duties themselves cease to be obligations. The reason is that these obligations hold only on the precondition that it is possible to fulfil them.

It should not require a special argument to show that "working conditions" refers to professional working conditions actually associated with a physician's function as a health care professional. Private contractual conditions such as fringe benefits, pension plans and the like are an entirely different—and professionally irrelevant—affair. It will also be clear that emergency conditions may also constitute exceptions. But we have already touched on that point above.

8. Physicians have the right to preserve their ethical integrity as persons

This clause is almost a mirror image of clause (2): If there is an obligation to respect the moral autonomy of the patient because the patient is a person, then there must also be an obligation to respect to autonomy of the physician. The physician is also a person. Therefore both considerations draw their moral justification from the same source.

The right to preserve their moral integrity is not compromised by the fact that physicians enter into a contractual agreement to provide health care. In this they are like other professionals. Lawyers do not lose their right to autonomy because they enter into a contractual agreement with their clients. To be sure, physicians and other health care professionals voluntarily agree to subordinate some of their rights to those of their patient in exchange for certain returns. However, this is not and cannot be an agreement to divest themselves of their right to moral autonomy. No-one can have a duty to violate their conscience or to do something that is otherwise unethical. That is an inalienable right even for physicians.

Consequently, any professional factor that violates physicians' right to personal autonomy in this ethical sense and that infringes on their integrity as persons is a trespass to their ethical being. The only exceptions that might arise are restrictions that grow out of the nature of the profession itself and that require their action in emergency contexts. Here one could argue that when physicians agreed to become physicians, they agreed to subordinate their values in such cases.

However, we should distinguish between something that violates the integrity of persons as infringing on their right to moral autonomy, and something that goes against their wishes, expectations and interests. The former legitimately falls under this rubric and is of ethical concern; the latter is not.

It also follows from this that if the values of the patients or of their appropriate proxy decision-makers disagree fundamentally with those of the physicians, then all other things being equal,[74] the physicians have the right to withdraw from the case rather than compromising their own integrity. Again, unusual circumstances like emergencies constitute exceptions.

9. Physicians have the right to fair and equitable treatment and remuneration for their work

This clause is a direct derivative of clause (8), and of the principle that underlies (2). However, it, too, should not be misunderstood. It is easy to confuse equity with desirability, and fairness with what physicians would like to see. The two are not the same. What constitutes an equitable return can only be determined by a comparison with other professions, the nature of the work that is done, the amount, the responsibility that goes along with it, the training that is necessary in order to be able to do it, and so on. It may be difficult to do this for medicine and other health care professions. One thing, however, is clear. Equity and fairness cannot be measured in terms of scarcity. Considerations of supply and demand, therefore, are not germane when trying to determine what constitutes fair and equitable remuneration.

OBLIGATION OF THE PROFESSIONAL VERSUS OBLIGATION OF THE PROFESSION

Finally, we should say a few words about the relationship between individual physicians, the profession of medicine, and society.

Values

All of us have values that determine the course of our decisions and of our actions. Physicians are no exception. Canada is a multicultural society. The kind of values that are encountered differ greatly. Physicians differ in their values as much as do other people. However, if a physician contemplates associating or affiliating with an institution or clinic, the fact that he or she holds values that differ from the professed values of the profession as a whole should be made known to the other party prior to the inception of the contractual association. In that way, the institution or clinic can plan appropriately so as to avoid situations that would place the physician into a conflict of conscience. For instance, they might draw up different duty rosters, they might not schedule these physicians to perform certain operations, etc.[75] In certain cases, they might even decide not to offer a particular physician the opportunity to practise in that institution or clinic because the actions that are a normal part of the institution's or clinic's activities would violate the physician's values on a constant basis.

Similarly, physicians as independent practitioners should inform their patients of any difference between their own values and those that are normally associated with the medical profession as these are expressed in the professions formally announced standards and its code of ethics. Again, all other things being equal, physicians should do this at the very inception of the physician/patient relationship. Those physicians who fail to provide that sort of information at that time without good reasons—during an emergency for example—are withholding important information which might have influenced the decisions of their patients to choose them as physicians. Therefore, they would be violating the principle of autonomy and respect for persons.

Withdrawal of Services

We indicated above that, emergency and similar contexts excepted, physicians have the right to withdraw from cases that violate their autonomy and that interfere fundamentally with their basic values so long as appropriate alternate arrangements have been made for their patients.

However, not all situations that might conceivably result in a withdrawal of professional services can be handled in this fashion. Sometimes situations arise where a physician feels compelled to withdraw his or her services for reasons other than personally held beliefs or values. These reasons may be based on how the physician feels about the non-valuational aspects of the working conditions. For instance, the physician may feel that the conditions that characterize the relationship infringe on rights (7), (8), and (9) above. This might involve institutional working conditions, it might involve fee schedules set by the provincial ministry of health and the like. It may even happen that this feeling is shared by more than one physician.

Of course it is not necessarily a foregone conclusion that the physicians who feel this way will withdraw their services, either singly or together. The appropriate thing for them to do is to try to resolve the difficulties that they experience through appropriate negotiations. However, these negotiations may turn out to be fruitless. Under such circumstances, the physicians may well contemplate a withdrawal of services in a concerted fashion and as a group, so as to give force to their demands. In the Canadian context, the physicians' strikes in Ontario and Saskatchewan appear to have been examples of this sort of thing.

Physicians who find themselves in such a position face a difficult choice. On the one hand, clauses (7) to (9) appear to grant them the right to such action. On the other hand, the monopolistic position of medicine, combined with the individual physician's professional commitment to health care and the physician/patient relationship into which he or she has entered with individual patients apparently rules against it. Is there a resolution of the dilemma?

A possible resolution of this difficulty lies in the distinction that we touched on in (4): the distinction between the obligations that hold for the individual physician, and the obligations that hold for the profession of medicine as a whole. The two are not the same. No individual physician has an obligation of ubiquity and universality of service. That obligation belongs to the profession in virtue of its monopolistic position. Therefore, the profession of medicine cannot sanction a total withdrawal of medical services. While individual physicians may consider job actions such as strikes etc., the profession as a whole has a duty to provide those services that are necessary in order to sustain a certain minimum level of health care. To put it in more concrete terms, the profession as a whole, in terms of its relevant associations, has an obligation to designate certain of its members to function in that capacity

At first glance, this may seem unrealistic. It would appear to undermine completely any chance of success that such job action might have. If the physicians who are designated to provide the relevant services really do their job properly, those against whom the action was directed would not feel constrained to consider the demands of the striking group seriously. Furthermore, the fact that a certain minimum level of health care would be maintained would not guarantee that the health status of individual patients would not suffer. Finally, the physician/patient relationship of individual physicians would still seem to be violated by this move.

These are of course serious considerations. However, they do not militate against the right of the profession to withdraw its services under the conditions that we have indicated. Instead, these considerations suggest that we should add one further condition: Hand-in-hand with the obligation of the profession to provide this minimum service goes the right of the profession to ask for binding arbitration through a third party who is mutually agreeable to both sides. Not to recognize a right to binding arbitration is to place physicians in an untenable position. The only other option for them would be either to cease being physicians or to accept whatever society sends their way.

It is important here to remember that the peculiar position in which the profession of medicine finds itself is the result of the service-monopoly conferred on it by society. That monopoly carries certain obligations with it. In particular the obligation of service. However, acceptance of that monopoly is also based on certain assumptions. One of these assumptions is that society will deal fairly with the profession and that it will not hold it up for ransom. Society has remedies to enforce its part of the monopoly bargain on the profession. Equality and justice demand that the profession also have some way of having its demands heard and adjudicated.[76] The only way to do that is through binding arbitration.[77]

This leaves the individual physician/patient relationships. The long and the short of it is that when physicians become involved in this sort of collective action, they are not entirely free of their professional obligations. They still have a duty to make sure that the patients with whom they have entered into a physician/patient relationship have access to them or to another physician who is willing and able to provide appropriate health care. The reason for this lies in the rationale of the collective action itself. It is not directed against individual patients, but in a sense against society as a whole. Therefore their action against society cannot be transferred into an action against their patients. At least not entirely so. The patients are members of society, and as such they do have some degree of collective responsibility for the government that is in power and that bargains with the medical associations. Therefore a modicum of responsibility does attach to the individual patients. However, the existence of the relationship cannot be denied. That is why a minimum standard of care must be provided, even under conditions such as these, and those physicians who have patients whose health status would be seriously compromised by such a withdrawal of their service would have a duty to continue to care for these patients.

Conclusion

What we have just done is sketch, in simple outline, what a code of ethics for physicians might look like. Another way of looking at it is to see it as a sketch of some of the more important considerations that should be kept in mind when evaluating such a code. Whichever way it is interpreted, the important point is this: A code of ethics for physicians—or, for that matter, for any health care profession—must be grounded on principles. It must take into account those features of the profession that uniquely identify it in the social context in which it is embedded, and it must provide general guidance for the members of the profession for the conduct of their professional affairs. A code of ethics cannot be more than that, because it cannot become too specific. If it did, it would not longer have guiding value for the array of problems that face the health care professional. On the other hand, it cannot be less than that, because if it is not grounded on fundamental principles then it will be merely a statement of ethos or a quasi-judicial document. In neither case, however, will it be a code of ethics.

ENDNOTES

[1] For a somewhat different approach, see A. Jameton, *Nursing Practice: The Ethical Issues* (New York and Toronto: Prentice Hall, 1984), Chapter 2.

[2] This includes the Canadian Psychiatric Association, and the Association of Medical Technologists, etc.

[3] Because of the statutorily delegated authority mentioned above.

[4] Canadian Nurses Association *Code of Ethics for Nursing* (Ottawa: 1990) 5.

[5] The expression is due to Robert Veatch, "Models for Ethical Practice in a Revolutionary Age," (*Hastings Center Report*, 2:3, 1972): 5-7.

[6] Oxford English Dictionary.

[7] A good example is found in T.L. Beauchamp and J.F. Childress, *Principles of Biomedical Ethics* (New York and Oxford: Oxford University Press, 1979) 10: "A professional code represents an articulated statement of role morality as seen by the members of the profession.Beauchamp and Childress however do profess some misgivings about the adequacy of such codes. (see above text, at 11). See also Janet Storch, *Patients' Rights: Ethical and Legal Issues in Health Care and Nursing* (Toronto: McGraw-Hill Ryerson Ltd., 1982) 1–20. See also Talcott Parsons, *Essays in Sociological Theory* (Glencoe, Ill.: The Free Press, 1954) 372 and elsewhere.

[8] See Chapter 1.

[9] See also M. Bayles, *Professional Ethics*, (Englewood Cliffs, N.J.: Prentice Hall, 1985).

[10] For an interesting discussion from the point of view of a health care professional see H.E. Emson, *The Doctor and the Law: A Practical Guide for the Canadian Physician* (Toronto and Vancouver: Butterworths, 1989), Chapter 13.

[11] For more on this, see W.K. Frankena, *Ethics* (Englewood Cliffs N.J.: Prentice-Hall, 1973) and R.B. Brandt, *Ethical Theories* (Englewood Cliffs, N.J.: Prentice-Hall, 1959). See also Aristotle, *Nicomachean Ethics*. The legal discussions of competence are usually intended to sketch conditions of responsibility from a legal perspective.

[12] For a similar position, see Robert M. Veatch, "Medical Ethics: Professional or Universal? " *Harvard Theological Review* 65(1972) 531–559, and "Models for Ethical Practice in a Revolutionary Age," *Hastings Center Report* 2: 3(1972, 5–7) *A Theory of Medical Ethics* (New York: Basic Books, 1981). Seem also T.M. Garrett, H.W. Baillie and R.M. Garrett, *Health Care Ethics: Principles and Problems* (Englewood Cliffs, NJ: Prentice Hall, 1988) Chapter 1.

[13] This is simply an application of the Principle of Relevant Difference and the Principle of Equity and Justice.

[14] See M. Lalonde, *A New Perspective on the Health of Canadians* (Government Printing Office, Ottawa, 1974). For a different analysis, see *Securing Access to Medical Care*, Commission for the Study of Ethical Problems in Medicine and Biomedical and Behavioral Research (1983, U.S. Government Printing Office, Washington, D.C.) 3 volumes. For further discussion of this applied to nursing, see E.H.W. Kluge, "The Profession of Nursing and the Right to Strike," *Westminster Institute Review* 2: 1 (1982), 3–6.

[15] See Chapter 8 for a discussion of the nature of health.

[16] For a discussion of conflicts of obligation in the allocation of resources, see Chapter 9.

[17] We here have in mind situations involving brain-dead individuals whose biological functions are sustained in anticipation of transplantation, etc.

[18] See the discussion on the nature of death on pages 281f.

[19] This is reflected in Article 5 of the *Code of Ethics* of the CMA. A similar position is maintained in the *Code* of the CNA in sections 2ff.

[20] For a fuller discussion of this, see the discussion of informed consent on pages 121–22.

[21] See CMA *Code of Ethics*, article 13 for some recognition of this.

[22] CMA *Code*, article 5.

[23] See Chapter 6, "Proxy Decision-Making."

[24] See the recent case of *Malette vs. Shulman* for a legal recognition of this.

[25] See *Reibl vs. Hughes* and *Hopp vs. Lepp* for a legal recognition of this. See also Chapter 6, "Proxy Decision-Making."

[26] See CMA *Code of Ethics*, articles 6 and 11 respectively.

[27] Clearly, the release of de-identified information for legitimate epidemiological studies by appropriate persons would not infringe on this. Furthermore, patients have a *prima facie* duty to release such de-identified information because access to such information by the appropriate individuals is a necessary condition for being able to plan for health care in the first place.

[28] Professional acceptance of this is reflected in the Canadian Medical Association's policy that on AIDS.

[29] This of course means that the patient or appropriate proxy decision-maker has given informed consent to their involvement.

[30] See pages 121–140.

[31] See the discussion of allocation of resources on pages 205–236.

[32] Something like this was recognized by Canadian physicians in their *Code of Ethics* of 1945, where physicians were reminded that in a very real sense, they are social agents. Ironically enough, this clause was dropped from subsequent versions of the *Code*, even though the privileged role of physicians was retained.

[33] This does not mean that it occurs within an institution. Rather it means a setting whose nature is governed by formal (and something formalized) rules of interaction.

[34] See pages 77–110 for more discussion.

[35] That is to say, in the formalized setting like that of a hospital or a clinic by which she/he is employed.

[36] See CMA *Code*, article 12.

[37] These include at least the presumption of treating the physician as a professional whose services are being sought in a genuine fashion. If patients depart from this assumption, there is every right to re-examine the relationship. See *Code*, articles 11 and 15 for some recognition of this fact.

[38] Compare CMA *Code*, article 15.

[39] We are here assuming competence on part of the patient.

[40] See CMA *Code*, article 12. See also the good samaritan legislation of some U.S. states, and the suggestions of the Law Reform Commission of Canada in its Working Paper 46, *Omission, Negligence and Endangering* (Ottawa: Law Reform Commission of Canada, 1985) especially recommendations 3–6. Due professional standard of care, of course, is expected even here. See Picard, 45f; Nathan, *Medical Negligence* (1957) 36–40; Rozovsky, *Canadian Hospital Law* (1975) 63.

[41] See Douglas Walton, *On Defining Death* (Montreal: McGill-Queen's University Press, 1979) Chapters VII to X, for a good analysis. See also proxy decision-making, Chapter 6.

[42] This is implicitly recognized by the CMA *Code of Ethics* in its injunction that a physician may not refuse services in an emergency context: Articles 11, 12 and 13.

[43] But see the Quebec statutes and the recommendations of the Law Reform Commission, mentioned in note 40.

[44] The Association of Canadian Medical Colleges estimates that the cost of training an undergraduate medical student averages $25,000 per annum. Average tuition fees run in the neighbourhood of $2,000 to $2,500 per annum.

[45] This underlies the attempt by some provinces, notably British Columbia, to restrict billing numbers for physicians on the basis of a medical manpower analysis that takes into account location, number of people, prevalent health patterns, and so on. The attempt so far has been struck down by the courts as contrary to the Charter's guarantee of liberty.

[46] See CMA *Code*, clause 47.

[47] See Emson, (ref. note 10) Chapter 2.

[48] That is to say, it is the result of legislation that restricts the practice of medicine to only those who have been duly accredited by the provincial medical licensing authorities, and the continued insistence of the profession to pursue what it perceives to be any infringement of this exclusive right to practice.

[49] The degree of economic attractiveness may be perceived differently by those who already are physicians and who practice medicine from the way in which it is perceived by prospective members of the profession. The fact that the number of candidates for medical school exceeds the number of available places by several orders of magnitude in most medical schools attests to the fact that compared to other professions, medicine is still considered to be economically attractive.

[50] Despite the fact that physicians were sometimes paid in kind rather than by salary, most physicians were rather well off.

[51] The U.S. situation was similar in many regards.

[52] See CMA *Code*, articles 25–28, and articles 47ff..

[53] See the recent decision by the Discipline Committee of the Royal College of Physicians and Surgeons of Ontario, which struck down the validity of Section 12(4) of the Health Disciplines Act, R.S.O., Chapter 196.

[54] M. Lalonde, *A New Perspective on the Health of Canadians* (Ottawa: Government Printing Office 1974).

[55] This suggestion was recently reiterated by the Medical Manpower Committee of the Canadian Medical Association.

[56] CMA *Code*, article 47, may be interpreted in this way.

[57] This stands in opposition to the stance taken in recent years by the CMA on this matter. The CMA General Council in 1989 refused to accept a motion from the Committee on Ethics that HIV sero-positivity is not a reason for refusing medical services. In our estimation, this constitutes an abrogation by the profession of a duty of service it acquired when it accepted its privileged monopolistic position.

[58] In the language of traditional logic, this would be to commit the fallacy of division.

[59] For different perspective on what follows, see CMA *Code*, articles 27 and 29.

[60] This is what is generally referred to as the self-governing function of a profession. See M. Bayles, *Professional Ethics* (Englewood Cliffs, N.J.: Prentice-Hall, 1985).

[61] This is involved in articles 27 to 29 of the CMA *Code*.

[62] See CMA *Code*, article 2 for one aspect of this.

[63] See CMA *Code*, articles 4, 39, 41.

[64] See R. Paulson, "Fatigue in Medical Personnel," *Journal of the American Medical Association* 246: 2 (July 10, 1982) 124; R.C. Friedman, J.T. Bigger and D.S. Kornfeld, "The Intern and Sleep Loss," *New England Journal of Medicine* 285: 4 (July 22, 1971) 201.

[65] This means that a physicians cannot merely accept ethically objectionable conditions.

[66] See CMA *Code* article 6.

[67] See L. Rozovsky, *Canadian Hospital Law* (1975) 105; *Tarasoff vs. Regents of the University of California* (1976), 131 California Reporter 14, 529 p. 2nd 553 C.S.C.; *Regina vs. Gordon* (1923), 54 O.L.R. See also J. London "Privacy in Medical Context" in Gibson, ed., *Aspects of Privacy Law* (1980).

[68] See also CMA *Code*, articles 47 and 48, and the CMA policy paper on AIDs.

[69] See CMA *Code*, articles 25ff.

[70] This is recognized clearly in the earlier version of the Codes of Ethics of Canadian physicians.

[71] See Report of the Disciplinary Committee of the Royal College of Physicians and Surgeons of Ontario.

[72] This finds its ethical basis in the Principle of Impossibility.

[73] Something like this seems to be aimed at by the CMA *Code*, articles 30–33. However, our discussion of this goes further.

[74] See clause (4) above, pages 59ff.

[75] This is particularly important in matter such as abortion.

[76] See Bayles (1981) 23–25, 28ff. See also E-H.W. Kluge, "The Profession of Nursing and the Right to Strike," *Westminster Institute Review* 2:1 (Fall 1982) 3–6.

[77] It is interesting to note that the Ontario Medical Association dropped its action against the constitutionality of the Canada Health Act when it received assurances that binding arbitration in matters of conflict would be acceptable under the Act.

SUGGESTED READINGS

- The Canadian Medical Association. *Code of Ethics*. Ottawa, 1987 (see Appendix 1.).

    This is the code of ethics that is accepted by all members of the Canadian Medical Association. It is also the basis of the *Code of Ethics* of the Royal College of

Physicians and Surgeons of Canada, on which it is based and essentially identical with.

- The Canadian Nurses Association. *Code of Ethics*. Ottawa, 1985 (see Appendix 2.).

  This *Code* is binding on all nurses who are members of the Canadian Nurses Association and its affiliate societies.

- The World Medical Association, "An International Code of Medical Ethics," *World Medical Association Bulletin* 1: 3 (1949).

  A Code that was promulgated by the World Medical Association. It has more symbolic than binding power, but nevertheless it is indicative of what the international medical community thinks is ethically appropriate.

- World Medical Association: *Declaration of Helsinki*.

  An expansion of the World Medical Association *Code of Ethics*, focusing on biomedical research involving human subjects.

- Beauchamp, T.L. and L.B. McCullough, *Medical Ethics: The Moral Responsibility of Physicians*. Englewood Cliffs, N.J.: Prentice-Hall, 1984.

  This is an extended treatment of ethical considerations for physicians who are in actual practice, as given from the perspective of two utilitarian thinkers.

4
The Physician-Patient Relationship

This chapter introduces the reader to different models of the physician-patient relationship. These models differ essentially because they are based on distinct interpretations of the role of the physician as decision-maker and on different approaches to patient autonomy.

Some of the questions that might usefully guide the attention of the reader for this chapter include:

1. Who has the primary right or duty of decision-making in the physician-patient context? Are there exceptions to this? Of what sort are they and what is their underlying rationale?
2. What does the notion of patient competence mean in ethical terms, and what does it imply for decision-making?
3. What are some models of the physician-patient relationship? Which one is appropriate in the Canadian context? Why?
4. What is paternalism, and what, if any, is its justification in the medical setting?

Introduction

In the preceding chapter we sketched the ethical position of medicine with respect to its social position and mandate. We went on to suggest that with due alteration of detail, analogous considerations hold for other health care professions.[1] Our present discussion will focus on the ethical problems that arise when physicians actually practise their profession.

The practice of medicine, where physicians encounter and interact with patients, is characterized by several ethically extremely important features:

1. It is a person-to-person interactive context of a fiduciary sort with the physician as service-provider, the patient as service-recipient.
2. The physician is in a position of technical expertise, the patient not.
3. The patient is usually in some degree of emotional turmoil or has some emotional or psychological concern, the physician is not burdened in this fashion.
4. The patient claims a right to health care services, the physician has a professionally acquired obligation to provide these services.[2]
5. A decision has to be made on the basis of the technically, ethically, personally, and socio-economically relevant data concerning the direction the medical services shall take.

Models of Physician-Patient Relationships

The phrase "physician-patient relationship" refers to the relationship that comes into existence between a physician and a patient as soon as the physician enters into an association with the patient in a professional capacity. As long as their association has a professional component, it exists even when the physician and patient are friends. In other words, the physician-patient relationship arises as soon as the individual comes to the physician for help; because at that point the patient comes to the physician not *as friend* but *as patient*. This does not mean that their relationship may not be on a friendly footing. It merely means that the element of friendship is not the primary determinant of their interaction.

However, the professional relationship between physician and patient raises several issues. One of the most important is the issue of control.[3] Despite the fact that it is normally the patient who seeks out the physician, the fact that the physician is a professional with knowledge and services for sale—and what is more, with knowledge and services that the patient requires—makes it inevitable that the physician will find him- or herself in a position to make treatment decision. It is therefore not surprising that the nature and direction of the physician-patient relationship, its quality and the structure of the interaction, will be very heavily influenced by the physician's attitude about how treatment decisions ought to be made and about who should make them. After all, it is the physician who controls the process in practical terms. The question is, How should that process be controlled? What should be its guiding ethical parameters?[4]

The Paternalistic or Priestly Model[5]

The various models of the physician-patient relationship that we referred to above all give different answers. The most traditional one is called the paternalistic or priestly model.[6] We encounter it in Percival's *Medical Ethics*,[7] where the physician is exhorted to make the decisions for the patient by blending "firmness with kindness," but despite its antiquity it has not disappeared from contemporary practice.[8]

The reason it is called the priestly or paternalistic model is obvious. It portrays the role of the physician as not only that of technical expert but also as ultimate decision maker over the whole scope and extent of the physician-patient interaction. The physician decides what should be done and to what extent; what should be told to the patient and under what circumstances. In short, it sees the physician as deciding what Bora Laskin[9] called the whole scope and nature of the relationship as lying in the control of the physician.

We encounter this perspective in the example of the physician who does not tell the patient that his cancer is incurable because she thinks that this would lead to despair on part of the patient, and that the patient would not agree to try a particular form of therapy which the physician thinks might be beneficial. We also find such an example in the neonatologist who does not tell the parents the precise nature and degree of deficit of their baby, so as not to deprive them of hope. In other words, this model sanctions an approach that requires the physician to take over the decision-making role because it is the physician's duty to do what is in the best interest of the patient (or significant others);[10] it is the physician who decides what counts as "best interests" because she or he has greater expertise and understanding.

To sum up, according to this model it is the physician who has, and ought to have, the control of the physician-patient relationship, and it is the physician who ought to make whatever decisions have to be made. The role of patient is to obey "doctor's orders."

The Agency or Engineering Model[11]

If the priestly model stands at one end of the spectrum of control, the agency or engineering model stands at the other. This model is characterized by the thesis that the physician is simply a technical expert who is engaged by the patient, no more and no less. According to this model, the patient has complete power to decide what he or she wants the physician to do. The physician has the obligation to do what is asked.

On this model, the personal ethical or valuational scruples of the physician count for nothing. Even when what the patient wants done is against the better judgement of the physician, he has the duty to go ahead and do it anyway. In a sense, this model turns the physician into a mere tool of the patient. One might almost say that the physician is demoted to the status of a moral eunuch. An example here would be the sort of situation where the patient asks for some medically doubtful therapy—eg., laetrile—and the physician against his or her better judgement prescribes it; or the sort of case where the physician performs a needless piece of surgery because the patient has asked for it.[12]

The Collegial Model

The collegial model falls somewhere in the middle between the two extremes of complete physician control and no physician control at all. In this model the physician and the patient come together as equal partners in an enterprise that centres on the health care needs of the patient. That is why this sort of model might also be called a co-operation model.

But this relationship goes further than mere co-operation. Unequal partners can co-operate in a common enterprise. For example, the medical student and the medical professor co-operate when they are researching a particular problem in cell transport mechanisms, or the nurse and the physician co-operate when they are engaged in a clinical trial or investigation.

The collegial model, however, goes further than this precisely because it is collegial in outlook. It is predicated on the thesis that physician and patient are in fact true equals. To be sure, they are not seen as equals in terms of technical expertise, or in the statutory authority they have as to the kind of things that can be ordered in terms of support services or that can be prescribed in terms of drugs, for example. Rather, they are portrayed as equals in the sense that both have equal decision-making authority with respect to the direction that the health care service delivery ought to take, and that both are equal in the sense that both share a common interest and common goals. The analogy that has sometimes been proposed in the literature is that of co-adventuring in the realm of health care.[13]

The Contractual Model

If the collegial model tends towards the centre of the scale of authority and control, the contractual model tends to be somewhat left-of-centre, more towards the agency side. It portrays the relationship between the physician and the patient as being defined by the terms of the contract into which the two enter when the patient comes to the physician in a professional capacity. In the non-socialized health care setting, a good example of this kind of perspective would be the physician in a private clinic who performs a renal transplant on a patient where she knows that the patient will not benefit from the operation, because the indicators are just not appropriate for a good prognosis.[14] In a socialized health care system, this sort of model may easily lead to a can-do/must-do mentality.

In a sense, this model is similar to the engineering or agency model. However, there are differences. In an agency model the patient has complete control over the direction and extent of the services that the physician is to supply, and the physician has no right of moral scruples. Furthermore, in an engineering model there is some expectation that when an unforeseen problem arises and the patient is not in a position to give directives, the physician will extend the nature of the services required in the direction already indicated by the patient.

In a contractual model, however, the physician has the right to follow her or his own ethical scruples in deciding on whether or not to accept the contractual obligation to the patient in the first place. Furthermore, when an unforeseen situation arises the physician has the right to stick to the letter of the agreement, unless the situation is somehow already covered in the contractual arrangement in the first place, either directly or by implication.

There is also an element of trust in this sort of relationship—trust in the sense of a fiduciary relationship. However, that element is severely limited by the assumption that it extends only to the degree that it would normally be covered in a contractual sort of arrangement.

The Friendship Model[15]

The friendship model has a lot in common with the collegial and the priestly models. It assumes that the physician has an obligation that stems from the personal interest that the physician has in the welfare of the patient. In other words, the fact of professional obligation is not grounded solely in the fact of legal obligation. It is also grounded in the personal relationship that the physician has with the patient. It is because the physician and the patient come together as friends that there is an element of trust, of good will and of general looking-out for the best interests of the patient.

However, it is precisely because they are friends that there is also a certain amount of overriding of the patient's autonomy—in the way in which friends would do this sort of thing. Information may be withheld, or at least managed; proxy decisions may be made for the patient rather than allowing the patient to make a wrong decision or become exposed to what the physician feels would be too great a burden; and so on. But as is the case among friends, there will always be a readiness to account for what the physician has done, and a readiness to defer to the patient should he or she insist.[16]

The Fiduciary Model

As its name indicates,[17] the fiduciary model is a model of trust. It acknowledges that the position of physician and patient is not one of equals, whether that be with respect to knowledge, psychological control or legal authority in the service delivery area. It recognizes that the extent of duty for the physician cannot be measured by the precise wordings of a contract; that the direction of the patient's values play an important role, but that at the same time the physician is also a person with values and rights.

If we were to use another adjective to describe this model we would say that it is a model of balance. The right of autonomy of the patient is balanced against the knowledge and expertise of the physician and the rights of the physician both as an individual and as a professional. The patient has an ultimate and basic right to control the direction of the health care relationship, the physician has the right to determine what is appropriate under the values thus indicated—and whether to enter into the relationship on that basis. Of course, the right to purely professional decision-making power does not detract from the physician's duty to obtain an informed consent for procedures and undertakings. However, the limits here are somewhat wider than they would be under a strict contractual model.

Furthermore, as distinct from the engineering or agency model, the physician has the right to limit the type of procedure or service to the kinds of things that she can feel comfortable with on the basis of her own values, but of course she would have to tell this to the patient. The CMA *Code of Ethics* recognizes this component when it states that:[18]

> An ethical physician will inform the patient where personal morality or religious conscience prevent the recommendation of some form of therapy.

However, while the code recognizes this obligation, it does not go far enough. We would want to argue that if there is some factor of "personal morality" that would affect the physician's actions in this regard, then the physician has the obligation to inform the patient of this as early as possible, ideally at the beginning of their relationship.

The reason for this is that once a physician/patient relationship has been established, the psychological facts of the matter are that the patient will find it very difficult not to be influenced, possibly even coerced, by the position of the physician as then stated.[19] In other words, delayed disclosure may well lead to a severe compromise of the free will of the patient, a will that is usually extremely fragile to begin with. In this regard, the *Code of Ethics* for Canadian Nurses puts it somewhat better:[20]

> A nurse is not ethically obliged to provide requested care when compliance would involve a violation of her or his moral beliefs. When that request falls within recognized forms of health care however, the client should be referred to a health care practitioner who is willing to provide the service. Nurses who have or are likely to encounter such situations are morally obligated to seek to arrange conditions of employment so that the care of clients is not jeopardized.

However, even this statement does not go far enough because it does not require that the patient be told at the outset. This is a condition that we consider indispensable for a truly fiduciary relationship.

To re-iterate, the fiduciary model is a model of trust. The patient must be able to trust the physician, even to the extent of assuming that the physician will not interfere with the patient's autonomy. The physician must not betray this trust.

However, to be truly fiduciary it must be a relationship of a trust that is rooted in autonomy on both sides, in a free but balanced giving. The patient voluntarily engages with the physician in an interrelationship that retains the direction-giving power of the patient while at the same time respecting the physician as person. This means that the physician must also be able to trust the patient. The physician must be able to trust that the patient is telling the truth; that the patient withholds nothing that the physician wants or needs to know in a professional capacity; that the patient will co-operate with the physician's endeavours.

These will be some of the presumptions on which the relationship will be based from the physician's side. If they are deliberately, freely and knowingly violated by the patient, then the basic presuppositions of the relationship of trust will have been broken from the side of the patient. With this, the obligation that the physician would otherwise have towards the patient would be attenuated to the degree that such a violation would lie within the control of the patient. The physician then has the right to review the whole relationship and, if she wants, to end it.[21]

Of course, there are situations in which this will not hold. For example, when the patient is volitionally, conceptually or emotionally compromised; or when there is no other physician who can or will take over the burden of health care delivery. In these sorts of cases the obligation will remain, but not on the original terms of a fiduciary relationship. The physician then has the right to practise defensive medicine, and need no longer operate on a basis of trust.[22]

Analysis

We have now in effect stated the case for the fiduciary model of the physician/patient relationship. In our estimation, the priestly model fails because it compromises the autonomy of the patient—the right to self-determination—too much. While it is appropriate to acknowledge the expertise of physicians and their legal authority, it is inappropriate to carry this so far as to give physicians ultimate decision-making authority in all but the most unusual of cases.[23]

Furthermore, if the direction that health care is to take is a function of the values of the decision-maker, then the priestly model commits what as been called the fallacy of expertise.[24] It assumes that expertise in a particular technical modality, in this case medicine, confers authority over whether that expertise should be employed in the first place, and in what direction.

The priestly model also places far too great a burden on the physician. It saddles the physician with the obligation to make decisions, whether he or she wants to or not. Not only is this contrary to the *Code* of the CMA and against Canadian case law, it may also lead to burn-out.[25]

The agency or engineering model fails for exactly the opposite reason; it denies the autonomy of the professional as a person. Although by entering the medical profession the physician, *de facto*, accepts a certain limit on what otherwise would be the free and unhindered exercise of his or her decision-making power, this does not mean that the physician loses autonomy altogether. The physician still retains her integrity as a professional. The agency model therefore goes too far in this regard.

It also ignores the fact that as a professional, the physician has obligations towards third parties and towards society that derive from the fact of professionalism itself.[26] For example, these come into play when the condition of the patient constitutes a threat to another person;[27] or when the health care needs of the patient impact on the issue of resource allocation within the social context.[28] In other words, the agency model would have us ignore the fact that the physician is still both a professional as well as a person, and that is unacceptable.

As to the collegial model, its shortcoming is really quite clear. The physician and the patient are not equals who come together motivated by a common interest, in order to achieve a commonly held goal.[29]

First of all, the very nature of the situation entails that the two are not equals in that context—the compromising aspects of ill health and need are too well documented to allow that hypothesis even a shred of credibility. As Spiro puts it:

> The encounter is inherently unequal: the patient seeks help, knows less than the physician about what is wrong with him in the technical sense, and comes full of anxiety and foreboding, or at least incommoded.[30]

Secondly, the motivations are different. No matter how motivated the physician may be to advance the cause of health and to help the patient, the fact remains that one of the primary motivations in becoming a physician and in taking a patient is also to earn a living. That aspect of the relationship colours it profoundly from the side of the physician, and there is nothing like it from the side of the patient.[31]

The contractual model errs in that it neglects the human aspect of the physician-patient relationship.[32] This is not simply a relationship of *quid-pro-quo* ; nor is it confined strictly to the letter of the contract—whether that contract be tacit, as is usually assumed on this model, or explicit. This sort of model would be appropriate if there were no compromise or deficit on part of the patient; if the knowledge base were the same; if there were no unforeseen happenstances that might arise; and if the relationship could be therapeutic when both participants in the interaction behaved in a purely mechanical fashion. But that is precisely what cannot be the case in the physician-patient context. Therapy requires interaction on a personal level with trust and understanding. The human being is not a car. In other words such a model might be appropriate in the context of mechanics, but not here.

Finally let us consider the friendship model. In a way, this model is one of the most tempting. It connotes an element of personal concern that many would like to see enshrined in codes governing such relations. It seems to take us back to "the old days" when medicine faced no problems of public interference and the physician could do in an unhindered fashion what he or she knew the patient wanted and what was right.

However, this is really quite unrealistic. Whether we like it or not, the profit motive in medicine is a fact. While physicians may be motivated by a zeal to help humanity, they are also motivated by economic considerations. To put it simply, they charge for their services, and they charge at rates that are bargained for in a very serious and very determined way. However, friendship is not something that is for sale. Therefore, while the physician may also be the friend of the patient, or at least may come to be a friend, the relationship of friendship is incidental to the interaction between the physician and the patient as physician and as patient.

Furthermore, friends are emotionally involved with each other. Perhaps not to a very great depth, although in true friendship the depth will indeed be great, but there will be an emotional commitment. If that commitment is not there, then there is no friendship. However, not only would it be unrealistic to expect this from a physician towards his hundreds and even thousands of patients, or from the physician who fills in when on call, or who takes over a locum, it would also be to require too much from the physician on a personal basis. Like all human undertakings, medicine is attended by failure. Furthermore, sooner or later all patients die. When a friend undergoes a reversal in her or his fortunes, we are emotionally swept along—and suffer; and when a friend dies, we are deeply affected. To require that the physician operate on a friendship model would be to require that the physician be assailed by these emotional factors every time that something similar happens to a patient. That would be to set the stage for burn-out.

Finally on this model it would follow that if the physician could not feel friendship for a particular patient, then either there would be no physician-patient relationship, or the physician should not take the individual as patient. It seems to us that if that were to be taken seriously, very few medical practices would survive.

Physicians as Decision-Makers

We therefore believe that the fiduciary model provides the appropriate ethical perspective on the physician-patient relationship. However, it is one thing to be appropriate in theory; it is another thing for that theory to be followed in actual practice. And in actual practice, the fiduciary model is not always the one that is followed. In fact, we sometimes encounter the conviction that when all is said and done, decision-making is not only the physician's prerogative but also the physician's duty.[33] Whatever the decision that has to be made, that is, whatever the decision beyond the initial one to engage a physician in the first place,[34] it is most appropriately made by the physician and not the patient.[35]

The reasons that are given for this (insofar as reasons are given at all and the whole thing is not simply a matter of conventionally sanctioned practice) are varied. However, we can identify four kinds; first, reasons that focus on the very nature of the profession;[36] second, reasons that centre in the allegedly diminished (or even absent) competence of the public in matters of medicine and health care; third, reasons that revolve about the claim that the physician is the only appropriate decision maker in emergency contexts; and fourth, reasons that capitalize on the pragmatic expertise in decision making that is acquired by the physician in the course of his or her practice.[37] In order to examine the validity of these reasons, and to underscore the thrust of our reasoning in favour of the fiduciary model, let us examine these in turn.

Argument from the Nature of the Profession

This argument usually involves two components: one focuses on the logic of the professional activities of the physician as physician; and another centres in substantial ethical principles that supposedly govern the conduct of medical practice: the principles of beneficence and of non-malfeasance.

The first argument goes something like this. The socio-legal status of the medical profession mandates an obligation of service. That service can be provided only when physicians are allowed to make decisions. Consequently it follows that according decision-making power to the physician is simply a precondition to his being able to fulfil his obligation as a professional.

The same point is sometimes argued in somewhat different terms as follows: Ethically speaking, one cannot have an obligation to do what is impossible to do. This, so it is said, finds legal reflection in the principle that equity does not require the impossible. Therefore, to charge an individual with an obligation and then to remove from that person the very means necessary for carrying it out, would be to place the individual in just such a position. However the practice of medicine requires constant decision-making, whether that be to medicate or operate, counsel or consult, immunize or simply to let matters be. Therefore, to deny physicians decision making power would be to bind their hands and make the very conduct of medicine impossible. It is for this reason that the primacy of decision-making power belongs to the physician. It derives from the fact of professional obligation itself.[38]

The second component of this argument centres in the claim that the very nature of the professional obligation is characterized by two fundamental principles: The principle of non-malfeasance[39] and the principle of beneficence.[40]

The principle of non-malfeasance is traditionally expressed as the obligation to avoid doing harm: *primum non nocere*. Its thrust may be expressed in the following two statements: "Do not intentionally or knowingly injure the patient" and "Do not intentionally or knowingly expose the patient to unjustified risk."[41]

However, so this reasoning has it, if we were to allow ultimate decision-making power to remain in the hands of the patient we would be violating the principle on both counts. In the first place, it would be to expose the patient unnecessarily to risks. Being insufficiently trained to understand the parameters that go into the making of such a decision, and being emotionally compromised because of the position in which the patient is placed, he or she is virtually certain to make a wrong decision. To allow this to occur would be like giving a knife to a child.

Furthermore, there are many situations in which providing the patient with the data necessary for making an appropriate decision would itself be to produce harm. That harm might be produced directly by affecting the patient's health as a result of the disclosure, or by putting him or her into a situation where the demands of making the decision itself are emotionally and psychologically debilitating. Alternatively, it might be produced indirectly by frightening the patient so severely that he or she would not even consider, let alone opt, for certain treatment modalities.[42] To avoid this happening, the physician has no choice other than to assume the decision-making role.

The principle of beneficence has been characterized as the "duty to help others further their important and legitimate interest" when we can do so with minimal risks to ourselves.[43]

Here again we can distinguish two components: a positive duty to bring about the good for others if it lies within our power to do so without harm to ourselves,[44] and a general duty to attempt to bring about a balance of good over harm in situations that allow for various choices. On both interpretations, however, the principle is assumed to entail that physicians have a general duty to decide among the various treatment options for their patients (or even whether there should be treatment at all) whenever the patients' own decisions are likely to be out of step with the advancement of their welfare or important and legitimate interests.

Analysis and Evaluation

All of these considerations have an air of extreme reasonableness about them. Particularly when we consider situations where patients[45] make choices that are clearly out of touch with what is medically possible, or where the result of such a choice would predictably lead to severe and irreparable harm for the patient. All of the physician's training has been to attempt to produce the best result possible and to avoid an increase in harm for the patient. It seems only too clear that the physician cannot simply stand by and let harm occur by letting the patient make the choice.

None of these considerations, however, amount to an ethical justification for saying that physicians have *and ought to have* ultimate decision-making power. To be sure, the conduct of the health care professions in general and of medicine in particular requires that certain conditions be met. For instance, it requires that physicians have access to adequate and true information, that the working conditions under which they operate are appropriate to allow them to follow their skill, and that they be allowed to make technical decision touching the nature of what should be done.[46] That does not, however, entail that the right (or even the duty) of decision-making *per se*, in its total and general scope, belongs to physicians. Or that it ought to belong to them.

In the case of medicine as in the case of all other professions,[47] we have to distinguish between the right to decide how to proceed in a purely technical sense once the decision to employ the services of the professional has been made, and the decision to employ the services of the professional in the first place and in what direction. Within certain limits (which we shall sketch in a moment), the first sort of decision-making is indeed the prerogative of the physician. It is entailed by the nature of medicine as a profession. The second, however, is not. It belongs wholly to the patient. The fact that it does so even in mortal contexts[48] found its first legal expression in the 1935 Alberta case of *Mulloy vs. HopSang*.[49]

HopSang suffered from a gangrenous right hand, and amputation was medically indicated to save his life. He refused permission to amputate. Mulloy, however, amputated the hand anyway because he assumed that the threat of impending death allowed him to overrule HopSang's refusal. He saved HopSang's life—who refused to pay him. Mulloy sued for costs. HopSang countersued in assault and battery, and the matter progressed through the courts. Finally the Alberta Supreme Court (Appellate Division) decided in favour of HopSang. It ruled that there is a fundamental difference between the right to decide what technical modality of treatment is appropriate once a decision to treat has been made, and the right to decide whether and with what purpose to proceed. The former right belongs to the physician, so it said; the latter to the patient.[50]

The case of HopSang is not an isolated one. There are others.[51] In all of them, the fundamental position that the courts have adopted, and one that reflects the ethics that we have advanced, is that the right of informed consent/refusal is an expression of the principle of the autonomy of the patient. The right belongs to the patient; that is why, " ... in the ordinary course where there is an opportunity to obtain the consent of the patient, it must be had."[52]

Of course, *Mulloy vs. HopSang* is only a legal case. As such it expresses only a legal conviction. However, a deontological ethical perspective would agree wholeheartedly with this decision. It would agree that patients have a fundamental right to decide whether to accept a particular treatment or not. That right is simply an expression of the principle of autonomy. Of course there are various parameters that will influence the exercise of this right.[53] Chief among these will be the values that the patient holds. These may differ from those held by the physician. However, so long as they are competent, a matter to which we shall return later, and so long as they do not violate the rights of others when they are put into practice, patients have the right to express them in their decisions. The physician has no right to overrule them.

Furthermore, the right to express these values extends not merely to the question of treatment or non-treatment itself. It also extends to the determination of the direction that the treatment should take. The constraints on medical practice that hold in the case of adult and competent Jehovah's Witnesses with respect to blood transfusion are here a case in point.[54] A physician must follow the competently expressed wishes of someone who is a Jehovah's Witness even if that means that the patient will die. The same is true for Christian Scientists, and individuals of similar persuasions. In a sense this imposes a limit even on the physician's right to technical professional decision-making. As soon as it impinges upon a patient's values, the patient also has a say.

The second line of reasoning is centred in an appeal to the principle of beneficence and the principle of non-malfeasance. It also fails. In fact, it fails on both the theoretical and practical plane. It fails on the theoretical plane because neither the principle of beneficence nor the principle of non-malfeasance is compatible with the deontological perspective that we have taken as fundamental and that seems to be supported both by the courts and the *Code* of *Ethics* of the CMA.[55] While it may be true that the principle of beneficence would legitimate the advancement of the important and legitimate interests of the patient, and that the principle of non-malfeasance would enjoin the prevention of harm; and while it may well be that in order to fulfil these two injunctions the physician would have to overrule the will of the patient, the fact is that both principles are utilitarian in nature. As one recent commentator put it:

It is important to notice that [a] tension exists ... within [sic] deontology, if it admits of beneficence and non-maleficence. These duties are, indeed, a kind of fragment of utilitarianism inside of deontology, and conflicts can arise as well between the deontologist's other principles as between deontology as a whole.[56]

Neither principle can have any place in a consistently developed deontologically oriented profession; and whatever argumentation is based upon it must be rejected. Happily, as we have already seen, the law recognizes that fact. A doctor might well believe that an operation or form of treatment is desirable or necessary, but the law does not permit him to substitute his/her own judgement for that of the patient. "This is for your (his, her) own good!" therefore has no place in an ethically oriented health care professional context if that good is bought at the price of autonomy.

The fact that they are utilitarian in nature excludes them from any consistently developed and internally coherent medical ethics. This does not to mean that something like them cannot be included in such an ethics and that something like them should not guide medical practice. We shall try to clarify this later in terms of the fiduciary nature of the profession. However, as they stand, these principles will only lead to an unacceptable form of medical paternalism.

Turning now to the pragmatic strand of our critique. Even if we were to ignore the preceding, the principle of beneficence would face extreme difficulties in implementation. Its underlying assumption is that an outsider can, as a matter of course, correctly determine the important interests of another person. Furthermore, it assumes that the outsider can also distinguish between those that are ethically legitimate and those that are not.

Both of these assumptions may be questioned. To see the problem, we only have to look at the diversity of cultural and subcultural perspectives that exist and that are explicitly sanctioned as legitimate within our society. What is considered important and what is valued is a function of individual and cultural perspective. Unless the physician shares these values or is aware of them as cultural variables, the physician will not even perceive them. Nor will the physician be able to accord them appropriate weight.

It is also important to note that the health care professions in general, and medicine in particular, themselves constitute a mosaic of distinct sub-cultures with tremendous variations in what is considered valuable and what important.[57] These variations are as great as those encountered in society itself. Therefore, there is no guarantee whatever, not even an overwhelming likelihood, that even physicians themselves would share the same values and therefore would apply the principle of beneficence in the same way.

With due alteration of detail, the same thing holds true for the principle of non-malfeasance. If we add to this such factors as the statistically verifiable distinction between physicians and patients in general—the difference between perceived and expected values on fundamental questions like that of disclosure of patient condition and prognosis comes to mind[58]—the problem worsens.

Finally, even if there were agreement on values on a general level, there is no guarantee that this will result in a correct weighting of these values from the standpoint of the patient under the conditions in which he or she seeks medical help. The weighting of values is a matter of idiosyncratic and unpredictable preference. It depends on psychological variables of which the physician may not even be aware, and over which the physician certainly has no control.

This problem of weighing reaches critical proportions when we note that the modern physician has very little personal patient contact of an enduring sort that will allow the physician to ascertain the patient's value system and personal preferences. What contact there is, is usually in an institutionalized context with its attendant consent problems. As to the psychological training that is necessary in order to be able to asses the patient properly in that regard, it is usually lacking in the physician's formal training. The upshot is that physicians almost always would have to decide on the basis of their own or on the basis of some projected valuations. Ethically, this is worrisome.

If the determination of what patients would consider as being in their best interest (or even of what they would consider a good) presents a problem, the determination of what they would consider as constituting harm or unacceptable or unnecessary risk, and so on, fares no better. Several studies have shown[59] not only that the evaluation of risk/harm as conducted by physicians is frequently unique to the profession itself and reflects its own sub-culturally determined standards, but also that such a professional evaluation frequently is entirely out of line with what one would have expected on a purely factual basis.

For instance, in one study[60] it was found that 55% of the responding physicians thought that punch biopsy of the skin presented merely a minimal risk to newborns, whereas in actuality this treatment presents a 53% risk of permanent scarring; 8% thought arterial puncture presented minimal risk to neonates and 24% thought it represented minimal risk to 12–18 year olds, whereas in fact there is a 39% risk of minor complications—i.e., somewhat above minimal—even for adults; and over 55% thought that a bone scan constituted minimal risk to neonates, whereas the World Health Organization and the International Commission on Radiological Protection found that the risk involves something in the neighbourhood of 100 per million of substantial genetic anomalies developing in the exposed child.[61] Similar figures exist for other areas of medicine.[62] And they do not even begin to deal with how the harm that might result would be perceived by the patient from a valuational perspective.

All this casts serious doubt on the claim that as a matter of course, physicians are better judges of likelihood of harm and of the impact of whatever harm results on the value-system of the patient. It therefore seriously undermines the argument from non-malfeasance. We can add to this the fact that another study has shown a very high correlation coefficient (0.947) between risks assumed by the physician for the patient and by the patient for him- or herself.[63] However, both judgements bore very little relation to the actual risk. So, for instance, strokes and heart attacks were seen as less serious than meningitis, multiple sclerosis or uraemia; frigidity as more serious than pneumonia or appendicitis; a slipped disc as more serious than starvation.

If we may echo the words of one commentator,[64] while it is understandable that lay assessment of the seriousness of an illness such as meningitis may still be in the grip of horror stories rooted in a pre-antibiotic era, it is not understandable how this—or anything like it—could be the case among physicians. If physicians' assessment about diseases for which accurate statistics are available can be so out of line with reality, it is difficult to accept their argument that they should have ultimate decision-making power simply because only by having such power will they be able to prevent a choice of treatment that foreseeably will lead to harm, or involve the patient in unjustified and unjustifiable risk.

The Argument from Patient Incompetence

The second reason for saying that primary decision making power should belong to the physician was the claim that all other things being equal, the patient really has diminished competence in the health care setting.

On the surface, this claim is relatively straightforward and simple. However, when we consider it carefully we find that it involves at least three separate and distinct strands. The *first* of these focuses on the notion of volition. It maintains that patients are volitionally compromised and compliant. That compromise is then traced to the fact of their need, to the patient role that they have assumed, and to the institutionalized context in which health care itself is sought, and given, in our society.

The *second* strand centres around the concept of cognitive competence. It maintains that the cognitive competence of patients is absent or at least diminished because they do not really understand the various medical parameters involved in the case. From this it concludes that therefore even if the patients volitional competence were unimpaired, they could not really exercise it in an appropriate fashion. Their cognitive abilities would not present them with an appropriate domain of options from which to choose.

Finally, the *third* strand focuses on the emotional aspect of competence. It maintains that patients, by becoming patients, adopt a certain role: the well-known sick-role so exhaustively described by medical sociologists. Because they have adopted this role, and because they are in a state of need, they are emotionally so labile that their competence in an emotional sense is compromised. This may then be (and usually is) intensified by the psychological implications of the disease process itself. The upshot of all three strands together is taken to be that the patient, simply in virtue of being a patient, is compromised as decision maker. It is on this basis that it then concludes that to allow someone who finds himself in so compromised a position on any or all of these counts to make decisions, is to open a door to potential harm.

Competence[65]

These, then, are three of the major strands that are involved in the argument from patient incompetence. The obvious question that we want to ask at this point is, Are they really telling? However, before attempting to answer that question we should look a little more closely at the concept of competence itself. What exactly do we understand by that term? There are, of course, different ways of approaching even this question: it can be approached from a psychological, legal, or sociological orientation, and so on. From an ethical perspective, however, we can distinguish four parameters: conceptual, volitional, emotional and valuational.

Conceptual Competence

Conceptual competence concerns only what may be termed the reasoning or intellective faculties of a person.[66] Here again we can distinguish several components. There is a *cognitive* aspect, which consists in the ability to understand or grasp data and the ability to appreciate their significance. This component plays the greatest role in most legal evaluations of competence.[67] It surfaces very clearly in the words of the *Ontario Mental Health Act*, which states that it is "the ability to understand the subject-matter in respect of which the consent is requested."[68]

Then there is an *inferential aspect*, which centres in the ability to see connections among data and the ability to draw conclusions from them.[69] This is the component that underlies the question, "Do you understand the consequences of your decision to forego or accept treatment?" It also plays an important role in legal evaluations. It is again reflected in the *Ontario Mental Health Act's* requirement that a competent person must be "able to appreciate the consequences of giving or withholding consent."[70]

Finally, there is a *mnemonic component* : the ability to remember data or decisions that have been made. It is centrally involved in inferential processes that go beyond the psychological present, but for all that it is logically distinct. It is also part of what underlies what are sometimes called questions of orientation. The presumption here is that a person whose awareness is confined only to an extended present can hardly be called competent in the proper sense of the term

Clearly, given the varied components of conceptual competence, conceptual competence is not an all-or-nothing affair. Not only does it involve variations as to the presence or absence of the components we have just mentioned, their degree of presence (or absence) is also a significant factor. Levels of conceptual sophistication are here implicated, as are variations in depth of inferential structure, the extent of the time-consciousness involved, and so on.

Evaluations of conceptual competence are therefore never easy. Of course, there are clear-cut or at least relatively clear-cut and obvious cases. Someone suffering from Down's syndrome and having the functional intelligence of a one-and-a-half year old clearly will be cognitively incompetent. Such a person will be unable to grasp the concepts necessary for orienting him- or herself in the world; to understand the natures of his or her medical condition; and to comprehend the various treatment choices. Such a person will also be inferentially incompetent because she or he will be unable to initiate, follow or prosecute, a train of reasoning of sufficient depth to allow her or him to make a decision among the various options available, their implications, and so forth.[71] More than likely, the person will also be mnemonically incompetent with respect to the various data, their significance, previous decisions reached, and so on.

On the other hand, someone suffering from Alzheimer's disease and living wholly in the present, as sometimes happens in such cases, may well be conceptually and inferentially quite competent within that temporal framework despite overall mnemonic incompetence; or a child of nine may be inferentially and mnemonically quite competent and yet fail to be completely competent on the cognitive level.

There are also situations in which conceptual competence *per se* is only temporarily impaired, as for instance in the case of someone recovering from anaesthesia, medication or other transient causes. A claim of conceptual competence, therefore, always has to be carefully circumscribed, and always has to be treated with extreme care. Perhaps a useful rule of thumb is this: Assume conceptual competence unless there are reasonable and convincing grounds to the contrary rooted in the nature and/or condition of the individual and his or her situation.

Volitional Competence

Volitional competence may refer to two distinct things: the ability of the individual to *make* decisions on the basis of what he or she has understood or inferred; or the ability of the individual to *carry out* the decision that he or she has made.[72] The first sort of inability may be pathological, as in some forms of mental illness. However, it need not be. It may simply be the result of shock, the result of an emotional trauma induced by the circumstances or situation. The individual may understand perfectly well and may be conceptually competent. It is just that this person simply lacks all emotional drive to convert the understanding into a decision.

As to the second possibility, it may be that although the patient does make a decision, he or she is so caught up in a pattern of behaviour that he or she is constitutionally unable to translate the decision itself into practice. Psychological conditions (for example, drug addiction) again furnish good examples here, but there are other much more subtle sorts of cases that also fall into this category. For instance, there are some people who, either through internal psychological make-up or the pressure of the context in which they find themselves, are so compliant that they sacrifice their own autonomy and are completely unaware that they are doing so. They merge their will with the will of the persons they take to be in authority.

Institutional contexts tend to have that effect on most people.[73] Moreover, it should not be forgotten that the professional health care setting itself, even when the treatment is not formalized and the interaction occurs on the home ground of the recipient, has an aura of institutionality about it. The fact is that whatever the relationship of the professional to the recipient may be, the professional here appears and acts as professional. That fact transforms the situation into a quasi-institutional one. The professional functions as the personification of the group that is the profession. Through this, the whole institutional framework that imbues the professional with legitimacy functions as an intangible but nevertheless real force to produce compliance. The octogenarian in a home who agrees to a course of treatment against his life-long beliefs, therefore, may well be volitionally incompetent in this sense.

We shall not dwell on external and overt parameters like the rules of an establishment (for instance, of a nursing home) or the law of the land. These may also act in a freedom-impairing fashion irrespective of whether they manifest themselves in obvious coercion or as covert threats. These factors are too obvious and too well-known to require comment. Nor shall we consider the sorts of cases that involve overt psychological pathology: for example, the person who is psychologically unable to act on his or her decision to go through a door, or a resident who cannot choose what to wear, in short, the sort of individual who cannot bring himself or herself to choose or decide on a course of action at all, or only with extreme difficulty. Their very nature consists in being volition-impaired.

Emotional Competence

Emotional incompetence is the inability to reach a reasoned (and reasonable) decision because of emotional pressures, feelings, and so on. It is usually negative emotions that are implicated in this context: emotions such as grief, sorrow, or despair. Positive ones like joy, delight, and pleasure are rarely if ever considered in this connection. Why exactly that should be the case is not clear. Since moderate sorrow is not usually considered incapacitating, one could easily argue that it is not the quality of the emotion that is considered decisive here but the intensity.

However, if this is the case then, clearly, positive but extremely violent emotions ought to be considered just as incapacitating as negative ones. The fact that this is not taken to be the case suggests that the real reason intensive negative emotions are considered competence-impairing is because there is a fear that the values adopted under the pressure of the negative emotions will be deviant from those that are considered normal, either for society or for the individual. If that is true, however, then a claim of emotionally-based incompetence really reduces to a covert form of rejection of values.

Before considering this aspect, however, we should recognize that even if we accept the competence-reducing function of negative emotional states, we are neither consistent in our application of this as a general principle nor does it in fact always hold true even according to our own standards. The principle seems to hold only in the health care context. Nowhere but here are we excused from responsibility because of depression about ourselves or those we love. A stockbroker can offer no such excuse for giving bad stock advice or for making bad financial decisions for his clients; and a truck driver cannot point to overwhelming grief as an exculpating reason why she ran through a red light and smashed into the side of a car.

In the health care context, however, things are often taken to be different. For instance, it is sometimes argued that when someone is closely attached (bonded) to a particular person, tragic news about him or her, for instances, the fact that he or she has just died on the operation-table may precipitate such an emotional crisis that a rational choice by the bereaved might not be possible. Parent-child relations, wife-husband connections particularly come to mind here. At the same time, however, the fact which we alluded to above—namely, that overwhelming negative emotions are not taken to strip us of our autonomy and competence as decision-makers in other cases—raises the puzzle why this should be thought to so in health care contexts.

The puzzle deepens when we consider that when it is physicians who are the recipients of bad news regarding their health or are in a negative emotional state because of bad news they have received about the health status of a loved one, there is usually no presumption that therefore they are incompetent. And yet one could easily argue that it is precisely here that we should make such an inference.

More specifically, one could point to the greater depth of knowledge that the professionals have in this area and then argue that this very knowledge would only serve to intensify the turmoil; precisely because the difficulties and problems attendant on the situations are much better appreciated and known by the physician than by the ordinary person, therefore the emotional turmoil would be incomparably greater, and therefore make physicians better candidates for emotional incompetence than anyone else.

Finally, there is this sobering consideration: If the argument from emotional pressure carries any weight at all, then there is a whole array of situations in which it tells against and not for the health care professional as decision-maker. Statistical data indicate that the fear of death is more widespread and more intense among physicians than among any other population group. Therefore, if incompetence is functionally related to the degree of negative emotional turmoil, then physicians should be the last to be considered competent in this domain.

But in a sense these objections are mere cavils. What they point out is not that emotional turmoil is not a competence-impairing parameter. Instead, they point out that we are inconsistent in our application and use of this notion. For when all is said and done, this much seems perfectly clear: While incompetence need not be *entailed* by a lack of (positive) emotional equilibrium, it may be present in some particular cases.

The point of the preceding considerations could therefore by summed up in the following manner: we must never approach the issue of emotional incompetence from an unbending perspective and with a preconceived answer. We must never presuppose. We must always look and see. And whatever criteria we use, we must apply them equally to all. The principle of equality and justice demands no less.

Valuational Competence[74]

We turn to the last component of ethical competence: valuational competence. Valuational competence focuses on the appropriateness of the values selected by the individual to determine the direction of his/her conceptual and volitional efforts. It is the most difficult notion of the three and the most easily mishandled. It is the sort of incompetence that may be ascribed to someone who wants radical or bizarre procedures out of peculiar ideas of beauty, because he or she values certain ideas, and so on. A good example is the medical student from Chicago who reportedly castrated himself surgically for no discernable reason (and did so in a surgically exemplary fashion), except that he felt that such a state was better than one of sexual normalcy.

However, we once again have to distinguish between two kinds of cases: cases where the values in question merely deviate from the range of values that are commonly accepted in a given society, and cases where the values are either mutually contradictory or are in conflict with the nature of reality. Many aesthetically oriented values fall under the first rubric, for instance those that result in whole-body tattoos, styles of clothing or even distinctive and "alternative" lifestyles. Examples of the second would be the valuation (and attempt to achieve) unlimited physical power, and eternal biological life.

However, we must be quite clear that deviation from this social valuational norm does not necessarily amount to valuational incompetence,[75] any more than the fact of adherence to it implies competence. One look at the social valuational deviance of conscientious objectors, of those who were opposed to slavery in 18th Century or in favour of women's suffrage in the 19th should be sufficient to illustrate the point. Perhaps the concept of valuational incompetence can be summed up like this:

1. The values adopted by the individual must be in keeping with the facts of reality. They must not set up action potentials that can never be satisfied even in principle, for example, the value of eternal biological life, of unlimited physical prowess, and so on.[76]

2. The values adopted must reflect the autonomy of the individual as a person. That is to say, if—as we have suggested (and as we shall spell out in greater detail below)[77]—a person is someone who has the capacity for cognitive self-awareness, then the values of the individual must be consistent with the nature of the individual as a person. This entails that values that deny the status of the individual as a person—as an autonomous agent—must be rejected.[78]

3.. The valuationally incompetent individual is one who, in spite of the evidence of the valuational unreasonableness of a position, nevertheless continues to adhere to it because he or she is unable to change it.

The last clause is crucial. It allows us to distinguish between individuals who are self-destructive because they want to be, and those who cannot help themselves.[79]

Before leaving valuational competence, we should like to raise one further caveat. Valuational incompetence should not be confused with being unethical, or with being morally evil. To be unethical is to violate the legitimate and effective (moral) rights of others. The violation of a right *per se*, however, may be the result of incompetent values in the sense that we have just sketched—as, for example, when our values do not allow us to treat others as persons. Such a violation will be unethical, and therefore evil, only if whoever violates these rights knowingly insists on doing so or if he or she should have known that such a violation would be the reasonable predictable outcome. If the act is pathological as outlined above, then the violator will not be unethical but incompetent, and possibly ill.

In sum, then, competence may vary conceptually, volitionally, emotionally and valuationally; and there is no logical (or, for that matter, psychological) reason to suppose that incompetence in one area, or competence, carries over into another. Nor should we assume that incompetence in a given area is necessarily global: that it is complete. In fact, this last consideration may be expressed in terms of the notions of duration and degree.

Extent of (In)Competence

Degree:[80] Competence may vary with respect to degree in each of the parameters we have discussed. Once again, children provide a good example. A child may understand the nature and effects of a proposed medical procedure, but not completely; the child may be able to assent to it, but only to a certain degree given its dependence on its parents or relevant others. The child may also hold certain values, but not appreciate or understand their nature and import fully.

All this is illustrated by the case of a ten-year-old Jehovah's Witness boy who is asked whether he will consent to a blood transfusion, and he refuses; or by the case of the fundamentalistic Christian girl who, when asked in the presence of her parents whether she will consent to animal tissue in her body (a pig heart valve), says "No." In such cases, the refusal clearly has elements not only of volitional incompetence—there is the element of parental pressure—but also of conceptual: the comprehension of what is involved is not quite complete. Still, by no stretch of the imagination can it be said to be entirely absent. That is why some ethicists have distinguished between consent and assent, and have maintained that children and other semi-competent individuals should be asked for their assent as a guide to the deliberations of the proxy decision-maker.[81]

Duration: None of us are totally in control of ourselves all of the time. The pressure of circumstances, whether emotional or physical in nature, force us into periods of incompetence. Anaesthesia, fever, emotional shock and the like all produce this effect. However, there must be no presumption that because such a state obtains at one point, therefore it is permanent. That may be assumed if and only if there is a permanent disability that grounds this state.

Still, the practical reality of health care delivery requires that there be criteria and categories that allow us to decide variations in competence without length review in each case. Therefore, the general presumption must be that except for children who have not yet attained 14 years of age, competence is present unless there are clearly discernible signs to the contrary; but once it has been shown not to be, it must be presumed to be absent in that area until criteria to the contrary spontaneously manifest themselves. The principle of impossibility, when applied to real life, makes any other course inoperable.

That is to say, the pragmatics of interpersonal and social conduct entail that we cannot evaluate competence on each and every occasion. We require criteria and standards that are workable. Furthermore, anything less would be unfair to those engaged as professionals in the health care setting. The time spent on continually assessing competence would detract from time available for the conduct of the profession, and would infringe on the rights of others to health care.

Since overt external indicators of competence frequently are either lacking entirely or uncertain, the only sort of procedure that is workable is chronological age. Tying the assumption of competence to chronological age is based on the observation that maturation in the physical sense tends to be correlated with maturation in the cognitive and psychological sense in a more or less predictable fashion and that these tend to be correlated with chronological age. The ethical justification for such a procedure is the principle of impossibility, otherwise professional/client interaction will be impossible. At the same time, the criterion requires an escape clause to the automatic presumption because, in fact, it may be false. It must therefore include the rider, "unless there are clearly discernable signs to the contrary." It will be apparent that this safeguards the "mature minor" as well as the incompetent adult.

Analysis and Evaluation

Having adumbrated the concept of competence, let us now consider the tenability of the thesis that gave rise to the whole discussion: The thesis that decision-making autonomy should reside with the physician because of the diminished competence of the patient.

We can now say with some degree of confidence that such a blanket assertion is not only far too ambiguous, it is also far too sweeping. Of course, a particular patient may be incompetent. What is more, he or she may be incompetent in a particular direction. But we cannot merely assume this to be true because we have some schematic approach to the circumstances, or because we have some a *priori* notion of what we just know to be the case. We have to look and see. The rule of thumb—the ethical rule of thumb—is that unless there are clear indications along the lines that we have indicated, a patient must never be presumed to be of diminished competence as a matter of course.

And even upon examination we have to be careful. What may appear to be cognitive incompetence may simply be lack of information presented at a level appropriate to the patient. (We shall return to the point later).[82] What appears to be volitional incompetence may simply be a culturally (or even individually) determined style of acting. The appearance of emotional incompetence may in fact be nothing other than a culturally based perceptual difference about how emotions are or should be expressed; and the appearance of valuational incompetence may reflect no more than the fact that the patient's value system deviates from what the physician (or the profession of medicine as a whole) accepts as appropriate values.

Finally, we have to ask the question that really has been standing in the wings all along. Does patient incompetence, however defined, give the physician the right, or the duty, of making the decisions for the patient? The answer is that it does not. Even if on close and careful examination a patient turns out to be incompetent, and even if the various competence-impairing parameters that are traditionally adduced did in fact exert an overwhelming competence-diminishing force in this particular case, it would not follow from this that therefore decision-making authority ought properly to reside with the physician. At least, not unless the circumstances are very unusual indeed. That conclusion would require separate argument, and would have to be established on its own. Rather, what follows is that the individual who is the appropriate proxy decision-maker for the patient ought to assume the decision-making function. And here ethics, law and custom agree that it is not necessarily nor inevitably the physician who fills the bill.

The Argument from Practice

One line of reasoning that might be thought to do this is the third one that we identified in the beginning. It went something like this: Physicians make medical decisions all the time. Therefore they have greater practice and expertise in making them than the patient who usually is faced only rarely with the need to do so. Furthermore, physicians also have an incomparably greater store of medical knowledge than the patient. Because of this, and because physicians constantly deal with a greater variety of problems than any one patient could ever expect to encounter, they have a much better overview of the real significance of a particular situation. For these reasons alone, then, a physician's decision will be much surer.[83] Therefore decision-making power should reside with physicians.

However, even if we were to grant the factual basis of this line of reasoning, does the conclusion really follow? Does it really entail that it is physician who ought to have primary decision-making power rather than the patient? Does this line of reasoning even show that the conclusion is reasonable? Could we not reply in the first instance that neither frequency of decision-making nor acquaintance with a variety of cases offers any assurance that the decisions that were made were themselves correct—or were made in an ethically appropriate manner?

In support of such a reply could we not point to historical examples? the treatment of certain types of patients in Nazi Germany, in Manchuria, and in the U.S. South;[84] the treatment of the elderly even at the present time;[85] and the historical treatment of women with respect to abortions, for example?[86] Surely frequency of decision-making is no indication of anything other than frequency of decision-making; and the lack of objections to such decision-making need not establish that the decisions were made correctly. It may simply indicate an authoritarian society, a closed (and powerful) medical profession, or whatever. It may even indicate that the health care consumer is ill-informed: that he or she requires what used to be called "consciousness raising" and so on. There are many possibilities here.

Acquaintance with a variety of cases in and by itself only shows experience of variety. It does not entail that the various types of situations were in fact approached in an ethically correct manner. Of course, it doesn't show the opposite either, but that is not the point. The point is that neither frequency nor variety have anything to do with ethical justification of decision-making power. That has to be established on different grounds. As it stands, the reasoning begs the question.

Furthermore, following a suggestion made in our general discussion of professional ethics, we have to distinguish sharply between two things: a decision made in a professional capacity on matters involving technical expertise, and a decision about the direction that a course of action should take in order to be reflective of a particular value-system. The fiduciary model of the professional-patient interaction requires that when a decision is of the second sort, it must be the values of the patient that are decisive;[87] and that unless he or she is incompetent, it is the patient's right to express these by making the decision him- or herself. To deny this is not only to fail to appreciate the distinction between the two kinds of decisions that we have just mentioned, it is also to reject the fiduciary model of physician-patient relationship itself.

The Argument from Emergency

The last argument in favour of the physician's pre-eminence of decision-making power focuses on the notion of emergency. There are interactions, so the reasoning, where time is of the essence, and a decision must be made without delay. The emergency rooms of hospitals provide the most graphic sorts of examples, but there are a myriad of others. Any medical situation may turn into an emergency in a trice. But to insist that even here, in emergency cases, primary decision-making power belongs to the patient and may not be overruled is in effect to make the practice of medicine impossible. Physicians must have the power to decide here. Otherwise, they will simply have to stand by and allow harm to occur—and that is absurd.

By way of analysis, let us begin by admitting that this line of reasoning does have a point, but only so far as the emergency contexts are concerned. From this, however, it is a far cry indeed to the practice of medicine as such and the delivery of health care in general. Ordinary contexts are just that: ordinary. They are not emergencies. There is time to inform the patient, to consult, to reason, and for the patient to reach a decision. The two sorts of contexts simply cannot be conflated.

But even for emergency contexts, the breadth of the conclusion is unwarranted. For one thing, we must distinguish between situations where time is of the essence and where the chance that an emergency may arise is not reasonably foreseeable; and situations where time is indeed of the essence, but the situation could reasonably have been foreseen. The first kinds of situations are unforeseeable emergencies—an unexpected stroke would be a good example, or a berry aneurysm. The second kinds of situations are foreseeable emergencies—the arrest of a cardiac patient here comes to mind.

Only in unforeseeable emergencies will there be no time to consult beforehand in order to establish the direction or even precise nature of the patient's values and wishes in the eventuality that an emergency might occur. Here indeed, all other things being equal,[88] the physician must have, and ethically does have, primary decision-making power. All other things being equal, he or she not only has the right but indeed the duty to act in the appropriate fashion without obtaining informed consent. But not in the second sort of case. There the physician's obligation is to establish beforehand what the patient would want, should the emergency occur. For the physician not to do so—not to establish this evaluational direction beforehand—is for the physician to abandon the fiduciary role.

A second limitation on emergency decision-making powers obtains when an appropriate proxy decision-maker for the patient is available and can be consulted. Next-of-kin usually fall into this category, as do legally appointed proxies and the like.[89] They may not be ignored unless in fact the time is so precious that, the fact of their present availability notwithstanding, consultation is impossible. The doctrine of emergency once more applies.

Finally, the breadth of this conclusion is limited by the fact that a patient, when competent, may have made a clear and autonomous determination of what direction treatment should take if the patient were ever to be in an emergency and unable to indicate his or her wishes. Jehovah's Witnesses usually act in this way; but so do many of the elderly who do not wish to be resuscitated. If such determination is reasonably accessible to the physician, for example, on a signed (and possibly even witnessed) card of the sort frequently kept by Jehovah's Witnesses, and if the situation that has arisen is of the sort covered by that statement, then the physician must abide by it.[90] The recent Supreme Court of Newfoundland decision in the case of *Little*[91] and of the Ontario court in the case of *Malette vs. Shulman et al.*,[92] constitute clear legal recognition of this ethical fact.

At the present time it is legally unclear whether such a direction can apply to all aspects of medical emergency treatment in the Canadian setting. Ethically speaking, however, it certainly does. If there is a competent, previously executed determination, reasonably available in emergency context, then even here the patient's will (or that of the appropriate proxy) prevails. Priority does not necessarily—nor automatically—rest with the physician. If it were otherwise, the principle of autonomy would govern health care contexts only so long as patients are competent and able to insist on their will.

Conclusion

The health care setting is one of the most delicate and intimate of all human settings. Certainly this is true from the side of the patient. In order for the health care professional to be able to provide an appropriate service, the patient has to be open and truthful towards the professional. But by opening up, the patient becomes vulnerable. Frequently the disease process has also exercised its influence on the patient or the patient has assumed a patient role. This increases the vulnerability of the patient. Furthermore, the patient is almost invariably driven by a mix of motivations and feelings: the desire to receive help, the drive to remain independent and to retain autonomy and the acceptance of a dependency role together with a somewhat ambivalent rejection of what goes with it, and so on. These tend to complicate the picture.

From the side of the health care professional, there is an equally strong and complicated mix of driving forces: the desire to do best for the patient, the interest in the disease process itself, considerations of professional duty mixed with personal values and perception, and so on.

As we pointed out at the beginning of this chapter, in most cases the health care professional is in a better position to shape the relationship that will arise because the patient tends to enter the health care setting in a compromised fashion. That suggests that in most cases it is the health care professional who has the greater responsibility to make sure that the nature of the relationship remains ethically appropriate. To us, that means that the health care professional has a duty to try and structure this relationship from a deontological perspective, motivated not by calculations of the greatest good for the greatest number or by considerations of what will advance the position of the professional or of the profession, but by concern for the patient as person. The relationship between health care professional and patient is fiduciary. If the health care professional loses sight of this, then the relationship will become like that between a car owner and his mechanic.

ENDNOTES

[1] For instance nursing, physiotherapy, dentistry, etc. However, we want to emphasize that they will be analogous, not the same. Clearly, the material professional and administrative differences of the various health care professions will result in ethical differences as well.

[2] For an analogous legal point, see Margaret Somerville, *Consent to Medical Care*, Study Paper, Law Reform Commission of Canada (Ottawa, 1979). See also E. Picard, *Legal Liability of Doctors and Hospitals in Canada* (Toronto: Carswell, 1984) 4; and H.E. Emson, *The Doctor and the Law*. (Toronto: Butterworths, 1989). See also Chapter 5.

[3] We here do not mean control in the physical sense, but rather in the sense of determination of the direction that the relationship will take and of the decisions that are made. See R.M. Veatch, (see note 6) and C. Barber Mueller, (see suggested readings) for different discussion. For a good discussion of the various issues from a nursing perspective, see J. Storch, *Patients' Rights* (Toronto: McGraw Hill, 1982). For the U.S. context, see A. Jameton, *Nursing Practice* (Englewood Cliffs N.J.: Prentice Hall, 1984) and J. Muyskens, *Moral Problems in Nursing: A Philosophical Investigation* (Towanda: Rowman & Littlefield, 1982). J. Flaherty and L. Curtin, *Nursing Ethics* (Bowen, Maryland: Bradey, 1982) is not quite as successful.

[4] For physicians as having control, see John C. Moskop, "The Nature and Limits of the Physician's Authority," in Martin S. Staum and Donald E. Larson, eds. *Doctors, Patients and Society: Power and Authority in Medical Care* (Wilfrid Laurier U.P.: Waterloo 1981) 29–44; David L. Jackson and Steward Youngner, "Patient Autonomy and 'Death With Dignity,'" *New England Journal of Medicine* 301(1979) 404–408; Franz Ingelfinger, "Arrogance," *New England Journal of Medicine* 303(1980) 1509.

[5] See R.M. Veatch, (note 6). On paternalism, see Glenn C. Graber, "On Paternalism in Health Care," in John W. Davis, Barry Hoffmaster and Sarah Shorten, eds., *Contemporary Issues in Biomedical Ethics* (Humana Press: Clifton, N.J., 1981); Allan Buchanan, "Medical Paternalism," *Philosophy and Public Affairs* 7(1978) 370–390; Joseph Ellin, "Comments on 'Paternalism in Health Care'" in *Contemporary Issues in Biomedical Ethics* (see ref. above); Bernard Gert and Charles M. Culver, "Paternalistic Behaviour," *Philosophy and Public Affairs* 6 (1976) 45–47; Gerald Dworkin, "Paternalism," *The Monist* 56 (Jan. 1972); Joel Feinberg, *Social Philosophy* (Engelwood Cliffs, N.J.: Prentice Hall, 1973) 52; Joan C. Callahan, "Paternalism and Voluntariness," *Canadian Journal of Philosophy* 16: 2 (1986) 199–220; H.T. Engelhardt, Jr. *The Foundations of Bioethics* (New York: Oxford Univ. Press, 1986) 252–262.

[6] What follows is based on Robert M. Veatch, "Models for Ethical Medicine in a Revolutionary Age," *Hastings Center Report* 2 (June 1972) 5–7, and Michael D. Bayles, *Professional Ethics* (Wadsworth: Belmont, California 1981) Chapter 4, and James I. Childress and Mark Siegler, "Metaphors and Models of Doctor-Patient Relationships: Their Implication for Autonomy," *Theoretical Medicine* 5(1984) 17–30. For a different approach, see A. Chinen, "Modes of Understanding and Mindfulness of Clinical Medicine," *Theoretical Medicine* 9: 1(February 1988) 45–72, who advocates a mix of formal, hermeneutic and pragmatic modes. The formal approach, which is that of Veatch and Bayles, is here presented as focusing too much on the structure of obligations without giving due weight to the attitudinal aspects of the physician-patient relationship. It is said to "objectify" the individuals. This, so it is argued by some, is counterbalanced by a hermeneutic element, which involves a "subjectification" of the value-systems and a "being-with" of both parties. Since a purely hermeneutic relationship is said to run the danger of paternalism, Chinen, in the above-mentioned text, suggests that there should be an initial attempt to establish a "congruence" of values, and that this should then be applied in a pragmatic sense. We feel that Chinen's hermeneutic element will be accommodated for in a properly structured fiduciary relationship.

[7] Thomas Percival, *Medical Ethics: Or a Code of Institutes and Precepts, Adapted to the Professional Conduct of Physicians and Surgeons* (London: Russell and Bickerstaff, 1803). There is a 1927 edition by C.D. Leake.

[8] See John C. Moskop, "The Nature and Limits of the Physician's Authority," in Martin S. Staum and Donald E. Larson, eds., *Doctors, Patients and Society: Power and Authority in Medical Care* (Wilfrid Laurier U.P.: Waterloo 1981) 29–44. See also Veatch, under what he calls the "priestly" model, and Bayles, (see note 6). See also J.E. Magnet and E.W. Kluge, *Withholding Treatment from Defective Newborn Children* (Cowansville: Brown Legal Publ., 1985) chapters 1 and 2 for a discussion in the context of Canadian paediatric practice.

[9] *Reibl vs. Hughes* (1980), 14 C.C.L.T.I. (S.C.C.).

[10] In the sort of case mentioned above, it would be the parents—although strictly speaking they only function as proxies. See Chapter 6,"Proxy Decision-Making."

[11] The term "agency" is due to Bayles (see note 6) By and large, we prefer the term "agency" since most engineers we know would not abandon personal ethical convictions in their professional dealings.

[12] For a rejection of a complete agency model, see also Margaret Somerville, *Consent to Medical Care*, Study Paper for the Law Reform Commission of Canada (Ottawa: 1979) chapters 2 and 3.

[13] For co-adventuring, see Eric Cassell, "Autonomy and Ethics in Action," *New England Journal of Medicine* 297(1977) 33–34; Thomas Szaz and Marc H. Hollender, "A Contribution to the Philosophy of Medicine: The Basic Models of the Doctor-Patient Relationship," *Archives of Internal Medicine* 97(1956) 585–592.

[14] On contractual approaches, see, Veatch, and Bayles, (see note 6.). See also Roger Masters, "Is Contract and Adequate Basis for Medical Ethics? " *Hastings Center Report* 5(Dec. 1975)24–28; and R.May, "Code and Covenant or Philanthropy and Contract? " in S.J. Reiser, A.J. Dyck and W.J. Curran, eds., *Ethics in Medicine: Historical Perspectives and Contemporary Concerns* (MIT Press: Cambridge, Mass., 1977) 65–76; Ellen Picard, "The Doctor-Patient Relationship and the Law," in Staum and Larsen (ref. note 8) 45–57, and *Legal Liability* (ref. note 2.)

[15] For a brief discussion of the friendship model, see Veatch, and Bayles, (ref. note 6). See also P.L. Entralgo, *Doctor and Patient*, translation F. Partridge (New York: World U., Library: 1969); Charles Fried, "The Lawyer as Friend," *The Yale Law Review* 85(1976) 1060–1089 and *Medical Experimentation: Personal Integrity and Social Policy* (New York: American Elsevier, 1974) 76 and elsewhere.

[16] The model therefore assumes a very personal relationship between physicians and patients. One of the draw-backs, of course, is that it would facilitate professional burn-out.

[17] The word comes from the Latin "fides", meaning trust. See also Veatch, and Bayles, (note 6); and Picard, *Legal Liability* (ref. note 2).

[18] CMA *Code*, article 16.

[19] Somerville, (see note 2), mentions the psychological impact of the physician-patient relationship. See also Jay Katz, *The Silent World of Doctor and Patient* (Free Press: New York, 1984) I and II; Dan O'Hair, "Patient Preference for Persuasion," *Theoretical Medicine* 7(1986)147–164; and Andrea Farkas Patenaude, Joel M. Rappeport and Brian R.Smith, "Physician's Influence on Informed Consent for Bone Marrow Transplantation," *Theoretical Medicine* 7(1986) 165–179.

[20] CNA *Code*, Value V, "Limitations."

[21] See CMA *Code*, "Responsibilities to the Patient" article 15.

[22] Defensive medicine is justified under such circumstances because the co-operation parameter that is part of the presupposition of a fiduciary relationship can no longer be relied upon. In fact, it is essentially absent. In light of the statistics on patient compliance (compare M. Becker and L. Maiman, "Strategies for Enhancing Patient Compliance," *Journal of Community Health* 6 (1980) 113–132) this raises an interesting question about just how much medicine in fact should be conducted—may be conducted?—defensively.

[23] The physician appears to be legally protected in emergency cases by the so-called doctrine of emergency. See Picard, (note 2).

[24] The term was coined by Robert M. Veatch.

[25] See Bayles (note 6), p. 68 with respect to D. Rosenthal's study of the cost to physicians when they follow this model.

[26] See Bayles (note 6).

[27] The U.S. case of *Tarasoff vs. The Regents of the University of California* (17 Cal.Rep., 3rd. 425(1976)) is here instructive.

[28] It also requires an ethical impact analysis with respect to allocation at the micro-level.

[29] See H.K. Spiro, *Doctors, Patients and Placebos*, (New Haven: Yale Univ. Press, 1986) 47, 116 and elsewhere.

[30] Spiro (ref. above), p. 47.

[31] On the human aspect of the relationship, see David H. Smith and Lloyd S. Pettegrew, "Mutual Persuasion as a Model for Doctor-Patient Communication," *Theoretical Medicine* 7(1986) 127–146; Engelhardt (ref. note 36), and Chinen (ref. note 6).

[32] That is, until the advent of more consumer oriented health care delivery, beginning in Canada essentially with the 1980 Supreme Court decisions on informed consent. While there were previous legal cases insisting on the patient's decision-making powers (for instance *Mulloy vs. HopSang* and *Parmley vs. Parmley*) by and large they were ignored in practice. See also Somerville (ref. note 12) 14ff.

[33] Compare Magnet and Kluge (ref. note 8) 8–30 and elsewhere; D. Crane, *The Sanctity of Social Life: Physicians' Treatment of Critically Ill Patients* (New York: Russell Sage, 1975) 3ff. J.H. Guillemin and L.L. Holmstrom, *Mixed Blessings: Intensive Care For Newborns* (N.Y. and Oxford: Oxford University Press, 1986) 109ff., and elsewhere.

[34] Of course that decision belong fundamentally to the patient. For a recognition of this by the medical community, see article 5 of the CMA *Code*.

[35] This perspective, as we shall see later, may give rise to a paternalistic attitude. For a good discussion of some of the issues involved here, see D.C. Thomasma, "Beyond Medical Paternalism and Patient Autonomy: A Model of Physician Conscience for the Physician-Patient Relationship," *Annals of Internal Medicine* 98: 3 (February, 1983) 243–247, especially the discussion of "Limitations of the Autonomy Model"; Garret et al. (ref. note 41) 29; Beauchamp and McCullough (see note 40) 35, 97–103.

[36] See Beauchamp and Childress (note 39), Ch. 4, and H.T. Engelhardt Jr, *The Foundations of Bioethics* (Oxford and New York: Oxford University Press 1986), Ch. 3.

[37] See J. Shaw, "Dilemmas of 'Informed Consent' in Children," *New England Journal of Medicine* (1973) 805. This line of reasoning is also involved the position that health-care decisions are inherently and only medical decision. For a contrary view, see Magnet and Kluge, op. cit. 173f. See also, Beauchamp and McCullough, (ref. note 40) 34.

[38] See above, pp. 79f.

[39] For an extended discussion, see T.L. Beauchamp and J.F. Childress, *Principles of Biomedical Ethics* (New York and Oxford: Oxford University Press, 1979) Chapter 4. For a critique, see Nicholson (ref. note 56).

[40] Compare Beauchamp and Childress (ref. note 39) Ch. 5, and T.L. Beauchamp and L.B. McCullough, *Medical Ethics: The Moral Responsibilities of the Physician* (Englewood Cliffs, New Jersey: Prentice-Hall, 1984), 27ff.; A. Buchanan, "Philosophical Foundations of Beneficence," in E. Shelp, ed., *Beneficence and Health Care*, 33–62.

[41] Compare Beauchamp and Childress (ref. note 39) 106–147, especially at 108ff. Also T.M. Garrett, H.W. Baillie, and R.H. Garrett, *Health Care Ethics: Principles and Problems* (Englewood Cliffs, New Jersey: Prentice-Hall, 1989) 51–55.

[42] This is well catalogued in *Reibl vs. Hughes* by Bora Laskin, C.J.S.C.

[43] Beauchamp and Childress (ref. note 39), 136.

[44] Compare M. Sloate, "The Morality of Wealth," in H.D. Atkins and H. La Follette, eds., *World Hunger and Moral Obligation* (Englewood Cliffs, N.J.: Prentice-Hall 1977) 127. See also Law Reform Commission of Canada Working Paper 46, *Omissions, Negligence and Endangering* (Ottawa, 1985) 15ff. for general duty. For an extended discussion of the Principle of Beneficence, see Beauchamp and Childress, (ref. note 39) 5, "The Principle of Beneficence." For a negative perspective, see Frankena *Ethics* (Englewood Cliffs, N.J.: Prentice-Hall, 1973) 47ff., and Feinberg, "The Nature and Value of Rights," *Journal of Value Inquiry* 4 (1970) 243–57.

[45] Or relevant others acting on their behalf. We shall consider proxy decision-making in Chapter 6.

[46] Compare Law Reform Commission of Canada, Working Paper 26, *Medical Treatment and the Criminal Law* (Ottawa: Ministry of Supply and Services 1980) 10, mentioning the so-called "captain of the ship" analogy.

[47] Compare Bayles (see note 6) Ch. 4.

[48] See also *Medical Treatment* (ref. note 46) IV: 3.

[49] *Mulloy vs. HopSang*, (1935) W.W.R. 714 (Alberta Supreme Court App. Division).

[50] As above.

[51] (For example) *Marshall vs. Currey* [1933] 3 Dominion Law Report 260; *Malette vs. Shulman.* et al (1990),72 o.r. (2d)417 (C.A.)

[52] *Mulloy vs. Hopsang* (ref. note 49).

[53] See Engelhardt (ref. note 36), Ch.7; Magnet and Kluge (ref. note 8), 173f.

[54] Compare Beauchamp and McCullough (ref. note 40) 35–37; Engelhardt (ref. note 36), 91; Beauchamp and Childress (ref. note 40), 83. See also *Malette vs. Shulman* (ref. note 51).

55 That is to say, with article 5 of the *Code*. Principle I can be interpreted in a deontological sense if one assumes that the well-being of the patient is defined by and in terms of the values of the patient.

56 R.H. Nicholson, *Medical Research with Children: Ethics, Law and Practice* (Oxford: Oxford University Press, 1986) 68.

57 Compare Crane (ref. note 33), especially part II.

58 See Crane (ref. note 33). See also J. Katz and A.M. Capron, *Catastrophic Diseases: Who Decides What* (New York: Russell Sage, 1975).

59 Nicholson (ref. note 56), 104.

60 Nicholson, 105.

61 Nicholson, 89.

62 See M.L. Slevin, L. Stubbs, H.J. Plant, P. Wilson, W.M. Gregory, P.J. Armes, S.M. Dower, "Attitudes to Chemotherapy: Comparing Views of Patients with Cancer with those of Doctors, Nurses, and the General Public," *British Medical Journal* 300 (June 2, 1990) 1458–1460.

63 See Nicholson (ref. note 56), 106.

64 Nicholson (ref. note 56), 106.

65 For an interesting recent book-length discussion and analysis of competence, see Allen E. Buchanan and Dan W. Brock, *Deciding for Others: The Ethics of Surrogate Decision Making* (Cambridge and New York: Cambridge University Press, 1989).

66 This is the aspect traditionally emphasized in legal contexts. See *Johnston vs. Wellesly Hospital* (1971) 2 O.R. See also *Booth vs. Toronto General Hospital* (1910), 170. W.R. 118. For a more recent case, see *Steinback vs. Jaffe* [1988] O.J. No. 1081. See also Picard (ref. note 2), 55ff. and A. Linden, *Canadian Tort Law*, 3rd. ed. (Toronto: Butterworths, 1982), 60. See also Beauchamp and McCullough (ref. note 40), 123; Beauchamp and Childress (ref. note 39), 69.

67 Here we distinguish the purely cognitive from the performative parameter. For a view that combines both to some extent under the general heading of "rational competence," see Haavi Morreim. "The Concepts of Patient Competence," *Theoretical Medicine* 4: 3 (October 1983) 231–51, especially 234–36.

68 Mental Health Act, R.S.O.1980, c.262, s.1(g).

69 This is in part what appears to underlie T.S. Szaz, critique of the notion of mental illness. See T.S. Szaz, *Ideology and Insanity* (New York: Doubleday and Co., 1970) and *The Myth of Mental Illness: Foundations of a Theory of Personal Conduct* (New York: Hoeber-Harper, 1961).

70 Mental Health Act, R.S.O.1980, c.262, s.1(g).

71 This is similar to the evaluative component that Morreim (ref. note 67) calls "performance competence" (237 f.), although Morreim's notion also includes a volitional parameter.

72 This is known ethically as the phenomenon of the weak will.

73 This is especially clear in the prison-context. See also Somerville 95–103). See also D.C. Martin, J.D. Arnold, T.F. Zimmermann, R.H. Richart, "Human Subjects in Clinical Re-

search—A Report of Three Studies," *New England Journal of Medicine*, 279 (1968) 1426 and Jameton (1984) 128. On the compromising effects of illness and institutional and legal arrangements, see S. Ketchum and C. Pierce, "Rights and Responsibilities," *Journal of Medicine and Philosophy* 6 (1981) 271–279; and G. Annas, "The Emerging Stowaway—Patients' Rights in the 1980," *Law, Medicine and Health Care* [Feinberg, 1982] 32–35, 46. This lack of personal confidence may even affect nurses in the institution; See C.K. Hofling, E. Brotzman, S. Dalrymple, N. Graves and C.M. Pierce, "An Experimental Study in Nurse-Physician Relationships." *Journal of Nervous and Mental Disease* 143 (August 1966) 171–80.

[74] Compare Morreim (ref. note 67) with respect to several aspects of what she calls functional competence. See also D. Wikler, "Paternalism and the Mildly Retarded," *Philosophy and Public Affairs* 8 (1979) 337–392, especially 379.

[75] The notion of valuational competence appears to be central to T.S. Szaz, critique of the notion of mental illness. See T.S. Szaz, *Ideology and Insanity* (New York: Doubleday and Co., 1970) and *The Myth of Mental Illness: Foundations of a Theory of Personal Conduct* (New York: Hoeber-Harper, 1961). However, Szaz would probably not accept our analysis.

[76] While an attempt to increase life span, physical prowess, etc. may be reasonable, the value of unlimited life, etc. violates the principle of impossibility—if only because of the third law of thermodynamics.

[77] See Chapter 11.

[78] This holds even on a utilitarian approach. "Good" would here be defined in terms of good for persons. Therefore if an act resulted in or aimed at a reduction of personhood, it would be in conflict with the basic principle of utility. This raises the question, how far a hedonistic utilitarian approach can consistently be purely material in orientation. Presumably that is why Mill ranked pleasure and fixed on those that retain awareness as being properly utilitarian.

[79] For instances, this allows us to say that not all suicides are incompetent.

[80] Compare Morreim (ref. note 67), 236.

[81] R.A. McCormick, "Proxy Consent in Experimentation Situation," *Perspectives in Biology and Medicine* 18: 1 (1974) 3–20. W.G. Bartholome, "Parents, Children, and the Moral Benefits of Research; " Nicholson (1986) 140 f., 146–51; L.A. Weithorn and S.B. Campbell, "The Competency of Children and Adolescence to Make Informed Treatment Decisions," *Child Development* 53 (1987) 1589–98. See also *R. vs. D.* All England Law Review 2 (1984) 449–458. Although Lord Brandon uses 'consent', the meaning appears to be closer to our notion of assent. Also National Commission for the Protection of Human Subjects of Biomedical and Behavioral Research, Report and Recommendation: *Research Involving Children* (Washington, D.C. DHEW, 1977) 13 and elsewhere. The "mature minor" rule is also implicated here. See Picard (ref. note 2), 55–64.

[82] See Chapter 5.

[83] See R. Veatch, "Models for Ethical Medicine in a Revolutionary Age," *Hastings Center Report* 2 (June 1972) 5–7 for a classic discussion of the so-called "priestly model."

[84] See J.H. Jones, *Bad Blood* (New York: Free Press, 1981).

[85] I.e. the refusal to allow geriatric patients to make decisions for themselves. In part, the "living will" movement appears to be a reaction to this. See J. Hammerman, "Health Services: Their Success and Failure in Reaching the Aged Older Adult," in *Dominant Issues in Medical Sociology*, ed., H.D. Schwartz and C.S. Kart (Don Mills: Addison-Wesley, 1978) 407; J. Thornton and E. Winkler, *Ethics and Aging* (Vancouver: UBC Press, 1988); J. Storch (ref. note 3), 146–148.

[86] Not only historical. It is only in 1988, with the Supreme Court Decision in *Morgenthaler vs. The Queen* that the situation changed in any significant way.

[87] Of course this does not hold without conditions. For instance that the values must be competent, that they must be genuinely held by the patient, and so on. It also does not apply to congenitally incompetent persons, who cannot really be said to have values in a morally relevant sense. On the temptation to go from professional expertise to imposition of values, see R. Veatch, "Generalization of Expertise," *Hastings Center Studies* 1: 2 (1973), 29–40. See also J.C. Moskop, "The Nature and Limits of the Physician's Authority," in M.S. Staum and D.E. Larson, eds. *Doctors, Patients, and Society: Power and Authority in Medical Care* (Waterloo, Ontario: Wilfrid Laurier University Press, 1981) 29–43, and M. Bayles (ref. note 6), 68–69; Engelhardt (ref. note 36), 327 n. 53.

[88] That is to say, there having been no previous competently executed indication by the patient of his or her wishes about what direction health care should take should he or she be incompetent and unable to decide for him- or herself. See *Malette vs. Shulman*. On emergency powers from a legal perspective, see Picard (ref. note 2), 45ff.; Law Reform Commission of Canada, *Medical Treatment*, 41–5. Linden (ref. note 66).

[89] See Picard, (ref. note 2), Various provinces specify the devolvement of surrogate/proxy authority in terms of familial propinquity.

[90] See Linden (ref. note 66) 63; See also Law Reform Commission (1982) 90f. and *Malette vs. Shulman*.

[91] *Matter of C.P. Little*, Supreme Court of Newfoundland (1987) No. F87111 at 57.

[92] *Malette vs. Shulman*, (Ont. C.A.)72 O.R.(2d) 417,[1990] O.J. No.450.

SUGGESTED READINGS

- Bayles, M.D. "The Professional-Client Relationship," in Michael D. Bayles, *Professional Ethics*. Belmont, Calif.: Wadsworth, 1981, Chapter 4.

    Bayles' book deals with professional ethics in general. In this chapter, he explores the notion of the professional/client relationship in generic terms. It provides a useful comparison to the classic paper by Veatch.

- Gordon, Harry H. "The Doctor-Patient Relationship: A Judaic Perspective," *The Journal of Medicine and Philosophy*, vol. 8 (1983) 243–255.

    Philosophical discussions of the physician/patient relationship usually focus on purely rationalistic considerations. Gordon's paper departs from this by approaching the relationship from the perspective of the Judaic religion.

- Mueller, Barber C. "The Doctor-Patient Relationship: A Unique Covenant," from J.E. Thomas, ed., *Medical Ethics and Human Life*. Sanibel and Toronto: Samuel Stevens, 1983 72–83.

    This paper outlines the views of a Canadian physician of what the nature of the physician-patent relationship involves in the context of modern Canadian society. It is interesting in the emphasis it places on the contextual nature of the relationship within society.

- Veatch, Robert M. "Models for Ethical Medicine in a Revolutionary Age," *Hastings Center Report* vol.2 (June 1972).

    Robert Veatch's paper is a classic in the field. He examines several ways in which the physician-patient relationship can be understood and outlines their implications.

- Tomlinson, Thomas. "The Physician's Influence on Patients' Choices," *Theoretical Medicine* 7: 2 (1986) 105–121.

    Tomlinson examines the role that physicians' wishes, attitudes and perspective has on the way in which patients make their decisions about treatment. It is not juridical but practice oriented in nature.

6
Proxy Decision-Making

This chapter considers some of the difficulties that arise for the health care professional when the patient is incompetent, and yet a decision about treatment has to be made. This presents particular problems in the case of children. Special attention is paid to the questions of who should act as a proxy decision-maker, and what criteria a proxy decision-maker should use in trying to arrive at a decision.

Some questions that might usefully be kept in mind while reading this chapter include:

1. What is a proxy decision? Are all proxy decisions the same in nature? Why should proxy decision-making take place at all?
2. Who is an appropriate proxy decision-maker?
3. What criteria should a proxy decision-maker use? Should these criteria be the same for all types of proxy decision-making?
4. What is the role of health care professionals in proxy decision-making? of the Courts? of the next-of-kin?

Introduction

In the preceding chapter we touched on living wills and durable power of attorney. These, of course, are legal devices for people to make sure that their wishes will be followed when they are no longer in a position to make a decision themselves. In other words, they involve what traditionally has been called "proxy decision-making." But consider the following cases:

1. A fifty-three year old man with previous history of a stroke a year ago again suffers another stroke. This time he is left hemiplegic with elevated blood-pressure, completely aphasic with what appear to be intermittent periods of awareness but according to a psychiatric

assessment otherwise generally incompetent. He is fed by a naso-gastric tube which he has pulled out on occasion. On other occasions he has apparently assisted the nursing staff in replacing the tube, and at times "holds" it during feeds. In general, his behaviour is unpredictable. His wife tells the attendant GP that he has told her often that if he were ever left seriously compromised by another stroke, he would want to be allowed to die. His wife therefore wants the naso-gastric tube removed and wants him to be allowed to die.

2. A six-year old child, KLF, was admitted to the Hospital for Sick Children on February 26th to have a tonsillectomy and adenoidectomy. The surgery was performed the same day. Immediately after surgery, in recovery, the child suffered from recurring bleeding, which continued of and on until March 2 and 3. She lost about 200–250 cc. of blood in that time. She is suspected of having thrombocytopenia, which affects the ability to clot. So far, she has been stabilized without blood or blood-products—which is important to her parents who are Jehovah's Witnesses and who refuse to consent to medical treatment that would involve blood or blood-products. It is ten days since the surgery, and a critical time when secondary bleeding may occur. Shortly after midnight (March 6th) KLF does indeed suffer a rapid bleed and loses 80 cc. Her total blood loss before this bleed had been 40% of her blood volume. The attending physician wants permission to transfuse if more blood is lost. The parents refuse because the use of blood is against their religion. The Children's Aid Society is called in to seek a court order for custody, so that it can order a transfusion.[1]

3. A profoundly mentally handicapped sixteen year old girl requires 24 hour care from her mother. The girl tends to "smear" her stool, and will presumably do the same with her menstrual flow. The mother requests that the girl have a radical hysterectomy, and the physician, after due consultation with a psychiatrist and a gynaecologist, agrees and schedules her for surgery. A nurse on the ward notifies a pro-life group who picket the hospital. The physician quickly cancels the surgery and discharges the girl. The mother is frustrated and angry.[2]

These cases extend the range of our previous discussion of proxy decision-making. Further cases are the comatose person who is brought into the emergency department of a hospital, the octogenarian suffering from Alzheimer's disease or the teenager suffering from Down's syndrome with a functional intelligence of a three-year old and a corresponding emotional maturity. There is also the patient who has been given pre-op medication, the rest-home resident who suffers only occasional lapses of rationality but who is volitionally highly compromised, or the child who has not yet reached the stage of independent and mature judgement. The list of cases that involve proxy decision-making is almost endless. What we need is some overview of the general principles that should be followed in such situations.

The operative assumption that underlies all this is that proxy decisions should be made in the first place. However before we go any further perhaps we should take a closer look at this assumption. Is it really true?

Of course, the reason for asking this question is not that there is any doubt about whether incompetent persons should receive treatment. All authorities agree, and indeed the reasoning in our previous discussions should have made this clear. Incompetence is not a reason for withholding treatment from a patient.[3] Rather, the reason for stating it as a question and for discussing it explicitly is that it allows us to bring out some ethical features that will become important in our subsequent discussion of proxy decision-making itself.

First, the fact that someone is incompetent does not rob that individual of the rights which otherwise would belong to her or him. All persons have a right to health care. Incompetent persons are not excluded. This is clear both in case (1) and case (2) above. However, a right that is not exercised because of an inability on the part of the right-holder, ceases to be effective as a right. Now, it is one thing for someone deliberately to put her- or himself into a situation where he or she is no longer able to exercise the relevant right in question. This is true, for instance, when people deliberately and for purely personal reasons decide to remove themselves from the rest of society and live as hermits in an inaccessible region where there are no provisions for health care whatever. Under such circumstances they still have the right to health care, but all other things being equal they will be unable to exercise it. However, the reason for this is the result of a deliberate choice. This may be regrettable or even foolhardy, but it is not in itself a matter of ethical concern.

The situation is different in cases like (1) and (2) and the others mentioned subsequently. Here the inability to exercise the right is the result of circumstances beyond the individual's control. In such cases, to allow the right to become ineffective by failing to exercise it on that person's behalf would actually be to punish that person for being the victim of bad luck. Ethically, that is unacceptable.

On the other hand, to allow an incompetent person to decide would be to honour his or her decision-making authority, but in a perverse way. For example, suppose we allowed a severely mentally handicapped female person to decide that she should be sterilized so that she would no longer have to worry about becoming pregnant. By treating the person as though she were competent, and by honouring her wishes, we would be allowing her to decide without full awareness and understanding, possibly even subject to inclinations or wishes over which she has no control. In other words, we would not be making due allowances for her disability. That, however, would be like expecting a physiologically normal performance from someone who is physically handicapped. It would amount to discrimination.

The long and the short of it, therefore, is that not making due allowances, and not engaging an appropriate proxy decision-maker as and when it becomes necessary, is to punish the incompetent individual for her or his lack of competence. While the intent for this may be non-discriminatory, it would effectively be to discriminate. It would place a burden on the individual that he or she cannot really bear and it would therefore disadvantage that person unfairly.

Why should proxy decisions be made? We can now see that the answer really is that *not* to make them, *not* to provide for appropriate proxy assistance when this is necessary, is to violate the principle of equality and justice as well as the principle of autonomy itself.[4]

Possible Proxy Decision-Makers

However, the fact that someone should act as a proxy decision-maker raises two very important questions: "*Who* should make the relevant decisions?" and "*How* should they be made?"

There is no dearth of candidates for the job of proxy decision-maker. In case (1) above, the wife is identified as proxy decision-maker; in case (2), the parents are identified, as well as the Children's Aid Society. This is not surprising. Our society has traditionally identified three major players: the health care professional (usually the physician),[5] the next of kin, and the courts or their social agencies.[6] The reason for choosing the physician was usually the fact that the physician possesses technical expertise, and the assumption that health care decisions are essentially defined by technical and purely professional parameters.[7] The reason for choosing the next-of-kin was sought in the religious, emotional, or social and biological ties that were said to bind the incompetent into the web of social interaction.[8] The third option—the designation of the courts and social agencies—was usually defended in terms of the *parens patriae* role of the judiciary.[9]

None of these considerations can be dismissed out of hand. Ethically speaking, however, some are better than others. For instance, identifying physicians as the appropriate proxy decision-makers because they have technical medical expertise is acceptable in some circumstances. For example, it is acceptable when the valuational parameters under which the choices are to be made have already been clearly identified and the application of these parameters is now merely a question of considering the enabling medical aspects of the case. Certain types of living wills here come to mind.[10]

But when these valuational parameters have not been clearly identified and settled, and when the physician is chosen as proxy decision-maker simply because of technical expertise, then this approach commits the fallacy of expertise.[11]

The health care context calls for professional and technically competent decision-making. In fact, without this the whole thing would be a farce. However, the need for technical expertise and decision-making is not the same as the need for valuational decision-making. There are certain exceptions to this, for instance, in emergency contexts where the primary proxy decision-makers cannot be contacted and a decision must be made.[12] If the child in case (2) required an emergency appendectomy and the parents were not available, the physician would clearly be the appropriate proxy decision-makers, and he or she would be protected by the doctrine of emergency.[13] But even here, the values on which such a decision was made could not be those of professional. They would have to reflect the values and perspectives of the reasonable person.[14] The fact that the patient is incompetent would not alter the fundamental ethical features of the situation. It would merely complicate it.

However, the suggestion that the next-of-kin are the appropriate proxy decision-makers, all other things being equal, is correct.[15] The reason for this primacy of the next-of-kin does not, however, lie in biological considerations of consanguinity, at least not ethically speaking. It lies more in what we have called the principle of best action.

The point can be put in the following way. In our society, family dynamics and family ties tend to foster a close personal association. It is therefore legitimate to assume that the next-of-kin tend to know the incompetent person better than anyone else. Furthermore, because of the personal relationships between the members of a family unit, relationships whose existence and strength are fostered and nurtured by current social conventions, it is usually correct to think that family members have the incompetent's welfare closer at heart than does the rest of the world.

It is therefore both reasonable and appropriate to assume that the next-of-kin are in a better position than anyone else to exercise the right of decision-making on behalf of the incompetent. It is simply unrealistic to think that the physician who has a practice of 6,000 patients can know these patients as well as the members of that patient's family, or that the physician can have their welfare at heart as strongly as the family itself. Familiarity breeds more than contempt. It also breeds awareness, love, compassion and understanding.

There is another consideration that contributes to this conclusion. It is purely ethical in nature. The right that a surrogate administers by proxy does not belong to the surrogate. Assuming proxy decision-making power does not involve the *transfer* of a right. It is the *assumption of a responsibility.* Therefore, the proxy decision-maker has an obligation to exercise the right of the incompetent person in as close a manner as possible to the way in which the individual himself would have done so, had he or she been able. Next-of-kin usually know the incompetent person better than anyone else. That is why, as a matter of course, they are the logical individuals to act in a proxy decision-making capacity.

Of course, if next-of-kin are identified as appropriate proxy decision-makers and the matter is left at that, this may create more problems than it solves. Often there are several people who can legitimately claim that they are next-of-kin: parents, siblings, spouses or other relatives all fall into this category. Therefore, unless a ranking order of decision-making power is somehow specified, it may well happen that these next-of-kin will make conflicting decisions and the health care professional will have no way of deciding which decision should be followed. In the recent past, this has sometimes happened over such issues as to whether to continue life-saving and/or sustaining treatment, or whether to remove organs for donation, and the like.

In order to avoid problems like this, most jurisdictions have statutes that detail the ranking order of the various next-of kin with respect to proxy decision-makers. The order usually goes something like this:

1. the spouse, who may be of any age, provided that she/he is competent;
2. if there is no spouse, or if the spouse is not reasonably available, any of the children provided they are of age and are themselves competent;
3. if there are no children, or if they are not of age or are incompetent, either of the parents who is mentally competent, or the duly appointed guardian;
4. if there are no parents reasonable available or if they are incompetent, any of the siblings who have attained the age of majority and are competent;
5. if none of the above is reasonable available or is competent, any other next-of-kin who has attained the age of majority and is mentally competent.[16]

While this goes some ways towards solving the problem, it does not go far enough. For instance, suppose the children do not agree. Who is then to be given priority? For that matter, what if the parents don't agree? Or the siblings mentioned under (4)?

Another problem arises if the next-of-kin do not live up to the expectations that we normally expect of them in our society. This would be true, for example, if the wife in case (1) really wanted to be free of the burden of an invalid husband in hospital, wanted to pursue her own life plans, and therefore only pretended that her husband had told her what he had said. It would also be true if the parents wanted to have a certain operation for their child—for instance, sterilization—not because it was for the best interests of the child but because it would serve their own convenience. This would might well be a version of case (3) above.

In short, sometimes the assumption that the next-of-kin will operate as the best possible candidates for proxy decision-makers and safeguard the interests and rights of the incompetent persons may have questionable validity. Inheritance conflicts, personal animosities and convenience play a role even in families. Prudence and justice demand that there be some way to guard against this sort of eventuality.

Here the physician has to step in and assume an evaluative role. Not as an adjudicator. That role belongs to someone else. Instead, the role is, so to speak, that of an identifier. Of someone who detects that something has gone wrong or is about to go wrong unless certain steps are taken. This is the role of the physicians. It is rooted in the nature of the physician-patient relationship.

The incompetent person is the physician's patient. The physician therefore stands in a fiduciary relationship to the incompetent person. The fact that a third party enters the decision-making process does not mean that the elements of trust and care that are characteristic of the physician-patient relationship disappear. Nor does it mean that they are transferred from the incompetent patient to the proxy decision-maker. The physician must exercise just as much care when considering the decisions of the proxy decision-maker has he or she would when considering the choices of the patient him- or herself. In fact, the physician must examine these choices even more closely; specifically, with an eye to whether in her or his estimation they follow the rules that bind acceptable proxy decision-making. Not to be thus vigilant and careful would be to transfer the trust relationship wholly to the proxy decision-maker and abandon the patient to his or her fate.

We want to emphasize again that this does not mean that the physician should play an adjudicatory role, nor that it is actually the function of the physician to take over the proxy decision-making function itself. Instead, the physician must try to be sure that the decisions that are made by the proxy are the result of reflective and proper consideration, not the outcome of a hasty reaction. Furthermore, the physician must also try to make sure that the criteria used by the proxy in reaching a decision are not simply reflective of the proxy's own values, feelings and/or expectations, but are ethically fitting. Therefore, the physician must consider the way in which the proxy has reached the decision, and must assure her- or himself that the criteria used are appropriate.

To some degree, of course, whether the process has gone awry is a matter of subjective assessment. But not entirely. In cases where the patient once was competent but now is competent no longer, the physician will have to balance the quality of life that may be expected from the relevant treatment options against the wishes and expectations expressed by the patient when she or he was competent. The physician must then compare this with the decision reached by the proxy decision-makers. This will be the more difficult, the less contact the physician has had with the patient prior to the onset of incompetence. Of course the situation is helped greatly if the patient has executed a living will, even in cases where the physician has had no prior acquaintance with the patient.

It is also helped tremendously by consultation with other health care professionals. In particular with the nurses. In most cases, it is the nurses who provide care for the patient on a constant and on-going basis. Therefore, they are much more likely to be attuned to the nuances of the patient's expressions, the values that the patient might hold, the relationship that the patient has or has had with next-of-kin, and so on. The nurse and other health care professionals who have this sort of relationship with the patient should be drawn into the physician's evaluative process, and their suggestions and considerations should be given serious weight. In the end, of course, the physician will have to reach a decision about whether to go with the proxy decision that has been made or to challenge it. The physician/patient relationship imposes that duty on the physician and nothing can change this.

At the same time, it is important to keep in mind that the nurse also stands in a fiduciary relationship to the patient. That relationship is characterized and circumscribed by the professional functions of the nurse as nurse. Therefore it may happen that a nurse and a physician disagree in their assessment of the appropriateness of a particular proxy decision. In such a case the nurse is bound by the same duty as the physician. As a professional, she or he musty engage the appropriate judicial machinery so that the case can be properly reviewed.

As to cases where the patient has not previously expressed any wishes or inclinations and where these are not clear from the direction of the non-incompetent's life or a living will, physicians will have to base their evaluations on a reasonable person standard. In other words, physicians will have to base their considerations on what they understand to be the kinds of values and quality-of-life considerations that are generally accepted by society at that point in time.

The case of children follows similar lines. Physicians have to proceed on the assumption that the parents as proxy decision makers will supply the cognitive and judgemental want of the child. If the physician is convinced that the proxy decision maker has not proceeded in this fashion then the physician must challenge the decision by going to the courts.[17] Case (2) above illustrates this rather well. Here it seems to the physician that the parents have introduced their own personal values into the process and that these values differ fundamentally and radically from the generally accepted ones of society. Another example would be if there was a treatment modality that had a reasonable chance of success but which was ignored by the proxy-decision makers because of their own values or agenda. This would be illustrated by the following case:

> A six year old boy fell while playing in the school yard and broke his wrist. Both he and his family were members of the Church of Christ, Scientist. That meant among other things that they did not believe in using traditional medical services. Instead, they believed that prayer and faith would help any material ailment of the body. Consequently he asked to be taken to a Christian Science facility, where trained practitioners of the faith would assist him. However, the school has a policy that all injuries sustained during school supervised activities were to be referred to the emergency department of Riverside Hospital for assessment and disposition. The boy was transferred by taxi to the hospital. The parents have been notified by the school and are there to take the boy away. The emergency room physician is now faced with parents who, because of their faith, refuse to give consent to a medically appropriate treatment that has an excellent chance of successfully dealing with the fracture so that no deficit remains.

The situation here is relatively uncomplicated. The boy is not able to give or refuse either consent or assent. Normally, his parents would be the appropriate proxy decision-makers. In this case, however, child welfare authorities should be brought in so that the boy will not be disadvantaged because of the belief of his parents. The situation would become more difficult if he were, say, twelve years of age. Although he would not yet be considered completely competent in all regards, he could reasonably be said to have some degree of understanding.[18] He could therefore give assent or withhold it. However, in all of these cases the basic ethical obligation for the physician and the proxy remains the same.[19] While the assent may be considered guiding, it need not be considered determining, nor is it appropriate to treat it as the final word, especially not when the deviation from social norms is extreme.

To sum up, then. Sometimes, for one reason or another, the normal process of proxy decision making goes awry. A proxy decision-maker may have a vested interest in mis-administering the incompetent's rights; or the person may be unqualified to act properly in a proxy capacity; she or he may not want to, or may simply be wrong in her or his decision-making and yet refuse to correct the mistakes; and so on. However, the physician-patient relationship does not allow the physician to stand by idly. There must be something that the physician can do in these cases. Some recourse must available; and the most obvious recourse is the courts. Of course, it is neither necessary nor desirable that the courts be asked to become involved on every occasion. In fact, the need would arise only rarely. However, it must always be *possible* for the courts to become involved as a recourse of last resort. Anything less would be socially irresponsible.

Criteria for Proxy Decision-Making

The next question that we must address is, "What criteria should proxy decision-makers use in reaching their decision?"[20]

This issue does not present any difficulties when those who are now incompetent have given a clear indication, while they were competent, as to how such decisions should be made. Nor does it present a measurably greater problem when they have expressed opinions and beliefs that clearly indicate how the patient would make the relevant decisions if they were able to do so.[21] The "living will" that we talked about before would fulfil that role rather well. In these cases, the proxy decision-makers would have a rather clear indication as to how they should fulfil their role. The course they are to take has already been determined by the individual her- or himself.

The situation is more difficult when the now incompetent individual has given no such previous indication. There are here two possible situations: one, where the incompetent individual has never been competent, but will become competent in the fullness of time (all other things being equal), and another where the incompetent person was previously competent and now is competent no longer.

There are several ways we could proceed. For instance, we could say that the proxy decision-makers should be permitted to follow their own subjective standards. That, however, would be inappropriate. There is no guarantee that either this particular incompetent individual or anyone else would share the point of view of the proxy. To allow the proxy decision-makers to follow their own subjective standards would therefore be to treat their duty to make a proxy decision as though it were a matter of exercising their own right of choice.

Nor would it be proper to adopt a best-interest standard if "best interest" is defined solely (or essentially) in terms of the physical well-being of the patient, or in terms of what is possible in a purely medical sense. A best-interest approach of this kind might well conflict both with what the individual him- or herself had previously indicated or with what would be considered appropriate from an objective reasonable person standard.[22]

On the other hand, it strikes us that the following might be appropriate: the proxy decision-maker might assume that the incompetent person would want the decision to be made using the values that are shared by ordinary members of society who are similarly placed. Likewise in the case of the not-yet competent individual, i.e., the child. The proxy decision-maker might want to assume that the child would want the decision to be made using the standard values of society but adjusted to the situation of the child itself.

The reason for this suggestion lies in the mechanics of socialization. By and large, people within a given society or social grouping tend to share the values and expectations of the society in which they live. If they disagree, they usually give some indication to that effect. Children, on the other hand, tend to acquire the values of the society in which they grow up, simply as a matter of socialization. The principle of best action therefore demands that unless there are clear indications to the contrary, a prudent and conscientious proxy decision-maker should proceed on this assumption.

These last considerations provides us with another way of approaching case (2) above. Children do not always grow up sharing the values of society at large. Particularly in the Canadian setting, with its cultural multiplicity and its acceptance of the valuational variations that this entails. This means that rather than coming to share the values of society at large, it is much more likely that the children will come to share the values of their family setting and of the immediate socio-ethnic groping in which they grow up.

This poses a problem. If the purpose of having proxy decision-makers is to make sure that the rights of the incompetent are exercised as closely as possible to the way in which the incompetent would have chosen had she or he been able, then the criteria that should be used in these cases are the criteria of the parents (or of the ethno-cultural sub-group) not of the remainder of society.

It is important to remember that case (2) is only an illustration of a much more generic problem. The same problem arises with other groups, such as members of the Church of Christ (Scientist), native peoples and so on. In all of these cases, the fundamental question really is, whether an accident of birth should redound to a disadvantage to the child.

And in all of these cases the answer must be no. There are two reasons. *First*, the fact that people are likely to acquire the values of the social setting in which they grow up does not mean that they invariably will do so. These are merely statistical data. However, the individual person is not a statistic, especially when it comes to making personal decisions. What is true of a group of people cannot automatically be applied to this particular person. This person might be different. Especially since the statistics do not support the belief that children who are born into a particular social setting will invariably and without exception come to share in the beliefs and values of the group which defines that setting. There is no way of knowing, therefore, whether this particular child would in fact grow up to share the values of its immediate social setting and accordingly reject the relevant treatment. Since we have no certainty on that score, we would be taking a calculated risk by assuming that the child will come to share these values. What is more, we would be taking a risk that was based on a logical error. We would be assuming that what is true of a group as a group is also true of a member of the group. That is called the fallacy of division.

Second, the principle of autonomy and respect for persons says that everyone has the right of self-determination, subject only to the equal and competing rights of others. That right of self-determination includes the right to develop one's own values. An incompetent child, as in case (2), has not yet had that opportunity. It can only develop these values as it grows older. In order to grow older, it has to be alive. Therefore, its right to self-determination, as guaranteed by the principle of autonomy and respect for persons, entails that it should be given that opportunity. Which in turn means that it must have access to the sort of treatment that the values of the parents would deny it.

However, this does not mean that every and all life-saving and/or sustaining treatment modalities are therefore obligatory. The very same reasoning that argues in favour of providing the child with the relevant treatment even against the wishes of the parents also places a limit on the nature of this treatment and on the extent to which it can be employed. There must be a reasonable chance of success for the treatment in question.

Furthermore, degree of reasonableness may not be defined by the health care professions or by the parents. These are interested parties who have a position to defend. The degree of reasonableness must be a function of what members of society would normally agree to.

Also, we cannot automatically assume that the values normal members of society would hold under ordinary circumstances are necessarily the values on which they would base their decisions in life-and-death situations. Data are emerging that suggest the values that people actually hold when faced with life-and-death decisions involving life-saving and/or sustaining treatment, differ significantly from what both health care professionals and the general public believe.[23] This is an important issue that has to be explored and developed further. Otherwise the role of values in proxy decision-making for incompetents really lacks sufficient basis.

The Permanently Incompetent Patient

The difficulties that proxy decision-making faces in the case of children and of those who have become incompetent after previously having been competent are magnified in cases where we are dealing with permanently radically and congenitally incompetent persons.

The difficulties in such cases are magnified because the criteria that would otherwise be appropriate in normal proxy decision-making contexts from the perspective of quality-of-life may well be inappropriate for them. The subjective quality of the life of the persons for whom the decisions have to be made may differ so fundamentally from that of the normal member of society that neither the objective reasonable person standard, nor that standard as adjusted to the level of a child, nor finally the patient's own subjective expression (insofar as such an expression is available at all) can be used as a guide.

The objective reasonable person standard assumes a subjective life-experience that simply does not exist in these cases. Therefore, to use that standard as a guide would be to use something that by its very nature would be inappropriate. The same thing is true of the standard of the reasonable person as adjusted to the level of a child. Even here we can assume a fundamental commonality of quality-perception that is absent in the case of the permanently congenitally incompetent patient.

The individual's subjective expressions do not give much of a guide either. These expressions have to be interpreted. By definition, however, any interpretation will an interpretation by people who themselves experience the world through an objective reasonable person perspective. That means that the significance of these subjective expressions may be radically misconstrued because such an interpretation may be based on a world experience that in no way parallels that of the incompetent him- or herself.

As we said, this presents a serious problem for the health care professional whose ethical duty it is to monitor proxy decision-making in such cases. What criteria for decision-making ought to be applied, and what ought the physician to look out for when trying to decide whether the proxy has acted appropriately?

An initial answer was given by the 1983 B.C. Supreme Court decision in *the Matter of Stephen Dawson*:[24] In this case the court stated that

> It is not appropriate for an external decision-maker to apply his standards of what constitutes a livable life ... The decision can only be made in the context of the disabled person viewing the worthwhileness or otherwise of his life in its own context as a disabled person—and in that context he would not compare his life with that of a person enjoying normal advantages. He would never know of a normal person's life having never experienced it.[25]

In enunciating this position Mr. Justice L. Mackenzie, who decided the case, was adopting what had become known as a substituted judgement[26] approach to proxy decision making for congenitally incompetent persons. Superficially, what this involved was clear. It asked the proxy decision-maker to place him- or herself into the place of the congenitally incompetent person and make the decision from that perspective.

However, closer examination soon showed that this approach presents physicians as well as proxy decision-makers with insuperable problems. The demand that proxy decision-makers put themselves into the position of the incompetent and judge from that perspective was logically incoherent. If the incompetent person lacks sapient cognitive awareness (or, less severely perhaps, if that person lacks any standards or criteria) then the demand that the proxy decision-makers make a decision from the perspective of the incompetent person is a demand that the proxy decision-makers decide without assuming any vestige of sapient cognitive awareness themselves (or, correlatively, without using standards or criteria). Either that, or they will have to project some criteria or some awareness into the situation. In either case, however, that would be to treat the congenitally incompetent person as though that person were not in fact radically and congenitally incompetent. That, however, would be contradictory. The notion of substituted judgement in the case of congenitally incompetent individuals, of viewing the situation from the perspective of the incompetent person "in its own context", is therefore a pure fiction.

The problem was pointed out in the literature. It found judicial recognition three years later in the case of *re Eve*.[27] This was a case involving the request by a mother to have her mentally severely handicapped and aphasic child sterilized. In the process of winding its way through the courts, it had been suggested that the appropriate way to approach the case was for the proxy decision-maker and the courts to adopt a substituted judgement approach and reach a decision on that basis. When the case reached the Supreme Court for ultimate determination Mr. Justice LaForest, stating the majority judgement, rejected the very concept of substituted judgement roundly:

> ... choice presupposes that a person has the mental competence to make it. It may be a matter of debate whether a court should have the power to make the decision if that person lacks the mental capacity to do so. But it is obviously a fiction to suggest that a decision so made is that of the mental incompetent, however much the court may try to put itself in [the incompetent's] place. What the incompetent would choose if she or he could make a choice is simply a matter of speculation.[28]

Mr. Justice LaForest went on to speak of "the sophistry embodied in the argument favouring substituted judgement" and quoted with approval from *Matter of Eberhardy*—a U.S. case, in which the court had stated:

> We conclude that the question is not choice because it is sophistry to refer to it as such, but rather the question is whether there is a method by which others, acting on behalf of the person's best interests and in the interests, such as they may be, of the state, can exercise the decision.[29]

This, of course, left the proxy decision-maker who makes a proxy decision in such cases, and the physician who has to monitor the decision-making, with the original problem. How should proxy decision making in such cases proceed? What criteria should be used?

To date, the issue remains juridically unresolved.[30] Ethically, we can however offer the following suggestion. It is based on the fact that if proxy decision-making is appropriate at all, the individual for whom such decisions must be made will still be a person. This means that no matter how different the quality of life of that individual may be, it still must be assumed to have a person-oriented nature. That in turn entails that when deciding upon treatment or non-treatment or when deciding the direction that a particular treatment ought to take the proxy decision-maker need not attempt the impossible task of trying to put her- or himself into the

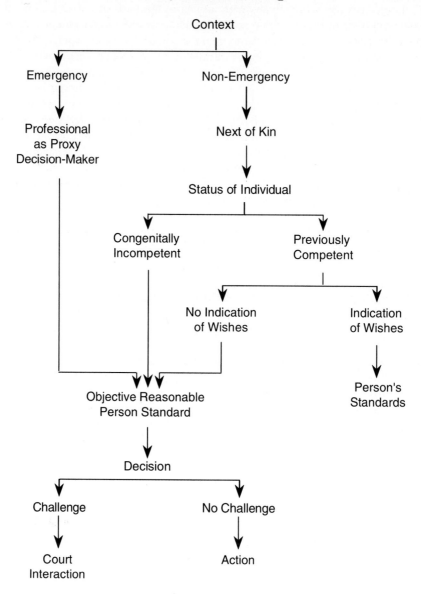

FIGURE 6-1
Proxy Decision-Making

position of the incompetent and decide on the basis of the quality of life that she or he would then (expect to) experience. Neither may the proxy decision-maker simply project what the ordinary person would do under such circumstances. That would be to ignore the very real difference between the congenitally radically incompetent and the ordinary person. Instead, the proxy decision-maker must focus on the type of decision that would be appropriate in the case of a normal individual with a similar degree of disability.

That is to say, using the state of disability as basic, the proxy decision-maker must consider the relative changes that would result in the quality of life of the incompetent individual if he or she were to be treated by the treatment options in question. Here any subjective expression of satisfaction with life, psychological affect and other evaluative parameters would have to be taken into consideration, and would have to be balanced against the likelihood of improvement, or simply retention of, sapient cognitive awareness, the possibility of meaningful social interaction, and the general cost of the treatment to the patient in purely human terms, irrespective of the individual's values(if any), and so on. These changes would have to be expressed in numerical terms. They could be called a comparative quality of life coefficient.

The proxy decision-maker must then perform a similar evaluation for an otherwise normal person with a similar medical problem and derive a similar comparative quality of life coefficient. The proxy decision-maker must then compare the two coefficients and consider the range of comparative quality of life coefficients under which the normal person would opt for treatment. If it turns out that on balance the comparative quality of life coefficient of the congenitally incompetent person under treatment would fall below the range considered acceptable for the normal person, the decision must be against treatment; in all other cases it must be in favour.

If we bring all of these factors together, we can represent the structure of ethically appropriate proxy decision-making as shown in Figure 6–1.

Conclusion

Proxy decision-making finds its roots in the principle of autonomy and respect for persons. The principle entails two considerations for those who are incompetent: they should not be harmed by the infringement on their liberty that the fact of their incompetence may imposes on them; and in those cases where the incompetents are capable of some choice, they should not be allowed to come to harm because of an unguided exercise of liberty on their part. Therefore, the fact of incompetence imposes on society an obligation to make sure that an appropriate proxy decision-making mechanism exists.

Children and congenitally incompetent persons present special problems that society has not yet resolved in a satisfactory fashion. It has recognized the special nature of the problem in the case of children by introducing the notion of *assent*. In the words of the Medical Research Council:

> A concept has developed that a child incapable of giving legally and ethically acceptable consent may give an "assent" which is significant in respecting a level of autonomy.[31]

But even this does not really solve the problem. For instance, the notion of assent comes without any quantifiable guidelines. It gives no indication how strong, or for that matter, how weak, an assent must be before it can be considered guiding. It also gives not indication of how a parental or proxy consent should be weighed against the consent of parents. It may be too simplistic simply to say that one or the other always carries the day.

Another problem about proxy decision-making in general centres on the role that values should play. It is again somewhat simplistic to say that society should make sure that socially acceptable values are followed when it comes to proxy decision making, because it ignores the fact that Canada is a multicultural society, where the differences between social sub-groups is defined precisely in terms of their respective values. How should this difference be given due weight? We could make a start by suggesting that the values of the sub-groups should be honoured just so long as doing that would not deprive the incompetent person of a right. However, that would only be a beginning.

There is also the fact that sometimes people who are incompetent are not static in their incompetence. Sometimes they change, and their values and perspectives evolve as they change in their capacities and in the degree and nature of their incompetence.

This is especially striking in the case of children. Traditionally, the problem of proxy decision-making in the case of children has been approached as the problem of how to scale adult values to the world of the child. This is appropriate, but only part of the story. The fundamental difference between children and adults is not simply that children have not yet had an opportunity to form values or to give an indication of how they would make decisions if they could. There is also the fact that the mental world of the child is evolving. That means that criteria that are appropriate for proxy decision-making at one point in time will not be appropriate for that very same child at some later date.

Any attempt to develop an appropriate methodology of proxy decision-making for children will have to take this problem into account. But at the same time, it will have to acknowledge what we said a moment ago: that the evolving values of the child will be influenced by the values of the parents and of the cultural sub-group in which the family unit of the child is embedded. We cannot ignore this developmental parameter. It is a fundamental feature of growing up in a family unit. For that matter, it is a fundamental feature of growing up in a human society. The question is, how to capture this without punishing the child for having been born to these parents.

Difficulties also arise in the case of adult patients who, so to speak, are in and out of competence: competent at one moment, incompetent at the next. Good examples are the episodic psychotic patients who require treatment either to make them competent, or to improve their life. Sometimes such patients give perfectly appropriate and valid informed consent to treatment when they are competent, but then resist that treatment when they are incompetent. What should the health care professionals do in such cases?

No universally accepted ethical protocol has evolved to handle such cases. However, our analysis of informed consent and therapeutic privilege provides us with the beginnings of an answer. It seems to us that it would be reasonable to assume that the consent given by patients when they are competent should carry decisive force. Not only is that consent in fact a competent consent, whereas the refusal by the patients when they are incompetent is by definition incompetent; to honour the request of the patients when they are incompetent in preference to the competently expressed wish would be to confirm them in that incompetence by withholding the treatment that would make them competent. In other words, that would be to withhold from them treatment that would allow them to become as autonomous as it is possible for them to be. Therefore, to proceed on the basis of the patients' wish when they are incompetent and respect their refusal would be to violate the principle of autonomy and respect for persons. In effect, it would be to punish them for their incompetent episodic occurrences.

ENDNOTES

[1] Adapted from "In the Matter of Kristie Lee F." P.C.C. (F.D.) Ontario (1072/88).

[2] Adapted from a Nova Scotia case that was resolved without court intervention.

[3] This is clearly reflected in the various declarations of medical, ethical and legal authorities that handicap is not a reason for discrimination, whether that be in medical or in legal, or for that matter in any other, matters. It is also clearly reflected in the non-discrimination clauses of the Canadian Charter of Rights and Freedoms.

[4] For a slightly different analysis from a legal perspective, see Harvey Savage and Carla McKague, *Mental Health Law in Canada* (Toronto and Vancouver: Butterworths, 1987), 121–124.

[5] Or the facility in which the individual may be. For instance, in B.C., the *British Columbia Mental Health Act* S. 8(1)(a)[amended 1981, c.21, s.44; 1985, c.12, s.2].

[6] See Edward W. Keyserlingk, *The Unborn Child's Right to Prenatal Care: A Comparative Law Perspective* (Montreal: McGill Legal Studies No.5, 1984) for a discussion of the various possible decision-makers on the paediatric context. For the non-paediatric context, see Picard, *Legal Liability of Doctors and Hospitality in Canada*, (Toronto: Carswell, 1984) Chapter 3, "Consent".

[7] See Savage and McKague (ref. note 4), 124.

[8] Savage and McKague (ref. note 4).

[9] For a good statement of these powers, see *Re Eve* (1986), 34 D.L.R. (4th),1.

[10] See Society for the Right to Die, *Handbook of Living Wills* (New York: Society for the Right to Die, 1987).

[11] See Robert Veatch, *Death, Dying over the Biological Revolution: Our Last Quest for Responsibility* (New Haven: Yale Univ. Press 1976) and Michael Bayles, *Professional Ethics* (Englewood Cliffs, N.J.: Prentice-Hall, 1985).

[12] See E. Picard, *Legal Liability of Doctors and Hospitals in Canada*, (Toronto: Carswell, 1984), Chapter 3, "Consent."

[13] See A. Linden, *Canadian Tort Law*, third edition, (Toronto: Butterworths, 1982), 63ff.

[14] This is what underlies the use of the objective reasonable person standard by the courts when they exercise their *parens patriae* powers.

[15] See Picard (ref. note 12), 60ff.

[16] This is based on the Ontario *Mental Health Act*, S.1(j). The legislation in most other provinces is similar.

[17] This derives from the fact that the physician's primary duty is towards the patient.

[18] The Ontario case of LDK is here a good example.

[19] This does not mean that the root of their obligation is the same.

[20] See Savage and McKague (ref. note 4), 119–124; see also W. Gaylin and R. Macklin, eds. *Who Speaks for the Child? The Problems of Proxy Consent* (New York and London: Plenum Press, 1982).

[21] *Bill 145, An Act Respecting the Public Curator and Amending the Civil Code and Other Legislation Provisions,* which took effect January 1, 1990, in Nova Scotia, allows individuals 18 years of age and over to mandate, by way of notarial deed or written document properly witnessed, someone to act on her or his behalf in the event of incapacity. Once the court has verified and approved the mandate subsequent to the incapacitation of the mandator, decision-making for that person becomes the legal responsibility of the individual indicated. See also the case of *Malette v. Shulman.*

[22] That is, unless "best-interest" is defined in terms of a duty to exercise the incompetent's right in a deontological fashion.

[23] See M.L. Slevin, Linda Stubbs, H.J. Plant, Peter Wilson, W.M. Gregory, P.J. Armes, S.M. Downer, "Attitudes to Chemotherapy: Comparing Views of Patients with Cancer with Those of Doctors, Nurses, and the General Public," *British Medical Journal* 300 (June 2, 1990), 1458–1460.

[24] *In the Matter of Stephen Dawson*, (1983) 3 W.W.R. 618 (B.C.S.C.) reversing (1983) 3 W.W.R. 597 (B.C. Prov. Ct.).

[25] As note 24.

[26] The concept of substituted judgement was introduced in the U.S. case of *Superintendent of Belchertown State School vs. Saikewicz*, 370 N.E. (2d) C 417 (Mass. S.C. 1977).

[27] *Re Eve*, [1986] 2 S.R.C. 388 (S.C.C.). The references that follow are to the original Supreme Court judgment pagination.

[28] *Re Eve*, page 64.

[29] *Re Eve*, page 65.

[30] For an interesting discussion of some of the variables involved from a judicial perspective, see Savage and McKague (ref. note 4), 121–122. See also Kluge, E-H.W., "After Eve: Whither Proxy Decision-Making?" *Canadian Medical Association Journal*, (1987) 137: 715-720.

[31] Medical Research Council of Canada, *Guidelines on Research Involving Human Subjects* (Ottawa: Minister of Supply and Services, 1987), 29.

SUGGESTED READINGS

- Brown, Barry F. "Proxy Consent for Research on Incompetent Elderly," in James E. Thornton and Earl R. Winkler, eds., *Ethics and Aging: The Right to Live, the Right to Die*. Vancouver: The University of British Columbia Press, 1988, 183–193.

  This is one of the few discussions that deals with the elderly incompetent patient. In light of the growing number of elderly in Canada in particular and the developed world in general, this discussion is of particular interest.

- Dickens, Bernard. "The Role of the Family in Surrogate Medical Consent," *Health and Law in Canada* 1: 3 (1980), 49–52.

  A somewhat dated but very good discussion of the legal status of next-of-kin in proxy contexts. It is complemented by the discussion of Savage and McKague.

- Medical Research Council of Canada. *Guidelines on Research Involving Human Subjects*. Ottawa: Minister of Supply and Services, 1987, 27–35.

  These represent the guidelines that medical experimenters must follow if they are to receive grants from the federal government. These guidelines are the basis of reviews of the ethical acceptability of medical experimentation on human subjects in Canada funded by the MRC. Most other institutions tend to consider these guidelines as basic.

- *Re Eve* (1987), 31 D.L.R. (4th) 1 (S.C.C.) 2 S.C.R. 388 (S.C.C.)

  The classic Canadian case dealing with proxy decision-making. It rejects the notion of substituted judgement. The case centres in the proposed sterilization of a mentally severely handicapped person, but its reasoning is transferable to other cases.

- Savage, H. and Carla McKague. "Competency and Proxy Decision-Making," from H.Savage and Carla McKague, *Mental Health Law in Canada*. Toronto and Vancouver: Butterworths, 1987, 114–124.

  The book deals with the general subject of the law as it applies to mental disorders in Canada. This section, from Chapter 4, deals with the notion of competence, ranking of appropriate proxy decision makers and the criteria that they should follow in reaching their decisions.

7
Experimenting with Human Subjects

Experimentation with human subjects, or research with human subjects, as it is also called, is increasingly moving into the forefront of public concern. This chapter familiarizes the reader with some of the more important aspects of the subject and indicates some of the considerations relevant in this connection. Its aim is therefore quite limited. It is not intended to cover all of the issues that arise in this context. The topic is far too specialized to be dealt with in a single chapter.

Some questions that might usefully be kept in mind while reading this chapter include:

1. What is a medical experiment? How does it differ from an ordinary health care procedure?
2. Is there a difference between therapeutic and non-therapeutic experimentation? If so, how could that difference be characterized?
3. What are some of the conditions that an ethically acceptable medical experiment would have to meet?
4. Is it acceptable to pay those who participate in medical experimentation?
5. What is the role of informed consent in medical experimentation?
6. What role, if any, should children and other incompetent persons play in medical experiments?

Introduction

Ever since the world became aware of the atrocities committed by German and Japanese physicians on captive populations before and during World War II, there has been general social concern about experimenting on human subjects.[1] This concern led to the formulation of the so-called Nuremberg Code in 1948, and to subsequent refinements and restatements of it by the World Medical Association.

At the centre of the issue stand several questions which cannot really be disentangled. One is the issue of informed consent. Who should give consent to participation in experimentation? Is such consent necessary? Always? What criteria should be used? These and similar topics have been hotly debated, and it is safe to say that there is really no universal agreement on how they should be answered. We have already dealt with informed consent in some of its aspects; therefore, we shall build on that discussion and suggest several lines of consideration.

Another issue is the need for experimentation itself. Do we have to experiment at all? Again there are opinions on both sides of the issue. And even when there is agreement on the need for human experimentation, there may still be disagreement over who should be involved, under what circumstances and to what extent.

Then there are issues like that of payment. Should those who volunteer to participate in medical experiments be paid at all? How much? Would this constitute undue enticement? What about compromised and "captive" population groups like institutionalized persons, children, foetuses and so on?

The distinction between therapeutic and non-therapeutic experimentation also demands some consideration. So does the question of what to do when it becomes clear that a new approach or intervention is superior to the standard treatment, but the strict scientific standards that have to be met before that approach will be approved by the authorities have not as yet been met. Then there is the whole complex of issues that surrounds the practice of randomization in clinical trials itself; or the question whether to follow scientific randomized, double-blind and controlled trial-procedures for drugs, treatments or procedures when these new treatments seem to be the only ones that have any chance of working.

We cannot touch on, let alone deal adequately with all of these subjects. What we will try to do is discuss briefly some of the major issue that we have mentioned and relate them to the other topics that we have already considered.

Experimentation and Consent

Let us begin with the issue of informed consent. As we saw in our earlier discussions, all other things being equal, informed, voluntary, and competent consent, directly or given by proxy, is an absolute ethical necessity in the delivery of health care.[2] To paraphrase a celebrated case, "if it can be had, it must be had." Informed consent is possibly of even greater importance in medical research and experimentation.

It was not always this way. One of the best-known examples of where appropriate standards of informed consent were not met involved the discovery of the vaccination against smallpox. Edward Jenner tried out his discovery on an eight year old boy without consultation with the boy and without proper informed consent from his parents. Louis Pasteur's experiments involving human beings would also be criticized extremely harshly by contemporary ethics review boards for their absence of informed consent, and there are many similar examples. In general, it is safe to say that until fairly recently:

> Individual ignorance, poverty and powerlessness would allow the researcher licence limited only by the researcher's power, conscience and religious beliefs of the times.[3]

In Canada, the issue of informed consent as such had already been broached in the celebrated case of *Mulloy vs. HopSang*. It affirmed the right of the patient to accept or refuse any treatment even if life hung in the balance. However, the situation for informed consent in experimentation did not become clear in a judicial sense until the case of *Halushka vs. The University of Saskatchewan*.[4] In this case, a university student had volunteered to participate in a non-therapeutic experiment involving a new anaesthetic. He had not been told that the drug to be used was new, that a tube would be advanced through a vein and into his heart, and that a certain amount of serious risk attended the procedure. The risk materialized, and Mr. Halushka was left half-paralysed. He sued the University and won. The case is famous for the judgement that focused on informed consent in experimental contexts:

> There can be no exceptions to the ordinary requirements of disclosure in the case of research as there may well be in ordinary medical practice. The researcher does not have to balance the probable effect of lack of treatment against the risk involved in the treatment itself ... The subject of medical experimentation is entitled to a full and frank disclosure of all the facts, probabilities and opinions which a reasonable man might be expected to consider before giving his consent.[5]

With this, Canada firmly recognized the legal duty to proceed only by means of informed consent in the experimental setting.

The Nature of Experimentation

However, informed consent is required not only for the sake of the law. Ethically, it is also absolutely essential. The reason lies in the nature of medical experimentation itself. Experimentation has been variously defined: in terms of the newness of the procedures employed,[6] the unproven nature of the methodology or therapy itself,[7] the absence of precise understanding of the regimen under the circumstances,[8] and so on.

Each of these definitions, taken by itself, captures a part of what is unique about experimentation. However, none of them on their own captures the whole. For instance, both the definition in terms of newness as well as the definition in terms of lack of precise understanding would not capture those procedures that are not new as such but used in a new setting, or treatments that are quite well proven in terms of efficacy, but where the technique needs refining. The definition in terms of the unproven nature of the methodology comes close, but even it does not quite fit. After all, the methodology is not exactly unproven.

However, it seems to us that if we combine the central ideas of these definitions, we can get a fairly good idea that what is so different about an experimental procedure, and what sets it apart from all others insofar as health care delivery is concerned, is the lack of scientific understanding and clarity. That is to say, to our mind, what distinguishes research and experimentation from all other forms of medical treatment and health care is the element of *uncertainty* that surrounds the nature of the activity itself and the intent to remove that uncertainty.[9]

To be sure, an element of uncertainty is present in every medical procedure. Every case is different, and our knowledge of patients themselves as well as of the causal laws of nature is never complete. However, when this element of uncertainty exceeds the usual norms of established practice, the situation becomes one of research and experimentation.

This uncertainty may be conceptual, technical, or systematic. In other words, it may manifest itself as a lack of understanding of the nature of the functioning of the treatment modalities on the subject to be treated, either in general or particular—e.g., in the nature and functioning of various chemotherapeutic agents. Alternatively, it may lie in the uncertainty of control over the functional variables that determine the outcome of a given procedure—e.g., in the use of brain lesions to control psychotic episodes. It may also involve a combination of these—e.g., in the use of drugs like AZT to retard the progress of AIDS.

When a physician intends to experiment, this intent may not ethically be withheld from the patient or the proxy. The reason for this is not that the absence of disclosure would necessarily deceive the patient or the proxy about the *material nature* of the procedure. The procedure may have been explained quite clearly. Instead, the reason would be that it would involve deception about how that procedure, treatment or undertaking is situated with respect to other approaches, and about the fact that the procedure is not in fact a validated one. It would also involve deception about the intentions of the physician: namely, that instead of using a validated procedure, the physician intends to use a non-validated one. Such information allows the patient (or proxy) to see the regimen in its true light. To withhold this sort of information, therefore, is to neglect to give the patient (or proxy) a piece of information that is essential if there is to be informed consent.

That is to say, there is a general and unspoken assumption that any health care procedure is conducted as a fulfilment of the patient's right to health care. It is normally assumed that a patient may not be used to develop or help to refine what may be uncertain procedures or parameters without the patient's consent. Furthermore, it is normally assumed that the medical procedures initiated will be of a standard and accepted nature. It follows that unless the patient is told otherwise, the treatment or procedures he or she consents to lie within the parameters of established health care practice. When that assumption is mistaken, the patient has the right to be informed of this. The physician has to inform the patient, unasked, if that presumption is not true. Otherwise the patient cannot give an informed consent.

With due alteration of detail, similar remarks apply to what are sometimes called innovative procedures.[10] These are procedures or modalities that are already known from another area but which are adapted to a new context without there being as much certainty as there is in their standard use. An example of this sort of thing would be the use of standard transplantation techniques to perform a new type of transplant surgery, or the use of an established pharmaceutical for a new ailment.[11]

The fact that these procedures have an established track-record in other contexts removes some uncertainty. In fact, under certain circumstances the uncertainty that surrounds the use of the technique or modality in the new context may be minimal. However, the fact remains that uncertainty is known to be present. In fact, the degree of uncertainty is greater than the degree of uncertainty that would normally attend a medical procedure. This is a crucial aspect of the treatment regimen under the circumstances. The health care professional is aware of it. The patient has a right to be aware of it as well.

Why Experiment?

All of what we have said so far has been based on the assumption that experimentation in the medical context is ethically appropriate. We should perhaps confront that assumption before we go any further. Why should physicians experiment in a scientific way at all? Why can they not simply continue with traditional and proven procedures and treatments, and simply expand on these as the occasion warrants and as they see fit?

If medicine as a profession has an obligation to provide medical services to society, then it must do so in the best way it knows how. That means it must test time-honoured regimens and procedures to ensure that they are effective and appropriate and that they are the best that can be offered. At the same time, it must determine that there are no other means that might provide a better treatment. The only way in which this can be done is by scientifically controlled experimentation that determines base lines and carefully plots deviations from these under carefully controlled conditions.

A great deal of research has been devoted to determining the best way this can be done. The same approach is not appropriate for all types of situations. For instance, in the case of competing traditional remedies, a statistical retrospective study may be more appropriate than a controlled double-blind placebo study; whereas a controlled double-blind placebo study (with or without cross-over) may be just the thing to determine the appropriateness and efficacy of a new drug for AIDS. But whatever method is appropriate, the fact remains that *experimentation itself* is appropriate. Otherwise, unless the parameters of a particular treatment modality are appropriately determined, treatment itself becomes experimentation—but in an uncontrolled fashion.

This does not mean that experimentation is appropriate in all situations. For instance, when the drug, treatment or procedure is well-known and has already proven itself as effective and appropriate for a particular condition, then clearly it would be ethically inappropriate to embark on a trial to test it. That might well deprive patients who are candidates for the drug or treatment of something they should have if they are to be treated in the best way possible. The principle of best action would be violated and the physicians would fail to fulfil their obligation to the patients. The potential benefit must always outweigh the potential risks.

Another example where trials would be inappropriate would be where the drug or treatment to be tested is no better than what is already available, has greater potential side-effects, or possibly is more expensive. Likewise, experimentation or more correctly perhaps, the continuation of an experiment, is inappropriate when it has become apparent during the course of the experiment itself that the modality under investigation is more effective or otherwise preferable to the modality against which it is being measured as a control.

The Medical Research Council of Canada has attempted to clarify the issue with a set of guidelines, and we shall take a look at them in a moment. The point is that the need for medical experimentation has to be gauged very carefully and with full awareness of the compromised state in which the patient enters the medical setting. For all that, however, the need is there.

Experimentation versus Research

This may be an appropriate point at which to indicate why we have remained with the term "experimentation" instead of using "research," as has been suggested by the Medical Research Council. The answer is very simple. "Research" connotes scientific activity, but in a rather aloof and disengaged sense. Collating records is just as much research as is investigating drugs with animal models or developing a new leg brace, and so on. The term "research" therefore does not highlight the fact that a great deal of medical experimentation consists of actions and procedures that involve patients directly and on a very personal level. These may be invasive or non-invasive, physical or mental, and so on. But whatever their nature, when they involve patients they are not aloof enterprises but involve the patients very directly, very acutely and with all the immediacy that a medical treatment can carry with it.

Furthermore, the term "experimentation" carries its own burden of associations. They are historical, and their emotional impact runs deep. For that reason the term may predispose us against experimentation simply because of these associations. The Medical Research Council of Canada characterized experimentation as "a deliberate and careful step into the unknown," and stated that it "generally involves uncertainty and ... risk."[12] We agree; and we think that it is only appropriate that the special ethical considerations that are associated with this should be retained in a way that makes it immediately evident to both the physician and the patient. To our mind, there is no better way of doing that than to use this historically and emotionally loaded term. It invites careful attention to the heightened element of informed consent that is necessary in the experimental/research setting.[13]

Therapeutic and Non-Therapeutic Experimentation

Another distinction that is fairly traditional is that between therapeutic and non-therapeutic experimentation. In a way, the distinction between the two is intuitively obvious. Therapeutic experimentation takes place when the primary aim of the protocol is to benefit the patient. An example of this would be the implantation of an artificial heart into someone suffering from complete cardiac failure where there is no suitable heart available for transplantation and when in any case the individual is not a good candidate for transplantation in the first place. Therefore, it follows from this understanding that therapeutic experimentation does not rule out the possibility of gathering data, of refining techniques, and so on. It is the intent that is defining.

Non-therapeutic experimentation could then be defined as experimentation where the

> primary concern is the advancement of knowledge, and there is a minimal, if any, immediate benefit to the subjects themselves.[14]

However, the fact that the distinction between the advancement of knowledge and benefit to the patient seems intuitively clear may not be very helpful in actual practice. It is difficult to gauge what the intent of someone is except by asking them. While we may want to assume that the answers we get will be essentially truthful, the fact of the matter is that even in scientific and medical circles this is not always the case. Professional careers sometimes hinge on the ability to conduct experiments and to show what are called "interesting" results. This pressure for results invites a blurring of the distinction between therapy and experiment. Particularly in institutionalized settings like intensive care units in teaching hospitals; and especially when the patients appear to be moribund anyway. Anecdotal reports suggest that at least sometimes this is the case.

Furthermore, it is possible in some cases to hide an intent to gather data behind a pretext of treatment if the protocol that would supply these data is appropriate for the kind of condition in question. This is particularly the case when the regimen might be considered appropriate for a particular condition but the researcher knows (or is convinced) that the likelihood of any therapeutic effect on this particular patient is essentially non-existent.

We would therefore suggest that the distinction between therapeutic and non-therapeutic experimentation should be defined in as objective terms as possible. There should be an objective correlation between an expectation of therapeutic effect and the experimentation in the first place. Therefore, if a particular protocol is appropriate for a particular condition; if, furthermore, it has as its intended purpose a therapeutic effect on the patient; and if, finally, that purpose is substantiated by acceptable data detailing an expected level or type of therapeutic effect, then the experiment may be considered therapeutic. Otherwise it should be considered non-therapeutic.

Guidelines for Disclosure

We began with the issue of informed consent in experimentation without going into detail as to what that informed consent should look like. The short answer is, that it should involve at least those factors that are necessary for informed consent in the non-experimental setting. In addition, it should involve patient knowledge and understanding of all those features of the situation that turn it into an experiment and that make it distinctive.

We have already outlined a theory of informed consent in previous chapters. Therefore the requirements that we mentioned then must also be met here—except in a more stringent fashion. Reality, however, is sometimes different from theory. The pressures that are operative in a particular situation may combine to weaken the thrust for informed consent that might otherwise exist. To escape this, it is very useful to have a fixed set of guidelines that constitute procedural requirements that must be met before any experimentation can take place.

The theoretical niceties of rigorous disclosure are difficult to attain in actual life. It is not always easy for the health care professional to work out precisely what should be revealed, in what detail, to whom and with what precision. The problems that arise here are magnified in the experimental context, which carries with it its own and special burden of anxiety for the patient.[15] The difficulties are compounded by the special problems that are raised by the fact of experimentation itself: by the deliberate, albeit well-meaning, venturing into what essentially is new territory.

In the past, it was usually assumed that any procedure undertaken by a health care professional was ethical as a matter of course. It was taken as a given that personal integrity, professional ethical considerations and the sheer nature of the profession would guarantee that this would be the case even in experimental contexts. However, as we have had occasion to observe, experience has shown that this is not necessarily true; nor is that experience confined to war contexts, such as Nazi Germany or Japanese Manchuria. Peace time contexts, whether in the U.S.[16] or other countries[17] have brought home the fact that physicians are no more ethical than anyone else. Canadian co-operation with the CIA in research involving psychotropic drugs,[18] or the U.S. example of the Tuskeegee Study[19] illustrate this only too well.

These remarks are not intended to reflect on physicians as researchers, although to be sure at times research careers certainly are at stake. Genuine humanitarian considerations usually play a fundamental role. However, the fact remains that experimentation is an ethically very sensitive and very difficult area in which the desire to improve the welfare of humanity may well outstrip the ethical concern for the individual patient. The individual physician may resent the intrusion of outside controls into this context. In fact, some have even gone on record as saying that the imposition of rules and regulations in general is "more likely to do harm than good," and that it will certainly not "curb the unscrupulous."[20] However, the fact remains that experimental situations easily lend themselves to a utilitarian approach for the delivery of health care at the level of the individual patient. This approach should be avoided if at all possible.

For this reason, society has embarked on a double venture. It has begun to develop guidelines for ethical experimentation, and it has begun to set up ethics review boards or ethics review committees whose function is to vet proposed projects as to their acceptability. The purpose of these is not to prevent experimentation and research. It is to try and make sure that if experiments are done and research is performed, it is done in an ethically acceptable fashion. Likewise, most medical and scientific journals have adopted policies that require explicit evidence that the experimental protocol is itself scientifically warranted, and that informed consent has been obtained from the research subjects, whether patient or otherwise.[21]

Canada has no national guidelines for setting up ethics review boards for institutions involved in experimentation. However, it does have some guidelines that deal with the protocols that experiments on human subjects should follow. Following the example of the Belmont Report in the United States,[22] the Medical Research Council of Canada proposed such guidelines, and it has up-dated them on a regular basis. Although they are binding only on projects funded through the Research Council, they are generally considered to be model requirements for medical research protocols in general. These guidelines require that a protocol for an experiment or a study should state:[23]

1. the reason for the study;

2. the research techniques that will be involved, such as randomization of treatment;

3. the reason why the prospective subject(s) is (are) being invited to take part in the study;

4. the reasonably anticipated benefits and consequences of the study itself;

5. the reasonably anticipated benefits and consequences of the study for the prospective subject(s); if none, these should be stated;

6. the foreseeable risks, including discomforts and inconveniences, to the prospective subject(s);

7. the foreseeable risks of the study itself;

8. complete details regarding confidentiality of prospective subjects;

9. the anticipated time commitments of the subject(s);

10. the intent to conduct a follow-up study in the future and retention of data (if applicable);

11. the rules for stopping the study and withdrawing the subject.

We would assume that the Council would want to see all of this information disclosed in a way and at a level that the individual participant can and does understand.

If the person is also a patient currently undergoing treatment, and if the progress of that treatment may be affected by participation in the experiment, the following should also be disclosed:[24]

1. the prognosis without any intervention;
2. the alternative interventions that are available, if any;
3. the experimental aspects of the intervention that is proposed;
4. the interventions that will be unavailable to the patient who participates in the research/study/experiment as a result of that participation;
5. an estimate of the likely success and failure of all the interventions that may be offered and withheld;
6. an estimate of the risks and possible side-effects of the interventions offered; and
7. a clear distinction between the procedures in the research protocol and those that would be a part of the usual patient care.

Of course these guidelines are not universally applicable. There are situations where they cannot strictly be followed because of the very nature of the experiment or research itself. For instance, it may happen the that an experiment by its very nature may require outright deception.[25] Some psychiatric contexts are clearly implicated in this connection. However, the Medical Research Council again has some very good suggestions on that score. It maintains that deception in research should be used only when:[26]

1. no other method will accomplish the same research objective;
2. It should not be used if there is a possibility of risk to the subject;
3. Nothing should be withheld which, if divulged, would/might cause the subject not to participate.
4. There should be an anticipated significant scientific advance expected from the project to justify even minimal deception.
5. Deception itself is permissible only when the subject may be "debriefed" without harm after the project is finished.
6. If the subject declines to participate after debriefing, the relevant data should be destroyed or surrendered to the subject.

Discussion

Useful as these guidelines are, they could be improved. In fact, we could point to two quite distinct shortcomings. One is pragmatic, the other ethical. Pragmatically, the guidelines dealing with deception assume that debriefing without harm is possible. That is not always the case.

More importantly still, it assumes that it is always possible to tell beforehand whether a subject can be debriefed without harm after the project is finished. This assumption is sometimes unwarranted. For instance, it may happen that in the course of an experiment facets of the participant's personality are revealed that the individual himself would not have wanted revealed had he or she been aware of them. The affront to a person's dignity occasioned by this may be irreparable. It may also happen that a participant develops psychological traits or tendencies which, but for the experiment itself, would never have developed or come to light and which the participant would not have wanted to know about had he or she known that they might come to light. There is no guarantee that "debriefing" would either solve the problem of affronted dignity or of diminished self-esteem.

In other words, in *any* medical procedure there is the danger that the procedure itself may introduce a new element or activate a latent condition which, but for the procedure, would not have arisen. This is true for experimental no less than non-experimental context. It also holds true for psychological aspects of the individual as well as for physiological ones. In the case of physiological experiments, the possibility of this sort of iatrogenic damage may usually be guarded against by proper controls on the parameters of the experiment, either in terms of cut-off points, quality-control or simply in terms of proper design. However, there is no such possibility in the case of psychological experiments that affect the very psyche of the individual. The very substance of such an experiment is psychological manipulation. Here debriefing may well be nothing more than an application of a band-aid to the wound that may have been artificially inflicted. Furthermore, not even condition (2), which says that deception should not be used if there is a possibility of risk to the subject, would be of much help. It assumes that it is possible to gauge accurately the possibility of risk itself. This is notoriously untrue in psychiatry and psychology.

Of course it is possible to read clause (5) of the guidelines differently. It could be read as saying that the debriefing itself must not produce harm. However, that would also be unsatisfactory. It would again assume something that neither psychiatry nor psychology comes even close to guaranteeing: namely, being able to tell beforehand whether a person will be harmed psychologically upon being told that he or she had been deceived and lied to.

The ethical shortcoming of the Council's approach is more global. Again it comes out in the Council's perspective on deception. Simply put, the Council seems to assume that if the only way it is possible to get certain information, then it is permissible get that information so long as the six clauses referred to above are met. In other words, what the MRC is saying is that under certain circumstances it is permissible to deceive people: not for their own good, but for the good of society.[27] This perspective is not negated by the Council's general concern with informed consent and its contention that before any experiment can be undertaken, there should be a careful examination of the risk-benefit ratio, and that careful consideration should be given to the question whether the probable benefits justify the risk. The fact remains that it is an inherently goal-oriented perspective according to which the end, sometimes, justifies the means. Of course, not any and all means, only those that meet the conditions set out; and not for all ends, only those that are considered worthy on balance. These conditions may rule out almost all deception. However, they do leave the door open to some. And this is the problem.

Both utilitarians and deontologists would agree that we have an ethical mandate to get information on one condition: that we can do so without acting unethically. For deontologists this means that if certain data become available only if we deceive, then these data must remain ethically beyond our grasp. This must not be misunderstood. It does not entail that deontologists would rule out all double blind experimental techniques. Such techniques can be made acceptable simply by explaining their nature to the experimental subject and then asking the subject to give consent to the experiment as explained. That would not interfere with the efficacy of the protocol, but it would safeguard the ethics. What deontologists would reject are experimental protocols in which truthfulness is abandoned, even if only rarely, but nevertheless as a matter of absolute principle.

Freedom and Autonomy

We have dealt with the "informed" in the requirement of informed consent. We have not yet touched on the parameter of consent itself. Essentially, what is involved here is the issue of autonomy.

In our previous discussion of informed consent we already indicated that the institutionalized context of modern health care delivery contains a heavy element of intimidation for the health care recipient. Patients are cut off from their usual lines of emotional support when the enter an institution. Even when interfacing with a health care professional in their own homes, the very fact that the professional operates as a professional reinforces the viewpoint not of the professional as person but of the professional as the embodiment of an institution. The normal patient feels overmatched in such a context.

These considerations apply with special force in the experimental context. The experimenter engages the participant on the experimenter's own turf. Any supposedly free informed and competent consent to experimental procedures must be evaluated from that perspective. The question, therefore, that arises is whether such agreement can truly said to be free. Especially if the subject of the procedure is dependent on the experimenter for treatment.

Of course there are cases where the answer has to be no. However, if careful attention is paid to the process of informed consent that we have indicated, and if the requirements that we have sketched are met, then in most cases the answer is yes. If, in addition to meeting the requirements that we have mentioned, the physician makes it clear that:

1. participation is strictly voluntary;
2. the right to appropriate medical care is in no way affected by whether the patient agrees to participate in the experiment or not, and the patient understands this;
3. the patient is aware that he or she may withdraw at any time unless withdrawal will have a negative effect on the quality of care that he or she can receive subsequent to the withdrawal as a result of having participated in the experiment in the first place;
4. what the implications of participation in the experiment are with respect to the availability of other forms of treatment; and so on.

The physician also has to ensure that such freedom-limiting parameters as physical coercion, attitudinal coercion and enticement are not present. As a final condition, we would add that the physician should disclose to the patient what benefit, if any, the physician as experimenter and as professional will gain from the experiment. It seems to us that it is unacceptable to hide this sort of datum from the patient. The patient is risking her or his health.

Coercion

Coercion of course is not an issue in the medical setting in general. As a rule, it is simply unacceptable. However, that rule may be breached under certain circumstances in the case of incompetent patients. Here it may happen that a proxy decision-maker agrees to a course of action that the incompetent rejects. This may especially occur with recalcitrant children or with difficult but cognitively incompetent adults; for instance, those who suffer from Alzheimer's disease. The situation becomes especially difficult if pain or discomfort is involved. Parents or appropriate others sometimes want their children to participate in therapeutic experiments that involve such things because they feel that this represents the best chance for the child. The surrogate decision-makers for the cognitively impaired adult may want that person to participate because there is no non-experimental protocol that allows even the possibility of alleviation or cure.[28]

For the experimental setting, the rule of thumb generally agreed upon seems to be that physicians should decline to enrol incompetent persons in non-therapeutic experimental protocols that require coercion. As for therapeutic experimental protocols, it is usually agreed that incompetents should not be involved against their will if

> the use of force would be inappropriate if the treatment were not experimental, there is another course of treatment that is available and is medically recognized as acceptable, or participation in the experimental protocol would in any way leave

the incompetent worse off than would have been the case under the normal regimen.

It goes almost without saying that the proxy or surrogate decision-maker should be given all the relevant information, options and opportunities that would normally be revealed to a patient if he or she were competent. Since the values of the incompetent subject represent an essential unknown in most of these cases, the surrogate should consent only to protocols that are scientifically better than alternative treatments available.[29]

Harm

Force or coercion, however, is only one aspect of experimentation with incompetents that has aroused interest. Another is the possibility that an experimental protocol, and in particular a non-therapeutic protocol, may produce harm for the incompetent patient. For instance, studies that attempt to identify disease markers in a particular patient group fall into this category. So do cold-water experiments that seek to determine the likelihood of survival of children and the speed with which they become subject to hypothermia.[30]

Some ethicist, like Paul Ramsay,[31] have argued that no experimentation involving any risk of harm should be allowed, and certainly none involving harm as well as requiring coercion. Others, like Richard McCormick,[32] have argued that all persons should be willing to participate in non-therapeutic experiments that represent no more than a possibility of minimal harm to them. From this McCormick and others have concluded that proxy consent is legitimate in these cases because it is merely the fulfilment of a social obligation shared by all.

A similar position has been adopted by the American College of Physicians. It has stated that "surrogates should not consent to non-therapeutic research that presents more than a minimal risk of harm or discomfort" to the incompetent persons who are in their charge. To this it has added the proviso that surrogates should not consent to procedures that they have reason to believe the subject would not have agreed to if competent.

We have some difficulty with the reasoning advanced by the American College of Physicians and Surgeons and by McCormick. In the first instance, as we have had occasion to observe, the notion of what constitutes "minimal harm" tends to be an extremely fluid and subjective one.[33] It is therefore not clear that it would provide any safeguard.

As to the reasoning advanced by McCormick, it may be true that all persons should be willing to participate in non-therapeutic medical experimentation to some degree. The fact is that everyone who receives health care is a beneficiary of centuries of medical development. This development has involved countless of patients and a great deal of social resources, both in terms of facilities, goods and services. It also draws on a broad scientific knowledge base that derives from many disciplines, none of which would have existed but for the fact of social participation and the existence of society itself. It could therefore be argued that all of this entails an indebtedness, and that it is legitimate of society to expect this indebtedness to be repaid.

However, even if that sort of argument were granted, and much more than what we have just sketched would be needed to establish the point, there is a difference between children and adults. That difference is here fundamental. Adults have a choice over whether or not they wish to avail themselves of the medical services offered by society. That is what the doctrine of informed consent is all about. Children have no such choice. Their position, and therefore what McCormick calls their indebtedness, is not of their own choosing. If someone is the recipient of a largesse for which she or he has not asked, then the fact that this person is a beneficiary in a material sense does not mean that she or he acquires an obligation in a moral sense of the term.[34] If it were otherwise, we could make others beholden to us simply by giving them a gift.

Of course, this leaves the problem that the medical knowledge that has been acquired in the context of adult patients cannot simply be transferred to children. The pharmaco-kinetic and biological functions of children are quite different from those of adults. Therefore, unless knowledge base-lines are developed in the course of non-therapeutic experiments, a very important part of medical knowledge will be missing, and a great deal of treatment of children will in fact reduce to uncontrolled experimentation.

What we have said does not touch on, let alone deal with, all the variations and possible problems that might arise in the context of medical experimentation. For example, we have not considered consider fetal experimentation,[35] experimentation on incarcerated or otherwise compromised subjects, and so on. However, we shall not pursue the matter further. The topic is so complex and so difficult that it should really be the subject of a separate discussion.[36]

Reward and Enticement[37]

Given what we have said about informed consent, the use of rewards and enticements in the non-therapeutic experimental setting here must be viewed with extreme caution. We say "here," because in the therapeutic context the very possibility of gaining an advantage from the experimental protocol itself constitutes an enticement whose subjective value is immeasurable in any real terms.

The non-therapeutic context is different. The potential participant can expect no reward like this. The variable of inducement should therefore be controlled much more carefully. That is why it has been argued that if someone participates in an experiment because of the reward that is offered, and if in the absence of such a reward the person would not consent, then the reward itself must be considered ethically suspect.

However, it has also been argued that this amounts to a limitation of freedom. All of us do things for reward that we would not do if no reward were offered. Working for a living falls normally falls into that category. Yet no-one would consider it unethical for employers to offer a salary to their workers for doing the work.

A possible way to resolve this disagreement might be found in the relationship between the reward offered and the freedom of the individual. We could say that a reward enticement becomes unethical only when it is freedom-constraining, either directly or in its effects. It is freedom-constraining only if the potential participant is in a socio-economic or other position where the welfare of the person depends (or is perceived to depend) on participating in the experiment and accepting the reward. Under such circumstances, consent would not be truly voluntary.[38] In more concrete terms, this would mean that offering a reward for participation in an experiment would not be unethical in and of itself. It would depend in the size and nature of the reward, and the context in which it is offered. The Medical Research Council states this limit as follows:

> Remuneration limited to compensation for expenses actually incurred and losses reasonably assessed, including loss of wages, is ethically acceptable, provided that it does not distort freedom of choice but facilitates collaboration by indemnifying subjects for their direct and indirect expenditures. Payments for time and inconvenience, if nominal, are similarly acceptable. Excessive remuneration, or other advantages or benefits, however, are an improper inducement to participate in a research project.[39]

We would agree. Limitations on autonomy should never exceed the minimal amount necessary under the circumstances. That means that the appropriateness of rewards for participating in any type of experimental procedure has to be gauged by considering the circumstances under which the experiment is conducted and the target population. *A priori* determination of that is impossible—and unacceptable. It would be as impossible and as unacceptable as an *a priori* determination of what workers should be paid for engaging in a dangerous profession.

Boards and the Health Care Professional

Finally, a few words about the health care professionals who are involved in medical experimentation. In a sense, they are really the primary players. While the people who participate in the experimental protocols are necessary as subjects, it is the professionals who initiate the whole thing and who determine its direction.

Health care professionals like to emphasize the fact that therapeutic experimentation has the possibility of benefiting the individuals who participate the therapeutic protocol, and that even non-therapeutic experimentation benefits someone: namely society. They rarely point out that the health care professionals themselves also benefit.

The fact of the matter is that the health care professionals themselves often stand to gain from the experimental protocols that they develop and in which they involve their patients. Most medical experimentation takes place in hospitals that are associated with universities, and most of the experimenters hold academic appointments. Careers, academic careers, depend on publications and on the development of new techniques methods, agents, devices and so on. Or on the discovery of knowledge. Experimentation, therefore, often has an undercurrent of self-interest associated with it.

This is not to say that the motivation will be entirely self-centred; but it is to say that personal interests and plans do frequently play a role. This may make the professionals whose plans are closely associated with the experiment's success unconsciously somewhat lax in their observance of the relevant ethical niceties.

It is here that the ethics review boards (or review ethics boards, as they are sometimes also called) that we mentioned above come in.[40] Ethics review boards are part of a surveillance mechanism that society has developed to ensure that human experimentation proceeds in as ethically acceptable a way as possible. Experimental protocols dealing with human subjects usually have to be presented to such boards for consideration, evaluation and approval. If, in the opinion of these boards, there is anything amiss in the protocol, or if the protocol could be improved in some fashion, the boards make recommendations to that effect. Permission to go ahead with the experiment is dependent on approval from such a board.

However, the mandate of such a board, when properly set up, goes beyond merely vetting experimental protocols in anticipation of approval. It is also to monitor the experiments that have been approved in order to see whether the conditions that have been imposed and accepted are in fact being followed. This is why approval of a protocol usually carries with it the minimal condition that at the conclusion of the experiment, a report has to be made to the board by the principal investigator(s) to see whether the conditions of the experiment have been complied with and nothing untoward has occurred. It lies within the nature of the boards that they should also be open to reports of untoward events during the life of the experiment.

Ethics review boards are variously structured. Some include a preponderance of health care professionals, others include a majority of people who come from other walks of life. In recent times, the tendency has been for such boards to lean towards a less professional composition. The reason is that health care professionals, and especially those who are also academics, tend to live and work in a sub-culture whose perspectives and values differ from those of the rest of society.

Furthermore, while these health care professionals are usually extremely well trained in their area of scientific specialization, they have very little training in ethics.[41] And given the fact that their professional views may well be out of step with the general values of society, the general feeling is that it is best to avoid problems by having lay representation on these boards, as well as by including people who are trained in the law and above all in ethics.

However, no matter how such boards are constituted, their effectiveness as monitoring agencies depends to a considerable degree on the willingness of the health care professionals who are involved in the experiments themselves to abide by the conditions of ethical medical practice in general, and by the special conditions on the experiments as and when these are imposed. We have already pointed to the Tuskeegee study in the U.S., where this was not done. Several generations of health care professionals knew that the study was unethical and there were reporting mechanisms available that would have brought the study under scrutiny. None of this happened because none of the professionals involved in the study, directly or indirectly, "blew the whistle."

The United States does not have a monopoly on unethical experimental protocols where no-one involved in the experiment or who knew of it "blew the whistle." The case of "psychic driving" and of "depatterning" experiments done by Dr. Ewen Cameron in Montreal, in the late 1950s and early 1960s provides a Canadian example. Dr Cameron was involved in developing psychiatric techniques which involved subjecting patients to rather unusual and scientifically apparently quite questionable procedures that included the use of psychotropic drugs like LSD, keeping the patients asleep for prolonged periods of time (over 86 days at a stretch) by the use of chlorpromazine and barbiturates, the use of sodium amytol combined with electroconvulsive shock treatments, and so on.

Cameron's colleagues were apparently aware that Cameron's treatments contravened usual medical practice, that they were experimental in nature, that they had dubious scientific value and that they were performed without informed consent either by the patients themselves or their next-of-kin. These colleagues also were aware that the procedures violated the traditional medical-ethical tenet: *primum non nocere!* (Above all do no harm!) and that they were therefore in contravention of what is sometimes called the principle of beneficence in one of its interpretations, or what has sometimes also been called the principle of non-maleficence.[42] It was certainly clear that they appeared to violate what we have called the principle of autonomy and respect for persons.

As one of the people who was involved with Cameron's patients put it:

> There was no shortage of contemporary critics of the work .... There were many sceptics, even in his department at McGill. Many psychiatrists in Canada and abroad considered the treatment methods extreme, overly risky and/or without proper theoretical foundation.[43]

That same person, however, went on to say:

> ... it is a valid criticism of [Dr. Cameron's] position that, as he became more and more convinced that his methods constituted valuable therapeutic innovations, his criteria for the selection of patients for these controversial treatments seemed to broaden. By the time I became personally involved with his patients (1961) it was my own view that many of the schizophrenic patients who were "depatterned" had not had adequate trials of appropriate phenothiazine medications that were then available and many of the psychoneurotic patients who received hallucinogenic drugs and psychic driving could have been helped by conventional psychotherapy. *Of course at the time I was quite junior in status and quite inexperienced in*

psychiatry; nevertheless, even in hindsight after more than twenty years of practising and teaching psychiatry *I still hold this view*.[44]

The reason we have highlighted the words in this excerpt is that to our mind, these words illustrate the danger we hinted at above. Review mechanisms, whether they consist of review boards or something else, will only work if they exist in the first place and use appropriate criteria; and in the second place, if those who are in a position to engage these mechanisms actually do so. There should always be such mechanisms, and they should always use appropriate criteria. But more than that, all physicians have a professional obligation that derives from the ethics of medical practice. This includes not only senior but also junior persons. They all have a duty to take appropriate steps when they have doubts as to the acceptability of a certain procedure or undertaking. This duty is the stronger, the more innovative or the more experimental the procedure. The prestige of a senior colleague, or even of a teacher, should not be allowed to obscure the ethical nature of the issue. Not to take these steps may be to fail the patient in an ethically unacceptable fashion. It may be to confuse what is ethically appropriate with what good manners or good etiquette would require.

Physicians and other health care professionals have an obligation to "blow the whistle" if they have reason to believe that the requirements of ethical practice are not being met. The same obligation applies to medical experiments and to "therapeutic innovations," except more so. Otherwise ethics review boards may function well in theory but work badly in practice. Apparently this was not done in the case of Dr. Cameron's work. Several people suffered an irreversible destruction of fundamental parts of their personalities. The fact that they did not die, as did many in the Tuskeegee experiment, is of little ethical consolation.[45]

Conclusion

We return to a question that we highlighted in the beginning. Should we experiment at all? One answer is in the negative. If experimentation requires the relaxation of otherwise strict ethical rules, then the price paid for the knowledge to be acquired is too great.

We acknowledge the correctness of the sentiment that speaks out of this position. However, we suggest that the spirit of this position can be maintained without falling prey to the danger that it mentions. We can avoid that danger. But also, if we do not experiment in a scientifically acceptable fashion and with suitable ethical safeguards, then every treatment itself becomes an attempt to refine parameters, and hence an experiment. Better to experiment under the controlled conditions with suitable safeguards than that.

From this perspective, therefore, the question is not whether we should experiment, or how, but what areas should be selected for experimentation. To answer this question requires that we consider the ethics of resource allocation.

ENDNOTES

[1] There is a growing group of people who are also concerned with the ethics of experimenting on animals. However, we shall leave discussion of that aside and concentrate on experimentation with human subjects instead. The ethics of experimenting with animals requires a separate discussion on its own terms.

[2] Clearly, there are exceptions. The emergency context here comes to mind. All other things being equal, the health care professional who comes upon an unconscious person in immediate need of medical assistance need not stop for informed consent. But even here, if it is reasonably possible for the health care professional to find out whether the person would agree to the type of assistance the professional intends to offer, then the professional must try and find out. And if the person has given an advance directive that rules out certain kinds of intervention, and if that advance directive is reasonably available to the professional under the circumstances, then the professional may not overrule this advance directive. *Malette vs. Shulman* provides a recent legal recognition of this fact.

[3] Medical Research Council of Canada, *Guidelines on Research Involving Human Subjects* (Ottawa: Minister of Supply and Services, 1987), 3.

[4] *Halushka vs. The University of Saskatchewan,* (1965), 53 D.L.R.(2d) 436. This is one of the few legal judgements in North-America that deals expressly with informed consent in the non-therapeutic experimental setting.

[5] *Halushka vs. The Univ. of Sask.,* 444.

[6] Compare B. Dickens, "What is a Medical Experiment? " *Canadian Medical Association Journal,* 113 (Oct. 4, 1975), 635–639.

[7] See MRC, *Ethics in Human Experimentation,* Report No. 6 (Ottawa, 1978), restated 1986. The MRC subsequently abandoned the notion of experimentation in favour of that of research. It defined research as "the generation of data about persons, through intervention or otherwise, that goes beyond that necessary for the person's immediate well-being." (*Guidelines on Research Involving Human Subjects* (Ottawa: 1987) 7.) One of the problems with this approach is that it does not pay due regard to the therapeutic/non-therapeutic distinction. The Council attempts to do so on p. 9 of the Report.

[8] *Ethics in Human Experimentation* (ref. note 7).

[9] See Medical Research Council of Canada, *Guidelines on Research Involving Human Subjects,* (Ottawa: Minister of Supply and Services, 1987), 7.

[10] We here differ from the MRC, which would appear to consider innovative procedures in a more relaxed fashion.

[11] For instance, the use of anti-rejection drugs like cyclosporin in transplantation. Some of these drugs were originally developed for another context.

[12] See ref. note 9.

[13] It is interesting to note that the Medical Research Council itself feels compelled to revert to the notion of human experimentation, rather than research, when it comes to the therapeutic-non-therapeutic distinction: "The interaction of therapy and research must be carefully considered. Although separate domains, often the two overlap in human experimentation … ." (*Guidelines on Research Involving Human Subjects.*)

[14] Report of the Consultative Group on Ethics, The Canada Council, *Ethics* (Ottawa: Minister of Supply and Services, 1977) 12.

[15] For a discussion of some of the issues, see G.J. Annas, L.H. Glantz, B.F. Katz, *Informed Consent to Human Experimentation: The Subject's Dilemma* (Cambridge, Mass.: Ballinger Publication Co., 1977). The distinction was recently reiterated by the American College of Physicians, in "Cognitively Impaired Subjects," *Annals of Internal Medicine* 111: 10 (Nov. 15, 1989), 843–848.

[16] See also H.K. Beecher, "Ethics in Clinical Research," *New England Journal of Medicine* 274 (1966), 1354–60.

[17] Implicated here is the Karelia study in Finland, experimentation with birth-control pills in France and third-world countries, and so on. For an historical account of experiments prior to World War II, see Jay Katz, "Prologue—Experiments Prior to 1939," in Jay Katz, *Experimenting With Human Beings* (New York: Russell Sage Foundation, 1972), 284–292.

[18] See *Linda MacDonald vs. Her Majesty the Queen*. This affair involved several Canadian citizens, who were subjected to brain-washing experiments by Dr. Ewen Cameron. Dr. Lowy, who later became Dean of Medicine, University of Toronto, and now who heads the ethics project at the University of Toronto and is a member of the Ethics Committee of the Canadian Medical Association "became involved with his [Cameron's] patients" in 1961 apparently as an intern (Cooper Report TAB 11, p. 10), and on that basis described his perception of the experiment at the time thus: " … his criteria for the selection of patients for these controversial treatments seemed to broaden. By the time I became personally involved with his patients (1961) it was my own view that many of the schizophrenic patients who were "depatterned" had not had adequate trials of appropriate phenothiazine medications that were then available and many of the psycho-neurotic patients who received hallucinogenic drugs and psychic driving could have been helped by conventional psychotherapy. Of course, at the time, I was very junior in status and quite inexperienced in psychiatry … "(TAB 11, p. 10)

[19] This was the longest study in the history of modern medicine. It took place in Tuskeegee County, Alabama over a period of thirty years, between 1932 and 1972. It involved following the course of untreated syphilis in order to see what would happen. Initially, at the beginning of the study, only Salvarsan had been available. As the study progressed, penicillin and other antibiotics became available. In order not to arouse the suspicion of the participants, they were given sub-therapeutic doses of these new drugs. The participants were not informed of the nature of the study, the treatments available, or anything else. The incentive was routine medical examination and free burial.

[20] H.K. Beecher, *Experimentation in Man* (Springfield, Ill.: Charles C. Thomas, 1959), 50, 52 and elsewhere.

[21] See the policies of the CMAJ, which will refuse publication of articles involving research or experimentation unless there is assurance that informed consent has been obtained from the subjects.

[22] National Commission for the Protection of Human Subjects of Biomedical and Behavioral Research, *The Belmont Report: Ethical Principles for the Protection of Human Subjects of Research* (Washington, D.C.: U.S. Government Printing Office, 1978) pub. no. 78–0012, App. 1–0013, App. 2–004.

[23] See ref. note 9.

[24] See ref. note 9, 22-23.

[25] Compare, for instance, the infamous Milgram experiment on obedience. Stanley Uligram, "Behavioral Study of Obedience," *Journal of Abnormal Psychology,* 67 (1963): 371-78. "Some Conditions of Obedience and Disobedience to Authority," *Human Relations* 18 (1965): 57-76. In this experiment, subjects were falsely informed that they would be administering electric shocks to other persons—who in fact were actors. The reason they were given for administering the shocks was learning protocol for the alleged subjects; The real reason was to test how far the people who were being deceived would go in obeying instructions to administer what they thought were powerful electric shocks. We are not of course endorsing the ethics of this experiment.

[26] See ref. note 9.

[27] See clause (5), ref. note 9.

[28] This is well illustrated by parents who consent to experimental protocols for their children. The case of the baby who had a baboon's heart experimentally implanted at Loma Linda hospital falls into this category.

[29] The Belmont Report. The recent expressions by the American College of Physicians does not depart essentially from this. It only specifies in great detail the duties of the proxy and the role that knowledge of the values and preferences of the patient—insofar as these are known—should play.

[30] Experiments of this sort were done at a University in British Columbia.

[31] Paul Ramsey, *The Patient as Person* (New Haven: Yale Univ. Press, 1978), 11-58.

[32] Richard McCormick, "Proxy Consent in the Experimentation Situation," *Perspectives in Biology and Medicine*, Vol. 18, No. 1 (Winter 1974), 2–30.

[33] See Chapter 4.

[34] For a somewhat different discussion, see T.H.E. Murray, "Gifts of the Body and the Needs of Strangers," *Hastings Center Report* 17: 2 (1987), 30–38.

[35] Compare R. Wasserstrom, "Ethical Issues Involved in Experimentation on the Non-Viable Human Fetus," National Commission for the Protection of Human Subjects of Biomedical and Behavioral Research, *Appendix: Research on the Fetus* (1975) DHEW No. (05) 76–128. There is a whole literature that has developed around the issue of experimenting with human foetuses. The Canadian government has recently struck a Royal Commission on New Reproductive Technologies, whose mandate will include fetal experimentation. See also E.-H.W. Kluge, and C. Lucack, "Experimenting Embryos and Fetus," in *New Reproduction Technologies: A Preliminary Perspective of the Canadian Medical Association* (C17A: Ottawa, 1991).

[36] Part of it will be given in our discussion of genetic engineering.

[37] See ref. note 9, 23.

[38] Compare Cohen, "Medical Experimentation on Prisoners," *Perspectives in Biology and Medicine*, Vol. 21, No. 3 (Spring 1978), 357–372 for a discussion of some of the issues that are involved here. We do not share Cohen's lenient attitude.

[39] See ref. note 9.

[40] See ref. note 9.

[41] Of course this is not surprising. It takes years of concentrated effort to become a health care professional; and it takes even more time to become a specialist and an academician. Given the amount of knowledge that these professionals have to absorb, there is very little time left over for becoming conversant with, let alone expert in ethical theory and reasoning. While in the last few years some efforts have been made to improve the situation—for example, by developing year-long courses in ethics that physicians who are on sabbaticals can take—these can provide only a superficial training in ethics. And given that during this time of training they have to keep current in their own discipline, it is not surprising that little actual professional training in ethics can be given or absorbed during that time. It would be like trying to turn someone into a physician by offering a year-long sabbatical training in medicine to them.

[42] See W.K. Frankena, *Ethics*, 2nd edition, (Englewood Cliffs, N.J.: Prentice-Hall, 1973), 43. See also T.C. Beauchamp and J.F. Childress, *Principles of Biomedical Ethics* (New York and Oxford: Oxford University Press, 1979), 97-134.

[43] Testimony of Dr. F.H. Lowy, Cooper Report, Appendix 6, p. 6.

[44] Cooper Report, Letter of Dr. F.H. Lowy to Mr. Cooper, January 9, 1986, p. 10 (italics added).

[45] Our analysis is in keeping with the public statement of the Board of Directors of the Canadian Psychological Association, Nov. 11, 1990, that "the practices used would not have been acceptable at that time, nor would they be acceptable now." The Canadian Psychiatric Association initially concurred when it said that "It may well be that certain patients admitted to the Allen Memorial Institute in the 1950s and 1960s were not offered sufficient disclosure, even by the current standards then applicable." (Letter of Q. Rae-Grant, Chairman of the Board. CPS July 6, 1990 to T. R. Berger).

SUGGESTED READINGS

- Beecher, H.K. "Ethics and Clinical Research." *New England Journal of Medicine* 274, 1350.

  One of the original articles that focused on the ethics of research with human an subjects. Beecher, then editor of the NEJM, pointed out several serious ethical inadequacies in certain experiments that had been performed. This is a classic work.

- The Declaration of Helsinki, World Medical Association, 1964.

  A somewhat up-dated version of the Nuremberg Code. See Frenkel for some analysis. Revised 1975 in the Declaration of Tokyo.

- Frenkel, D.A. "Human Experimentation: Codes of Ethic." *Legal Medical Quarterly* 1: 1 (1977) 7–14.

  A very good survey article in a Canadian journal that details some of the developments in international codes on human experimentation. Frenkel points out how the initially strong restrictions in the Nuremberg Code have been relaxed over the years.

- *Halushka vs. The University of Saskatchewan* (1965), 53 (2d) 436.

  This is the classic Canadian case outlining the legal requirement of informed consent in experimental contexts.

- Health Protection Branch and Pharmaceutical Manufacturers' Association of Canada. "Guidelines for the Conduct of Clinical Investigation." Ottawa: Health Protection Branch, Health and Welfare Canada, 1985.

  These are older than the MRC guidelines, but complement them in that, as the title suggests, they focus on experimentation and research in the development of pharmaceutical agents.

- Jonas, Hans. "Philosophical Reflections on Experimenting with Human Subjects," in P.A. Freund, ed., *Experimentation with Human Subjects*. New York: American Academy of Arts and Sciences, 1970.

  A view of human experimentation from the perspective of someone who is humanistically inclined.

- Katz, J. *Experimenting with Human Beings*. New York: Russell Sage Foundation, 1972.

  A thoughtful book with many examples, written prior to the disclosure of the Tuskeegee experiment. It anticipates some of the reasoning that has since become standard.

- Medical Research Council of Canada. *Guidelines on Research Involving Human Subjects*. Ottawa: Ministry of Supply and Services, 1987.

  These guidelines are the Canadian bench-mark against which research protocols in the health care field are measured. They contain the minimum requirements that a research protocol must meet if it is to be federally funded.

- National Commission for the Protection of Human Subjects of Biomedical and Behavioral Research. *The Belmont Report: Ethical Principles for the Protection of Human Subjects of Research*. Washington, D.C.: U.S. Government Printing Office, 1978, pub. no. 78–0012, App. 1–0013, App. 2–004.

  This three volume report not only states what essentially has become the position of the U.S. government on research with human subjects, but also contains a good collection of analytical papers presented to the Commission. The papers are noteworthy for their breadth and general clarity.

- Nuremberg Code: *The Trials of War Criminals before the Nuremberg Military Tribunal*. (Washington D.C.: U.S. Government Printing Office, 1948.

  The first modern international code dealing with human experimentation. The clauses contained in it were what underlay the prosecution of Nazi physicians and health care professionals by the Allies.

8
Health Care and Health

This chapter considers the question of the right to health care. We begin by investigating the concept of health itself and then try develop a value-free definition. Next we discuss briefly the notion of a right, apply this to the notion of health care, and then place the whole issue into a social perspective. Our conclusion is that there is a right to health care, and that although how that right is expressed may be social-context-dependent, it nevertheless is universal in nature.

It will be useful to keep the following questions in mind when reading this chapter.

1. What is health? Why is it sometimes claimed that the concept is value-laden?
2. How do we state and evaluate the definition of health in terms of the homeostatic balance and proper function of a biological organism?
3. Is a judgement of ill health (disease) in and by itself a mandate to treat?
4. What is the relationship between social deviance and ill health?
6. How could one defend the claim that there is a right to health? The claim that there is no such right?

Introduction

Most Canadians believe that they have an equal right of access to all medically necessary health care services irrespective of their condition or their financial resources.

Canadians have not always felt this way. Until the 1930s they agreed with the citizens of many other countries that health care is a matter of privilege that has to be earned, and that those who could not afford to pay for it did not have a right to it. The experiences of the 1930s fostered a change in this perspective, and by the 1940s the outlook had changed fundamentally. First in the prairie province of Saskatchewan and then in other provinces the now prevailing attitude emerged. It led to the establishment of universal health and hospital insurance in Saskatchewan in 1944[1] and successively in other provinces. It was reflected in the Hall Report of 1964,[2] the Lalonde Report of 1974,[3] and led to the Canada Health Act of 1984, which was proclaimed in 1985.[4] Today, all Canadian provinces and territories have a universal health care system where physicians and hospitals provide services according to province-wide schedules, and where only certain services have to be paid for by patients themselves.

The belief that there is this right of equitable and universal health care is not something that all countries share; nor is it shared to the same degree even by those who accept the general principle. For instance, although the Scandinavian countries have the same outlook as Canada, the United Kingdom differs in some important respects. It accepts the general principle of social responsibility for health care, but it also believes that society does not have an obligation to provide all medically possible, or even all medically indicated, services to all of its citizens. It therefore allows the growth of private clinics and private hospitals for those who are able to pay. To take another example, somewhat closer to home, the U.S. has traditionally maintained that health care is a service like all other services, and that it should therefore be available only to those who can pay for it. The following statement reflects this attitude rather well:

> The concept that "Health Care is a Right" is demonstrably false, but its wide acceptance has had the effect of destroying true rights.[5]

While in recent years the United States government has moved towards a more socially responsible perspective by establishing Medicare and Medicaid programs, the fact remains that there are over 35 million uninsured people in the United States who have either inadequate access to health care, or who have no access whatsoever.[6]

All of this raises a series of fundamental questions. Is there a right to health care? Assuming that there is, how is such a right grounded? What exactly does it amount to in terms of its nature and extent? How does it compare to other rights in society?

There is a wide variety of opinions on these matters. However, before addressing any of this, we have to have some clarity on two even more fundamental issues. What is the nature of health? and, How does the right to health care differ from the right to health? Without clarity on the notion of health, our whole discussion will be plagued by a fundamental ambiguity that has important practical implications; because depending on how the notion of health is defined, different kinds of services will be included in the right to health care. And depending on whether we distinguish the right to health from the right to health care, the orientation of health care services that are mandated will be different.

The Definition of Health

Let us begin with the notion of health. In a way, of course, we know what health is. It is what is provided for by nurses, therapists, physicians, clinicians, and what hospitals, clinics, nursing homes and so on, seek to promote. But to define "health" in this way—so to speak by enumeration—really assumes that we already know what we are talking about. Otherwise, we would run the danger of excluding what should be included, and vice versa. It also runs the danger of not allowing us to deal with health issues that were not recognized as such in the past; mental health issues, for example. More importantly, however, it would make health a matter of political decision by turning it into what governmental agencies set up to provide the various services and what professional organizations who actually provide them decide it is.

Therefore, what we really need is a definition that somehow tries to get at the logic of the underlying concept itself. Perhaps something like what used to be called an analytical definition. There are no shortages of candidates. The best known is the definition offered by the World Health Organization.

> Health is a state of complete physical, mental and social well-being and not merely the absence of disease or infirmity.[7]

However, as a whole series of authors have pointed out,[8] this definition is extremely vague. For instance, what does "well-being" mean, or "infirmity?" It is also circular; because it defines "health" in terms of its correlative, "disease." The notion of disease, however, can itself only be defined in terms of health; so this gets us nowhere. Furthermore, the definition is far too inclusive. It would have us classify social and moral problems as health problems.[9]

Other definitions have been suggested to overcome these problems. For instance: Health is "a state of physiological normalcy," a "proper working order of the human body,"[10] "the general condition of the body with respect to efficient or inefficient discharge of conditions," as "spiritual, moral or mental soundness or well-being,"[11] the ability to function "in a given physical and social environment,"[12] the "well-working of the organism as a whole ... an activity of the living body in accordance with its specific excellence,"[13] or simply "a state of physical well-being."[14]

Health and Values

But such definitions have also run into criticism. In fact, the very attempt to define health at all has been criticized. On a general level, the criticism has been that a proper definition is impossible because concepts like those of health and disease are inherently value-laden. They include not only descriptive components but also normative ones. Tristam Englehardt, Jr. focuses on these normative components when he says that:

> To say that something is a disease commits us to saying something about human nature and the nature of human well-being. Further, such talk involves choices among human goods ... In short, discussion about what counts as health and disease involves considerations of what counts as the proper human state, and the latter is caught up with value judgements which are both explicit and implicit.[15]

and more clearly still: "To call someone ill is a social judgement."[16] This critique is echoed by Joel Feinberg, albeit from a somewhat different perspective:

> It may seem ... that the ascription of functions to components parts or subsystems is a wholly factual matter consisting of, first, a description of a part's effect and, second a causal judgement that these effects are necessary conditions for the occurrence of some more comprehensive effects. But the illusion of value neutrality vanishes when we come to ascribe functions to the organism itself.[17]

When the reasoning that underlies this perspective is taken to its conclusion, it leads to something like the position of Peter Sedgewick. Sedgewick claims that:

> ... illness and disease, health and treatment, (are) social constructions ... Outside the significance that man voluntarily attaches to certain conditions, there are no illnesses of diseases in nature.[18]

The position of Thomas Szaz is similar, although it is not quite so extreme. Szaz focuses on the concept of mental illness. He admits that there is such a thing as organic brain disease, defined in terms of physiological dysfunction. However, he maintains that the concept of mental illness is a "myth." It is the legacy of a religious mythology and heir to the notion of witchcraft, according to which "mastery of certain problems may be achieved by means of substitute symbolic-magical operations."[19] The value concept that Szaz sees buried in all of this is that of a smoothly functioning social order where deviant behaviour of a divisive sort does not exist. He therefore characterizes mental health judgements as nothing more than expressions of society's current disapproval of certain ways in which individuals may try to cope with the pressures of modern life. He maintains that we can see the ultimate denouement of accepting this sort of notion in countries who imprison political dissidents as mentally ill precisely because they are dissidents: i.e., deviant.

What we have just sketched will give some idea of the range of positions that exist on the very notion of health itself, and of the criticisms that have been levelled at any attempt to define it. However, the question we should asks ourselves is, whether these criticisms are justified. Do they really show that the attempt to define health and disease in a value-free fashion is doomed to failure?[20] The issue is important, because if we cannot give a value-free definition of health, then we will always have to ask ourselves whether the health services that are provided by our society are so coloured by our values that they in fact amount to a cultural agenda. This would have to be of particular concern to Canadians because Canada, by choice and by Charter, is a multicultural society.

Judging and Evaluating

Is it possible to give a value-free definition of health? At one level, the answer has to be no. We can define something only by using concepts. However, the concepts that we use when we give a definition are part of the overall conceptual framework by means of which and through which we see the world. To borrow a metaphor from the philosopher Immanuel Kant, they are like a set of irremovable glasses. Without them we can respond to stimuli at a reactive level, but we cannot perceive.[21] It is these conceptual glasses that allow us impose meaning and significance on what would otherwise be completely meaningless and uninterpreted sensory data.[22] To perceive is to judge. Not necessarily in a conscious or deliberate fashion, but it is to judge nevertheless.

The metaphor of the irremovable glasses is fortunate because it leads to the next point. How a pair of glasses is ground, the colour and nature of the glass, condition what we perceive. They may distort, colour, enlarge, make smaller and so on. The parallel to concepts lies in this: Linguists, psychologists, anthropologists and sociologists have pointed out on innumerable occasions that the concepts that form our conceptual framework are culture-bound and even language-related.[23] Therefore there is no such thing as a conceptual framework that does not in some way condition the perceptions and the understanding of the people who use it. All concepts that form part of a conceptual framework are related to each other in some way or another, if only by the associations that surround them because they are learned as part of the life-style that defines the culture itself.

That is why we said that on one level, the answer to the question whether we can give a value-free definition of "health" has to be no. If by "value-free" we mean a definition that is completely independent of the sort of conditioning that occurs because a concept is part of an overall conceptual framework, then that is clearly impossible. To look for that sort of definition is to look for a definition without concepts. That cannot be done.

However, the fact that all concepts are embedded in conceptual frameworks, and the fact that they are interrelated by the associations that tie them together does not necessarily mean that they are value-laden. Nor does it mean that every time we use a concept we are in fact making a value judgement. We have to draw a distinction a between making a judgement, evaluating something and putting a value on it. To return to what we said a moment ago, every time we perceive something in the world or say something about it we are making a judgment. This may not be a conscious process. In fact, it usually isn't. However, without such judging the sensory data would remain without cognitive significance. In fact, it would be highly doubtful whether they could be considered at all.[24]

Judging then, in this sense of the term, consists in bringing sensory data and concepts together. Evaluating is a special form of judging. It is not simply interpretative, as for instance when we perceive something to be a cow. For example, when we say something like "This cow is larger than that one"; or even when we say, "This cow is not a particularly representative member of the species bos bovis holsteinensis," the basis is comparative.

Valuing is very similar to judging. However, it goes beyond it. Valuing involves attaching a value to that which is judged, apprehended or perceived. It therefore essentially involves values. The notion of values can be approached in various ways: psychologically, logically, ontologically and so on.[25] Their precise epistemological and ontological status is unclear.[26] This is not the place for discussing the various interpretations that have been offered. The only reason it is relevant here is that if there are values that are attached to the notion of health, these values would affect the nature and direction of health care. It is really this aspect that is relevant to the claim that the concept of health is value-laden. And from that perspective, we can characterize values as action potentials: as psychological gradients that move people into action.

Even in this sense, values are not independent things. We cannot be motivated to do something if we do not understand or have no idea of what we are supposed to do. Therefore values depend on the concepts that permit understanding. However, people do not acquire concepts in isolation. They are not programmed like computers, where each new datum can be entered independently of all other data. People learn their concepts in a social context.[27] This context not only influences the way in which the concepts are learned but also the emotional and valuational significance that the person attaches to them. This in turn influences the sorts of actions that persons find appropriate (or inappropriate). The traditional way of putting this is to say that to learn concepts or to learn a language is to learn a way of life.[28] When we learn a concept, therefore, we also acquire a set of values. To use a metaphor, these values surround concepts like a halo. Whenever a concept comes into play, the values that surround it are called up as well.

Therefore, logically speaking, when we make a judgement we are not necessarily making a value judgement. We may simply be understanding what is going on—perceiving, so to speak—with out any action potentials or psychological gradients coming into play. This would be the case when we are saying something like, "This is an aardvark"; or "The boat is moving rapidly towards the English Channel."

Even though judging, valuing and evaluating are logically distinct, in reality they work together. As we said, concepts are learned as we learn a language with values attached. Therefore, when a concept is applied, the values associated with it also come into play. This may be very obvious, as for instance when we say something like "Insider trading is reprehensible." On the other hand, it may be quite covert; for example when we make statements like "That is a democratic process." Here all the values that surround the purely epistemic concept of democracy are called up and come into play in the attitude that we adopt.

However, despite this close connection, the fact remains that logically at least the values and judgements can be distinguished from each other. Furthermore, not all values are ethical ones. For example, the value attached to the speed of a car, to the colour of a glove or the to size of an egg are quite real despite the fact that they are not ethical in nature.

This can be applied to the health care context. When we determine that a heart-valve is mal-functioning and we say, "This valve is not functioning properly," we are identifying something as a heart-valve and we are looking at its functioning. Furthermore, we are looking at its functioning within a certain context—as installed in a specific heart—and we are saying that it does not meet a particular standard of operation. We are therefore making a judgment, and we are making an evaluation. However, we are not necessarily making a value-judgement; and certainly not an ethical one. It is a strictly operational evaluation. It becomes a value judgement only if we attach a value—that is to say, an action-potential—to the "proper" or "trouble-free" operation of the valve. And it becomes an ethical value-judgement when the values that we attach are ethical in nature.

Health as an Evaluative Concept

Let us return now to the definition of health. Some commentators have suggested that health can be defined in a value-free fashion if we define with reference to proper biological function. The proper biological functioning need not be construed in valuational terms, but simply as a standard to which bodily states can be compared.

However, here we run into the objection raised by Englehardt and Feinberg. They maintain that the standard we pick as basis of our judgement is a function of the social norms within which we are operating. Consequently it contains an ineluctable bias and it is not value-free. The question we have to ask is whether that is really true. Why can we not define health and disease without this? Must the basis always reflect socially determined norms?

Let us look at a few cases. Consider the object we normally call a knife. Irrespective of what we value or perceive, it has a certain shape and physical make-up. That shape and that make-up may be described differently in different languages and in different cultures; however the fact remains that even if there were no culture, and even if all langauge speakers ceased to exist, there would still be something, and it would still have the properties it has, no matter how they are described.

The knife can be used for certain purposes. These range from driving nails into a wall to serving as a paperweight to functioning as an objet d'art. The person who made it, however, or at least the person who designed it, intended it for a purpose, cutting, to which it is more or less well suited by nature of its design. If its manufacture is flawed and it cannot be used for that purpose, then it is justifiably said to be dysfunctional.

An internal combustion engine can be used as an anchor and even as a planter for petunias. However, what it is best suited for by virtue of its design is to act as a power source. Furthermore, it is that use which serves as the basis of evaluating its functionality as an internal combustion engine. If it cannot operate as an internal combustion engine because of some internal impediment to its operation, then it is said to be dysfunctional.

With due alteration of detail, we can apply this reasoning the realm of living things.[29] Biological organisms are complex entities whose unimpeded function is in keeping with the genetic code contained in their DNA. This should not be misunderstood. We are not suggesting even for a moment that biological organisms are designed or that they have a teleology. All we are saying is that they function in accordance with a pattern laid down in their genetic code.

All biological organisms, whatever their nature, function this way. They differ in the specific ways in which they function because their DNA's differ. However, the ultimate functioning of all biological organisms involves reproduction. This is true whether we consider a virus, a unicellular organism or something much more complex. To put it captiously, biological organisms are DNA's way of making more DNA. Survival is a necessary precondition of reproduction. A biological organism that cannot survive cannot reproduce. The functional quality of a given organism can therefore be evaluated in terms of how well or how ill its internal constitution and the operation of its constituent parts (if any) and its integrated functioning as a whole allow that organism to fulfil its genetically determined manner to survive and reproduce.

Which brings us to the concept of a homeostatic balance. Every organism has an internal constitution whose basic nature is determined by its genetic make-up. However, organisms also exist in an environmental context. In order to survive and have the capacity for reproduction, they must be able to interact causally with the environment. They must be able to respond to the challenges of the environment while at the same time maintaining their functional integrity. We refer to such a state as a state of homeostatic balance. Therefore we would like to define health as the state of complete homeostatic balance of an organism that gives it the capacity to fulfil its genetically determined manner of survival and reproduction.

This definition of health applies to all biological organisms and it also applies to human beings, for whatever else human beings may be, they are also biological organisms. However, human beings are also social animals with understanding and volition. It is these last two qualities that give the concept of health as applied to human beings such a peculiar flavour. The fact that humans have both a psychosocial and a material side must be reflected in the relevant notion of health. The concept of the homeostatic balance of the human person must therefore be open to psychosocial as well as biological considerations.

As to biological considerations, we can distinguish two aspects: the homeostatic balance within a given subsystem or organ, say the liver; and the integral homeostatic balance of the organism as a whole. The homeostatic balance of the one does not entail a homeostatic balance in the other. For instance, while the liver of someone who suffers from brain cancer may be in homeostatic balance, the person's body as a whole will not be in homeostatic balance. On the other hand, while the pancreas of someone who suffers from diabetes is not in homeostatic balance, the body as a whole may be in balance because of dietary regimen and medications.

The same thing holds true for the psychosocial aspects of human beings. These include reasoning ability (understanding), emotions (feelings), and volition (will). Finally, the integrated complex of biological and psychosocial parameters can be dealt with in the same way. This is shown in Figure 8-1.

This way of approaching the notion of human health allows several conclusions.

1. Ill health (illness, sickness, disease) may be brought about (caused) in three ways: genetically, functionally, or through a combination of both. Homeostatic balance may be absent either because of a genetically determined condition,[30] like haemophilia, Tay-Sachs or cystic fibrosis; or because of external (environmental) influences on the functioning of the individual, for example because of pollutants like heavy metals in the water, or disease factors like rubella, AIDS or malaria; or because of a combination of both, as for example in the case of PKU, certain forms of cancer, allergy reactions or certain types of alcoholism. Further, homeostasis may be absent at all levels of integration of the individual, right up to the way the individual functions in the social context. Figure 8-2 shows the possibilities.

2. The fact that someone deviates from a physiological or psychosocial norm does not necessarily mean that the person is ill, any more than the fact that a person fits the norm means that the individual is healthy. In fact, it may happen that a whole population is ill and that the illness is the norm. The prevalence of malaria or of other parasitic diseases in certain parts of the world, or the prevalence of nutrition-associated diseases, illustrate this only too well.

3. The fact that a certain state is considered unacceptable within a certain society context does not necessarily mean that it is a state of ill health. What is acceptable is a function of social values. To identify the two is to turn health assessments into value judgements.

4. It is impossible to state specific, absolute and universal criteria for what constitutes health. What constitutes homeostasis can be determined only within a socio-physical environment. What constitutes ill health in one context may be the acme of functional adaptability in another and may have supreme survival value. Differences between groups of people in their ability to metabolize proteins is an example of this.

5. The fact that someone suffers from ill health is not a mandate for medical treatment. A decision to treat is a decision about how to react to a health status assessment. It is not something that is inherent in the assessment itself. To go from the one to the other requires a premise that connects an absence of homeostasis with a duty to treat or with a duty to receive or seek treatment.

FIGURE 8-1
Health

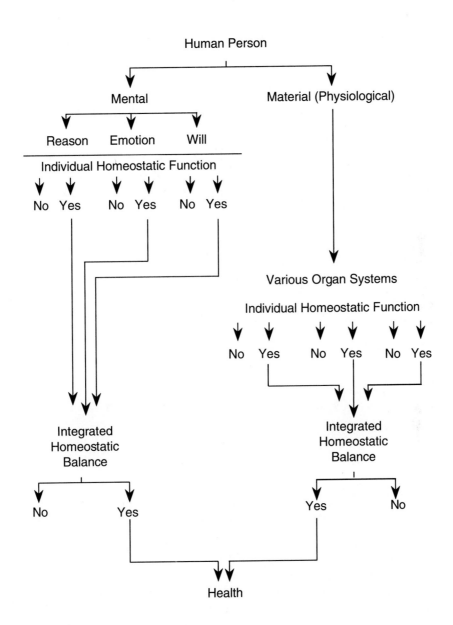

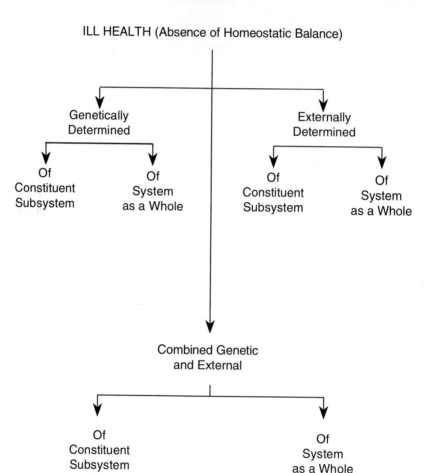

FIGURE 8-2
Ill Health

Right to Health versus Right to Health Care

Now that we have sketched a definition of "health," we want to turn the claim to the questions that have been standing in the wings: Is there a right to health? Is there a right to health care? Is there a duty? Is this an unconditional right? Does it have limitations? If so, what are they? How are they drawn? and so forth. But once again, before we can deal with these issues directly, we have to do a bit more analytic work. We have to distinguish between the right to health as opposed to the right to health care.

So far, we have used phrases like "right to health" and "right to health care" interchangeably, as though they meant the same thing. But they don't. As we shall see in the next chapter, the fact that they don't has tremendous implications for the delivery of health care services at the macro- and the micro-level.

To put it bluntly, no one has a right to health. The reason is simple. One cannot have a right to something if the fulfilment of that right lies essentially outside the capabilities of anyone to guarantee. This follows from the principle of impossibility.[31] No matter what we do, we cannot guarantee that people will be healthy, any more than we can guarantee that they will be happy. The most that we can do is guarantee that we will make every effort to ensure their happiness; or, as in the present context, to try to provide for their health. We can guarantee the attempt, but we cannot guarantee the outcome.[32] For instance, we may be unable to do anything about people's genetic make-up;[33] and all other things being equal, we certainly cannot force people to take advantage of the health care opportunities that we offer them. People may insist on leading imprudent lifestyles by smoking, immoderate alcohol consumption, lack of exercise, and so on. In these cases their health will suffer, no matter what we do. Furthermore, we cannot prevent all accidents. The human condition simply rules this out. Finally, we cannot guarantee that there will be sufficient resources to provide all necessary health care services to the degree that may be necessary in each case.[34]

Therefore, people do not have a right to health. What they do have is a right to health care. However, this immediately raises two questions. One is somewhat theoretical, whereas the other has profound practical import: What is the basis of this alleged right to health care? What is its extent?

Origin and Nature of the Right to Health Care

The right to health care has been defended in various ways. For example, it has been argued that health itself "is a primary good" and that it "generally helps people to carry out their life plans, whatever they may be."[35] It has also been suggested that health care "expresses and nurtures bonds of sympathy and compassion," and that therefore "a society's commitment to health care reflects some of its most basic attitudes about what it is to be a member of the human community."[36] In a similar vein, some authors have suggested that the right to health care is rooted in "a basic obligation of charity or beneficence to those in need."[37] Still others have suggested that access to health care is rooted in society's obligation to provide for equality of opportunity for its members.[38]

The sentiments expressed in some of these considerations are certainly laudable. Charity and beneficence are virtues that should be encouraged. We would also agree that the commitment to providing health care would be a social expression of care and concern. However, the fact that something is a virtue does not turn it into a duty, and the fact that something would be an expression of care and concern does not make its observance into an obligation. Therefore, these considerations may not be the most fortunate ones for establishing a universal and equal right to health care.

The principle of equality fares better in that regard. If equality and justice are fundamental principles that govern ethical conduct, then society itself, in its actions, must seek to fulfil this principle. Therefore, when it comes to providing services, society must attempt to maximize equality of opportunity for all of its members. The ability to take advantage of the opportunity that society offers to a considerable degree depends on the health status of the person in question. People who suffer from malaria cannot take advantage of schooling to the same degree as all other persons; people who suffers from cystic fibrosis, measles, or abscessed teeth are similarly disadvantaged; and so on.

However, while the principle of equality fares better, it is insufficient. It applies only to those health care problems where in fact there are societal differences. It does not impose an obligation on society to provide health care services in matters where every member of society is affected equally or where everyone is likely to be affected in the same way. This is especially important in matters of public health, in preventive health care programs, and so forth. These programs do not provide those who are disadvantaged with equalizing assistance, nor can such programs be construed in that fashion. Their purpose is to raise the general level of health in society. Therefore they tend to help everyone in the same regard and to the same degree.

This does not mean that the principle of equality cannot be used to ground a right to health care. All it means is that the principle of equality cannot be considered its only ground. We would like to suggest that another ground lies in the nature of human society and in the way in which it arises. As Thomas Hobbes[39] so aptly put it, life in a state of nature and outside the context of formalized social institutions[40] is apt to be "solitary, poor, nasty, brutish, and short." People form societies in order to ameliorate that condition. However, in order for societies to be possible, social interactions have to be integrated lest the structure fly apart. There have to be some limits on unbridled and uncontrolled actions by members of society. These members must necessarily limit their right of freedom of action: not entirely, but sufficiently in order for society to be able to function.

However, this limitation of freedom is conditional on the expectation that society will try to provide for the fundamental needs of the individual to the best of its ability; and that it will do so in balance with the competing rights of others and the resources available. Finally, there is also the expectation that society will try to provide an opportunity for self-realization on the part of the individual person.

All of this has important implications. One of the most important is clearly that society undertakes to provide for the necessaries of life of its members. This involves two parameters. One is external, the other internal. The external parameter comes into play when the individual's life is threatened from the outside. In this case, society has an obligation to provide against things like aggression, natural disasters, and so on. The internal parameter comes into play when the individual's life is threatened from the inside in ways that involve the individual's ability to maintain itself as a human organism. In other words, the internal parameter comes into play when the health of the individual is threatened. Various social services are here implicated. Health care is one of them.

Duty versus Right

The right to health, therefore, flows from the principle of equality and justice and the basic presuppositions that underlie the existence of society itself. However, a right is something very special. It is a claim which people may exercise if they wish, but they do not have to. Therefore, if there was only a right to health care, then the members of society would never have any obligation to use the health care services available in a given society. It would always be a matter of choice.

However, this raises serious problems when we come to communicable disease, public health measures and the like. If health care in these contexts were wholly a matter of choice, these measures could never be really effective; and when governments make the use of such measures mandatory, they would be violating the autonomy of the individual persons. At the same time, the fact that some people objected to inoculations or vaccinations would demonstrably put other members of society at identifiable and serious risk. These factors have to be reconciled.

Our suggestion is that the right to health care has a correlative: the duty to be responsible in one's social behaviour. As we said in the beginning, the principle of autonomy and respect for persons does not mean that everyone can do what she or he pleases under any and all circumstances. It means that everyone has the right to freedom of action subject to the equal and competing rights of others. When the rights of others are threatened, society is entitled to interfere in keeping with the nature of that threat. If, as in the case of communicable diseases, the life and welfare of others is threatened by the irresponsible behaviour of others, society has a mandate to interfere. Otherwise it would not respect the principle of autonomy and respect for persons in regard to those other individuals. They would be affected by this irresponsible behaviour. Furthermore, their right of equitable access to the available health care resources would be threatened. The irresponsible behaviour of these other persons would create a need, or a shortage, where otherwise no shortage would exist.

Therefore, the duty to be responsible may entail that people must submit themselves to validated public health measures. To measures that are intended to control the spread of infectious diseases and the like. This duty derives from the very same principles that ground the right to health care itself, and it is supported by the same presumptions that govern equitable access.

This does not mean that there are situations when the right to health care becomes a duty. Logically, rights and duties can never be the same. What it means is that under certain circumstances the social obligations that people have because they are members of society involve the use of techniques, procedures or resources that fall into the area of health care and that normally would be open to them as a matter of choice.

There is also another context in which the issue of right versus duty might be raised. It concerns situations where people have access to health care but refuse to use it, only to ask for health care later on. The sort of situation we have in mind is may be illustrated by the following case.

> Marfa B. had been diagnosed as suffering from essential hypertension. Her pressure was 120/170 when at rest. An echo-cardiogramme showed a thickening of the ventricals, which was consistent with the diagnosis, and her kidney function was somewhat impaired—a finding that was also consistent with the sort of end-organ damage that one would expect from someone suffering from essential hypertension. Her physician suggested she take an angiotensin enzyme inhibitor, and Marfa did so on a trial basis. It proved to be effective in lowering her pressure to 90/130. However, Marfa decided not to continue with the medication because of the inconvenience it presented to her. She was just unwilling to take her medication regularly and every day. She was told that unless she controlled her hypertension, she could look forward to severe heart damage and probably also kidney damage. That would be resource intensive, and could threaten her life. Marfa persisted in her refusal.[41]

In principle, Marfa of course has the right to accept or to refuse any health care regimen. However, such a refusal is not without its consequences. If, as a result of such a refusal, she later needs health care resources that she would not have need had she accept help in the first place, then she has voluntarily brought about a preventable need. That does not mean that she should not have access to the resources at all. However, it does mean that when there is a competition for health care resources, her refusal has to be taken into account as one of the factors that led to the shortage in the first place. And that in turn means that anyone who wants to have an equal access to health care resources has an obligation to accept appropriate health care when it is warranted.[42] In that sense, while there is no duty to health care in any absolute sense, there may be said to be a conditional duty, conditional, that is, on future expectations.

The Rights of the Incompetent

If the distinction between a right and a duty to health care presents problems in the case of competent individuals; it becomes even more difficulty when we are dealing with people who are incompetent. The situation sometimes arises when we are faced with someone who is comatose and the question is whether to continue life-saving and/or sustaining measures, or whether to discontinue them. This becomes especially troublesome when the person is someone who is congenitally incompetent: someone like a child, who has never had the opportunity to express any values, who has never even held any values, and where all decision-making has to be made without the possibility of guidance from that person her- or himself. What happens to the right to health care then?

The principle of equality and justice, and the principle of autonomy and respect for persons would suggest that even though it might be difficult to do so in practice, the very same sorts of considerations should be applied here as anywhere else. "The rights of the incompetent should not be less than the rights of the competent."[43] But consider the following case.

> Marcia was a six-year-old girl who, as a result of meningitis, was hydrocephalic with a rather small asymmetric head with grossly enlarged ventricals, a porencephalytic cyst on the left frontal lobe, atrophied optic nerves and skull sutures closed for over three years. She also suffered from cerebral palsy, incontinence, a chronic nasal discharge, had only a slight response to auditory stimuli, no reflex movement except a stereotypical response to pain, unorganized random movements of head, eyes and limbs, and no real discernible cognitive function. She had a shunt (to drain accumulation of cerebral fluid) replaced and the shunt had again become plugged, requiring "revision." Some "coning" [44] had already occurred, and the situation was life-threatening with a high probability of fatal outcome unless the shunt was revised. The question was whether her parents could refuse permission for this revision, or whether they had an obligation to agree to it.[45]

This case presents all sorts of issues. For instance, there is the question whether the parents are the appropriate proxy decision-makers. Then there is the question of what criteria they should use in arriving at a decision; the question of the role of the health care professionals in all of this; of the social service agencies, and of the courts.

In the present context, the question mentioned at the end of the case is the most important. In cases like these it is sometimes assumed that the parents (or appropriate other proxy-decision makers) cannot refuse permission for treatment because that would mean that the child (or incompetent person) would die. If that were to happen, it would be a violation of the right to health care of the child.

However, that logic does not follow. Under normal circumstances, a patient may refuse any treatment that she or he does not want;[46] otherwise the right to health care would not be a right but a duty. Therefore, the proxy decision-makers, in this case the parents, must be able to consider the same range of options as would be open to Marcia were she competent. Their choice cannot be artificially constrained in such a way that "the presumption must be in favour of life." If it was, then Marcia would be punished for the fact that she is incompetent.

Therefore, the parents must be able to take the option of non-treatment seriously. This does not mean that their decision should necessarily go in that direction. Marcia might profit as a person from having her shunt revised. Alternatively, not revising it might do more harm to her than good, and would therefore violate the principle of best action. There may be all sorts of reasons why we would want to say that the parents should decide in favour of a revision. However, the important point is that this cannot be a foregone conclusion. The choice, the deliberative process, must be real; and the option of non-treatment must be a live one. Otherwise what is a right to health care in the case of competent persons becomes a duty for those who are incompetent. This would affect the conduct of health care delivery at its very core.

Conclusion

We began with the statement that most Canadians believe that they have an equal right of access to all medically necessary health care services irrespective of their condition or their own financial resources. We have tried to show that this belief is ethically correct. It is grounded in the very presuppositions that underlie membership in a society and in the principle of equality and justice. We should also point out that our argument had nothing to do with the peculiarities of Canadian society. It therefore follows that our conclusion holds for societies in general. If that means that societies who do not accept this are not fulfilling their societal obligation, then we have to accept that inference.

It is an easy step to go from this to the conclusion that therefore society has an obligation to make all possible health care services available to all of its members under any and all circumstances. However, that inference would be mistaken. In the next chapter, we shall explore why.

In the course of our discussion we also looked at the notion of health itself. We attempted to arrive at a definition that was value-free. For this, we looked at the notion of the functioning of an organism, and at the concept of a homeostatic balance. We insisted, however, that the judgement that someone is ill does not amount to a mandate for treatment. At least, not under normal circumstances. All other things being equal, so we said, health care is a right, not a duty. There are exceptions, of course. However, these have to be justified in terms of the equal and competing rights of others. The principle of autonomy and respect for persons is here at stake. By the same token, we insisted that the fact that people are incompetent or otherwise unable to exercise their right to health care does not mean that therefore that right should lapse. Even in their case, the right should not become a duty. That inference should come as no surprise, because it takes us back to something that was central to our discussion in Chapter 6—the rights of the incompetent should not be less than the rights of the competent solely because they are incompetent.

ENDNOTES

[1] Saskatchewan Hospitalization Act, 1946, which followed the Health Services Act of 1945. The program outlined in this legislation did not become fully operative until an agreement was reached with the College of Physicians and Surgeons of Saskatchewan with the so-called Saskatoon Agreement of 1962. See also Mr. Justice Emmett Hall, *Report of the Royal Commission on Health Services* (Ottawa: Queen's Printer, 1964) for a discussion of the evolution of health services in Canada.

[2] The Hall Report, see note 1, above.

[3] The Honourable Mr. M. Lalonde, *A New Perspective on the Health of Canadians* (Ottawa: Minister of Supply and Services, 1974).

[4] Canada Health Act, R.S., 1985, c. C–6.

[5] R.M. Sade, "The Patient's Right to Choose," IATROFON 10: 1 (1990).

[6] See D.W. Light, "Corporate Medicine for Profit," *Scientific American* 155: 6 (December, 1986), 45. See also Report of the Council on Scientific Affairs of the American Medical Association, "Societal Effects and Other Factors Affecting Health Care for the Elderly," *Archives of Internal Medicine* 150: 6 (June 1990) 1184–1189.

[7] WHO, *The First Ten Years of the World Health Organization* (Geneva: World Health Organization, 1958).

[8] The best known is Daniel Callahan, "The WHO Definition of Health," *Hastings Center Studies*, 1: 3 (1973), 77–87.

[9] Callahan, see ref. note 8.

[10] Joel Feinberg, "Disease and Values," in Joel Feinberg, *Doing and Deserving: Essays in the Theory of Responsibility* (Princeton: Princeton University Press, 1974), 253–55.

[11] Oxford English Dictionary.

[12] René Dubos, "Health as Ability to Function" in T.L. Beauchamp and L. Walters, eds., *Contemporary Issues in Bioethics* (Belmont: Dickenson Publ. Co., 1978), 99.

[13] Leon Kass, "Regarding the End of Medicine and the Pursuit of Health" in Beauchamp and Walters, ref. note 12, 108.

[14] Callahan, "The WHO Definition of Health," see ref. note 8. A somewhat more theoretical and developed analysis is offered by Ellen Idler, "Definition of Mental Health and Illness and Medical Sociology," *Society, Science and Medicine* 3A, 723–31. She claims that these and other definitions are based on a Parsonian model of illness and disease: one that defines it as "an abstract, biomedical conception of pathological abnormality in people's bodies, where this is indicated by certain abnormal signs and symptoms which can be measured, recorded, classified and analyzed." To be quite correct, so she argues, the concept should be modified so that "subjective reality plays a role in determining whether an individual becomes ill in the first place."

[15] H. Tristam Englehardt, Jr. "Human Well-Being and Medicine: Some Basic Value-Judgements in the Biomedical Sciences," reprinted in T.A. Mappes and J.S. Zembaty, *Biomedical Ethics* (New York: McGraw-Hill, 1981), 214.

[16] Englehardt, "Human Well-Being and Medecine," see ref. note 15, 216.

[17] "Disease and Values," 254, reprinted in Mappes and Zembaty, ref. note 15, 211.

[18] Peter Sedgewick, "What is Illness?" *The Hastings Center Studies* 1: 3 (1973) reprinted in Beauchamp and Walters, ref. note 12, 114.

[19] Thomas Szaz, "The Myth of Mental Illness," in Mappes and Zembaty, ref. note 15, 227.

[20] For other attempts to define "health," see President's Commission for the Study of Ethical Problems in Medecine and Biomedical and Behavioral Research, *Securing Access to Health Care: A Report on the Ethical Implications of Differences in the Availability of*

Health Services. (U.S. Govt. Printing Office: Washington D.C., 1983) 3 vols., vols. two and three.

[21] Immanuel Kant, *Critique of Pure Reason*. (Hartknoch: Jena, 1792).

[22] See N. Swartz, ed., *Perceiving, Sensing, Knowing* (New York: Doubleday, 1964) for the controversy between sense-datum vs. percept theory. In this connection, see also R. Chisholm, *Realism and the Background of Phenomenology* (New York: Glencoe, 1960); D.C. Dennett, *Content and Consciousness* (London: Routledge and Kegan Paul, 1969); J.M. Hinton, *Experiences* (Oxford: Clarendon Press, 1979)

[23] See Ludwig Wittgenstein, *Philosophical Investigations* (Oxford: Blackwells, 1954).

[24] See Chisholm, and also Dennett, ref. note 22. The position is of Greek and medieval origin, but finds its classic modern expression in Gottlob Frege's theory of judgement. For modern commentary on this see, the work of Michael Dummett.

[25] For a recent discussion of the ontology of values, See the work of Roman Ingarden, especially his *Man and Value* (trans. A. Szylewicz) (Dordrecht: Philosophia, 1984).

[26] For a somewhat different investigation into the emotional aspects of values, see Robert M. Gordon, *The Structure of Emotions: Investigations in Cognitive Philosophy* (New York: Cambridge University Press, 1987).

[27] See Wittgenstein, ref. note 23, for a classic discussion of this from an ordinary language perspective.

[28] Wittgenstein, ref. note 23.

[29] Compare Dubos, ref. note 12.

[30] The reason why we do not say "congenital" is that, unless the condition is genetically determined, it will be at least in part a result of external influences. The genetic-congenital distinction is here important if only for the sake of conceptual clarity.

[31] Compare Robert Veatch, "Just Social Institutions and the Right to Health Care," *Journal of Medicine and Philosophy*, 4: 2 (1979) and J.S. Millis, "Wisdom? Health? Can Society Guarantee Them? " *New England Journal of Medicine*, 283 (July 30, 1970), 260–61.

[32] This must be taken with a grain of salt. Obviously, we can do so in a sense and to a degree: by genetic screening, abortions for fetal indications, etc. For more on this, see Chapter 13 of this text.

[33] Not even with the advent of contemporary germ and somatic cell line therapy. For more on this, see Chapter 13 of this text.

[34] For an approach that is somewhat different from the one we have adopted, see Mark Siegler, "A Right to Health Care: Ambiguity, Professional Responsibility and Patient Liberties," *Journal of Medicine and Philosophy*, 4: 2 (1979), 148–57. See also Robert Sade, "Medical Care as a Right: A Refutation," *New England Journal of Medicine*, 285: 23 (Dec. 2, 1971), 1288–92. Compare *Securing Access to Health Care*, President's Commission for the Study of Ethical Problems in Medicine and Biomedical and Behavioral Research (U.S. Government Printing Office, Washington, 1983). 3 vols., vol. I. See also Chapter 8 of this text.

[35] President's Commission for the Study of Ethical Problems in Medicine and Biomedical and Behavioral Research, *Securing Access to Health Care*, 3 vols., "The Ethical Implica-

tions of Differences in the Availability of Health Services," (U.S. Govt. Printing Office: Washington D.C., 1983) vol. 1, 16.

[36] See ref. note 35. vol. 1, 17.

[37] Allen Buchanan, "The Right to a Decent Minimum of Health Care," in *Securing Access*, ref. note 35, 232. See also David Gauthier, "Unequal Need: A Problem of Equity in Access to Health Care," in *Securing Access*, ref. note 35, vol. II, 179–105.

[38] Norman Daniels, "Equity of Access to Health Care: Some Conceptual and Ethical Issues," *Milbank Memorial Fund Quarterly*, 60: 1 (1982) reprinted in *Securing Access*, ref. note 35, vol. 2, especially 41–47; and Daniel Wikler, "Philosophical Perspectives on Access to Health Care: An Introduction," *Securing Access*, ref. note 35, vol. 2, especially 219ff.

[39] Thomas Hobbes, *Leviathan* I: 13.

[40] As John Rawls has pointed out, this formalization need not be explicitly codified or even explicitly entered into in a formal way. It may merely exist *de facto*.

[41] This is based on a case communicated to the author by Dr. Mark Ujjainwalla, whose help is gratefully acknowledged.

[42] For more on this see Chapter 9.

[43] *In the Matter of Colyer*, 660 P. (2d.) 738 (Sup. Ct. Wash. 1983).

[44] The accumulation of fluid depressing the lower brain centres associated with vital functions.

[45] This case is based on a series of cases related to the author by Dr. Campbell, Sheffield, England.

[46] We are here assuming that we are not dealing with some of the exceptive circumstances that we identified above.

SUGGESTED READINGS

- Boorse, C. "Health as a Theoretical Concept." *Philosophy of Science* 44 (1977) 542–573.

    A somewhat difficult but theoretically very interesting study of the concept of health that has had some influence on U.S. policies.

- Brown, W.Miller. "On Defining 'Disease'." *Journal of Medicine and Philosophy* 10: 4 (1985) 311–328.

    An attempt to wrestle with the value parameters inherent in the notion of disease and illness.

- Burns, Chester R. "The Nonnaturals: A Paradox in the Western Concept of Health." *The Journal of Medicine and Philosophy* 1: 3 (1976) 202–211.

    As its title suggests, this is an attempt to take a closer look at what is meant by "natural" and its cognates.

- Callahan, Daniel. "The WHO Definition of Health." *The Hastings Center Studies* 1: 3 (1973).

  One of the first and certainly one of the best-known critiques of the WHO definition of "health."

- Goosens, W. "Values in Health and Medicine." *Philosophy of Science* 47 (1980) 100–115.

  Like the article by W. Miller Brown, it considers the notion of health and illness in terms of value considerations. However, it expands the discussion somewhat my including reference to the notion of medicine as a discipline.

- Klerman, Gerald L. "Mental Illness, the Medical Model, and Psychiatry." *The Journal of Medicine and Philosophy* 2: 3 (1977) 222–243.

  Most discussions of the notion of health and disease focus on physiological functioning of the human body. This article is an attempt to place the notion of illness and disease into the psychiatric context.

- Nordenfelt, Lennart. *On the Nature of Health.* Dordrecht and Boston: D. Reidel Pub.Co., 1987.

  A relatively recent full-length work devoted to a discussion of the nature of health. It builds on many traditional definitions and concepts.

- World Health Organization. "The Concept of Health," *The First Ten Years of the World Health Organization.* Geneva: World Health Organization, 1958.

  This contains the classic definition of "health," which has become the operant definition for many departments of health throughout the world.

9

Health Policy and the Allocation of Resources: The Ethics of Discrimination

This chapter deals with the right to health care under conditions of limitation. It distinguishes between macro-allocation, meso-allocation and micro-allocation and suggests some ways in which the conflicts that arise at the various levels of health care resource competition might be resolved.

The following questions might be useful as a guide when thinking about the various issues:

1. What does the notion of a basic level of health care mean? How would such a level be determined?

2. What does the distinction between hetero- and auto-induced health conditions amount to? Does it have any relevance when it comes to allocating health care resources?

3. What is the difference between macro-allocation, meso-allocation and micro-allocation of resources?

4. How could one defend the claim that there are limits to society's obligation to provide health care services? Would that limit be the same for all people?

5. Are there any reasons why health care professionals themselves should become involved in the allocation process? If so, how would that square with the ethical positions of their profession?

Introduction

Health care resources are limited. The responsibility for this does not lie with politicians, but in the nature of human society itself. Societies have only a finite number of people. Furthermore, the material resources available to societies are also limited. Therefore, no matter how technologically advanced a society may be, the amount of goods, services and other things that a society can produce is finite. This finite amount has to be divided among the various services that society has to provide to its members as a matter of social obligation. Health care is only one of these obligations; education, transportation and defense are others. All of them have to be funded from the same limited resource pool. This means that although the proportion of the overall resources that each social service receives may be adjusted differently, the amount will be finite.

The fact that societal resources are limited may not pose much of a problem when the types of health services that are available are relatively cheap, and when the demands that are placed on them can be met within the existing allocation framework. However as the services become more expensive, as the number of people who demand them increases, and as the number of requests for the services themselves go up, so does the cost to the system and the relative drain on the health care resource pool itself. Sooner or later, the limits of the resource pool are reached, and society has to make a decision. Who shall have when not all can have? What shall be available when not everything can be made available? These are the questions that stand in the wings. What is then the extent of the right to health care, particularly when resources are scarce?

The issue is of increasing concern for Canadians. The fact is that Canadian society is changing demographically: it is aging. With increased age, there comes an increased consumption of health care resources. This means a correspondingly greater drain on the health care resources that are available.[1] Canadian society therefore has to come to grips with the problem of health care resource allocation.

However, the problem is not simply due to such demographic factors as aging. The increasing technological sophistication of medicine and of health care itself is an important contributor. The introduction of transplantation has saved thousands of lives, but at a tremendous cost to the public purse in terms of capital and operating costs for transplant centres, treatment and follow-up costs for transplant patients, and so on. The development of medical imaging technology such as computer assisted tomography (CAT scans), magnetic resonance imaging (MRI) and positron emission tomography (PET scans) has improved the diagnostic abilities of physicians but at tremendous capital expenditure costs, as well as in terms of hidden down-stream costs entailed by the more accurate and earlier detection of diseases. People who would previously have died because their illnesses were detected too late are now being diagnosed early enough that they can undergo treatment. This has to be paid for, and demands a commitment of resources where previously none were required.

Death is cheap, but even such simple techniques as amniocentesis have to be paid for. While it may not cost much to perform such a test on a specific occasion, when such tests become routine they add up to a considerable total. Or we could look at the development and increased use of surgical procedures such as by-pass operations. They also have developmental costs attached to them and their availability has to be funded. Such funding has to include not just the material costs and salaries for physicians, nurses, technicians and so on, but there are also the additional costs generated by the fact that people who are very ill have been given a renewed lease on life.

We mention these things to emphasize that no matter how beneficial a particular health care service may be, it has to be paid for. It is easy to lose sight of this fact when we only look at the person who benefits from the service. When we lose sight of the overall cost implications, we lose sight of the fact that when resources are limited, what is given to one person is unavailable to another. When both have an equal right to health care, how can one, how should one, decide whose right should be served? And by what? For how long? Under what circumstances?

These questions become particulary difficult when, as in the Canadian context, we believe that everyone has the right of equitable and just access to health care. Providing such a level of health care takes money: lots of money. In most provinces, the health care budget is the largest single item of public expenditure. This money has to come from somewhere.

Canada is in the difficult position of having a constitution that makes the providing of health care services a matter of provincial jurisdiction,[2] while the money needed for governmental expenditures is usually collected by the federal government in the form of taxes.[3] The federal government returns to the provinces some of the tax money that it collects. These are called transfer and equalization payments. These payments are calculated according to a complicated formula that involves the number of people in a province, the socio-economic capabilities of the province, the types of services needed, and so on. It is at the level of transfer and equalization payments that the federal government attempts to exercise some control over the provision of health services in the various provinces. Among other things, it makes the payments conditional on the provinces ensuring universality of health care inclusive of certain types of services, and on the provinces not permitting extra-billing. That is to say, the provinces must make a certain level of health care universally available, and they must not allow physicians to charge fees higher than the set fee schedule agreed to by the professional medical association of the province and the provincial government. If a province allows extra-billing, its transfer payments will be reduced to the amount that such billing is estimated to amount to.[4]

This relationship between the federal and provincial governments has led to a considerable amount of friction. Nevertheless, the underlying theme of universal and equitable access to health care is not something that any province would nowadays wish to challenge. It is too firmly entrenched in the minds of Canadians. We have attempted to justify this belief in our discussion of the previous chapter.

Global Issues

Putting matters this way may have created the impression that the allocation problem only concerns competition between individuals—that it is only a problem of micro-allocation. Unfortunately this is not true. The problem is much more complicated. It also involve the question of how much of its resources society should devote to health care in the first instance. How should society balance the competing demands on its resources in terms of its duty to provide other social services? How should the global health care resource pool be determined? And given that there is a resource pool of a certain size, what orientation ought health care services take in order to fulfil the citizens' right to health care?

Health Care Budgets[5]

The question of the global size of a health care budget has received scant attention. Since there is no explicitly formulated and generally accepted schema for determining health care budgets, we would like to propose the following for consideration: Any global budget determination should take the following factors into account: the socio-economic capabilities of the society at that time; the prevailing state of medical sophistication; the average health profile of members of society; the competing areas of social endeavour; and the values of society as a whole. These factors can then be fleshed out in the following ways:

The Socio-Economic Capabilities of Society

The socio-economic capabilities of society set the overall limits within which any social allocation must occur. These limits need not be defined solely in terms of actual production capabilities of society. They may include the ability of society to mobilize capital by borrowing on the credit side. On the debit side, they may also include such factors as the actual disposable resources left to society in terms of spending power. But in any case, the capability to mobilize resources constitutes the outer resource limits.

The Prevailing State of Medical Sophistication

The prevailing state of medical sophistication does not refer to what is medically feasible *in a particular society* at a given time, but what is medically feasible as such. Adjustment to what is medically feasible within a given society occurs later, when the resources actually allocated to health care are known.

Average Health Profile of Members of Society

Once the overall resource framework has been settled, and once it has been determined what is medically feasible, the next step is to develop a statistically valid averaged health profile of the members of society. Among other things, this should include the health conditions that people in the society are likely to develop, and so on. Medical sociology and epidemiology can here provide invaluable assistance.

Competing Areas of Social Endeavour

The parameters we have indicated have to be integrated in to a global matrix and weighted with respect to each other. This is probably the most difficult task of all. It is also the area of allocation policy determination that is the least well developed. We suggest that it should have several components. First, it should involve the development of a multidimensional matrix that correlates the types of services available as such with the epidemiological groups identified from the average health profile of society with the expenditures necessary to reach a certain level of health status in these identified groups. This would provide the fiscally responsible social party with a variable scale that would allow it to determine at what level of expenditure a particular statistically average level of health care would be available at what cost.

The next step would be to identify the other areas of socially mandated expenditure and do something similar for them. With this in hand, it would then be possible to develop a comparative matrix that would make it possible to read off what expenditure in one area would have what implications in terms of social expenditure in the relevant areas: For instance, education versus health care versus defense versus transportation, and so on. This might be called an *expenditure impact analysis* for varying levels of expenditure in the various areas of social endeavour.

Values of Society

However, an expenditure impact analysis gives only the material possibilities of allocation. It does not provide any way that someone can decide what point in the multi-parameter matrix an allocation decision should be made. The reason is that such a decision is not a material decision. It is a value decision. The material facts carry no values in and by themselves. They are decision-theoretically neutral. Another way of putting this is to say that they lack action-potentials because in and by themselves they carry no action-gradients. These gradients have to be superimposed or added to the matrix. The only place from which they can be imposed is from the outside: by people who look at the facts, who bring their values to the facts and who see them in terms of more or less strongly weighted action-potentials.

All of this is merely a theoretical way of saying that the material facts have to be evaluated in terms of the values and value-strengths of society as a whole. That again involves several steps. First, those who make their allocation decisions have to know what the fundamental values of society are and with what strength these values are held. For example, is health a fundamental value? Is security? Mobility? Education?

The second step is to find out the strengths of these values and to determine their strengths relative to each other. The outcome of this investigation will be a series of relative value-strength coefficients. These relative value-strength coefficients will be numerical expressions of the weighted action-potentials that we mentioned a moment ago. When these relative value-strength coefficients are superimposed in the expenditure impact matrix, the decision-makers can get an idea of how much society is willing to allocate to what area of social endeavour given its fundamental values.

However, this is not all. As it stands, the proposal we have sketched would allow a society to decide that it would prefer to devote the majority of its resources to aggressive warlike efforts rather than to health care. Therefore, those who need appropriate health care in order to live decent lives or to have an equal opportunity to fulfil their life-goals would be penalized for their ill health. This would be unjust. Therefore, there has to be a requirement that the fundamental values entering into these calculations must be defensible in terms of the fundamental principles of ethics. This would allow societies to take due account of their individual differences in social and valuational perspectives without becoming unethical in their global allocations.

The proposal we have just sketched sounds complicated; and it is. It is also quite idealistic. It assumes that society is willing to proceed rationally in its global allocation procedures. However, this is something that anyone who is concerned with ethical considerations really has to assume.

Orientation

Once an overall global health care budget has been determined, the decision-makers face another task. They must decide what proportion of the resources available to health care should go to research, what proportion for emergency funds for unforeseeable happenings, for preventive efforts and for acute care and so on.

Preventive services (inclusive of public health measures) are designed to minimize as far as possible the need for crisis services. They include undertakings directed towards encouraging a healthy lifestyle, improving living standard and so on. It has frequently been suggested by medical sociologists that society is not doing enough in these areas; that to place the major emphasis in health care delivery on preventive is both cost-inefficient and allows the quality of life of the ordinary member of society to deteriorate too far before action is considered necessary.[6]

The central thrust of this suggestion has been that an emphasis on acute care ultimately leads to an artificial resource shortage and therefore to a forced problem of allocation. Forced, that is, because the shortage of resources could have been ameliorated, if not prevented, if the proper preventive steps had been taken. Therefore, according to this perspective, an acute-care orientation ultimately contravenes the principle of best action. It also contravenes the principle of respect for persons (autonomy). Because, by bringing about an artificial stringent resource crisis, it limits the choices open to members of the public later on. Furthermore, it is better not to let the quality of life of persons deteriorate if it can be avoided. To do otherwise is to treat human beings as objects to be weighed against convenience.[7]

Limitation

However, to settle the issues of global allocation and of orientation is not to settle the question of how to allocate the resources that are available in a given area. In other words, the issue that still has to be addressed is that of the internal limits within each of the funded areas of health care. This issue can be distilled into the following question: What are the limits to the distribution of health care services in a vertical sense—which is to say, with respect to the kinds and areas of services that are available; and what are the limits to the distribution of health care resources in a horizontal sense—which is to say, with respect to right to health care of particular persons?

This matter has received a great deal of attention over the last few decades. Not surprisingly, it has generated a variety of opinions. For example, Janet Storch has maintained that:

> One philosophy of distributive justice proposes that, when there is not enough money to provide the services everyone wants or needs, society's least advantaged should be taken care of first. If this philosophy were implemented on a government program level, greater attention would be paid to human services and less to programs that benefit the corporate structure; if implemented at the health program level, more monies would be spent on programs for the aged or for native people, and less on exotic lifesaving technologies or on white middle and upper class abortion services. Those with the greatest need for services, although they might have the fewest financial resources, would have access to health services equal to the services available to those who can pay.[8]

Robert Veatch has argued that:

> It seems ... reasonable that people would have a right to an opportunity to the health care services offered in the institution in proportion to their need to reach some particular level of health.[9]

Gene Outka suggested that all persons should have equal access, "as needed, without financial, geographic or other barriers, to the whole system of health services,"[10] and contends that if such equality cannot be attained then that particular type of service ought to be interdicted entirely and for all:

> The formula's allowance for no positive treatment whatever (in these sorts of cases) may justify exclusion of entire classes of cases from a priority list.[11]

Not surprisingly Charles Fried, who is a lawyer, has objected to this. He has proposed that instead, in each case and for each person, there must be a right to services designed to attain

... decent minimum of health which accords with sound ethical judgement ... The decent minimum should reflect some conception of what constitutes tolerable life prospects in general ... On the other hand, the notion of a decent minimum should include human and, I should say, worthy surroundings of care for those whom we know we are not going to be able to treat.[12]

In the Canadian context, the Hall Report (Royal Commission on Health Services in Canada, 1964)[13] held that there is a right to "universal" and "comprehensive" medical care. While the Lalonde Report of 1974 (A New Perspective on the Health of Canadians)[14] amended this somewhat, it still insisted on an "equality of opportunity." That perspective was maintained by the federal government in its Canada Health Act. While the Act met with considerable opposition from organized medicine, led by the Canadian Medical Association and the Ontario Medical Association, it was not the equitable-and-universal-access provisions that sparked their opposition, but the fact that they perceived the Act to interfere with the autonomy of physicians and patients.

However, no matter how these issues are ultimately resolved, the fact is that resources are limited. This means that elective allocation has to occur. The fact also remains that selective allocation is discriminatory allocation. Therefore, what is really needed is an ethics of discrimination. We shall discuss the issue under three headings: macro-allocation, meso-allocation and micro-allocation.

Macro-Allocation

Primary Macro-Allocation

Macro-level of allocation is concerned with competition between types of services within a given area. Central questions here include the following: Is there some ethical mechanism for distinguishing between types of health care services that should be funded, and is there a limit on the extent of allocation for a given area since it has beaten out the others?

Various answers have been proposed. Some have suggested that cost/benefit analysis provides the answer,[15] others have focused on cost/effectiveness coefficients,[16] on quality-of-life years gained (QALY's),[17] and so on. So far, no clear favourite has emerged. However, there is a tendency on the part of health care funders (provincial governments, hospital districts and so on) to assume that efficiency and effectiveness are the primary determinants of just and fair allocation. As several commentators have pointed out,[18] this is not necessarily true. Therefore, perhaps it would be useful to reiterate some of the considerations we raised in our discussion of society's obligation to provide health care.

The first consideration is conceptually simple but pragmatically very important. Ethically speaking, no-one can have an obligation to do the impossible. The principle of impossibility rules that out. Therefore, society cannot have an obligation to devote resources to types of situations, conditions and illnesses that are incurable. Diseases like Huntington's chorea or the various trisomies here come to mind. This does not mean that society should not fund research into these diseases. Nor does it mean that resources should not be allocated for palliative or other appropriate measures. Since palliation is something that we can do, it follows that by definition it is not impossible. Therefore, it does constitute a legitimate area of allocation.

Possible versus Available

Within the realm of what is possible we should distinguish further between the fact that something is possible and the question whether it ought to be available. It is tempting to argue that availability of types of resources should be decided in a democratic fashion on the basis of communal preferences or in some way that reflects the professed values of the community. However, as we suggested in our discussion of global allocation, that would be to confuse of ethics with ethos. There is no guarantee that such values reflect what is ethically correct. Equity and justice demand that society provide for the basic needs of the individual insofar as that is possible and fair, not simply insofar as it agrees with the will of the majority or their professed values.

Another important factor is that not all levels of allocation are meaningful. Every area of health care has a certain basic level that must be reached before the services that can be provided become effective, a quantum level of effectiveness so to speak. If this minimal level is not reached, then the allocation will be essentially wasted. For example, allocating funds to a nuclear diagnosis program or buying diagnostic equipment for case rooms that are insufficient to cover the cost of training and employing the necessary personnel to run it leaves the whole program ineffective. Or again, allocating only enough funds to cover vaccination programmes in urban centres without allowing enough funds for rural areas threatens the effectiveness of the whole program.

Statistical Needs

If we now turn to macro-allocation itself, we can see that it is possible for social planners to know that certain health care related events are likely to occur and that certain expenditures will be required. The statistical data dealing with the level health and types of health care needs of the average member of society make that sort of knowledge possible. Therefore, an ethically acceptable macro-allocation pattern would provide for the types of services that are necessary on the basis of the medical profile of the population. For long-range planning, it would be adjusted to make due allowances for shifts over time. Furthermore, it would be functionally related to the number of individuals likely to be involved.

However, if macro-allocation were based on this alone, it would encounter several objections. First, considered from a purely practical standpoint, it would virtually guarantee that individuals whose health care needs fall outside the social norm would never have their health care needs satisfied. In effect, therefore, it would deny universality of health care.

Second, one of the primary drawing cards of this sort of approach is supposed to be the fact that it provides a way of calculating levels of expenditure. However, for that to be possible we have to treat individual persons and their rights as calculable quantities. This not only misconstrues the nature of rights, it also contradicts the deontological orientation we have advocated. People are not quantifiable entities, and rights are not calculable quantities. They cannot be added together, divided, or otherwise manipulated in an arithmetic fashion. For instance, the fact that there are more people who need an appendectomy than there are people who need myringotomies does not mean that therefore the right of those who need myringotomies weighs any less or merits less attention, even if myringotomies are more expensive than appendectomies. From a deontological perspective, the effectiveness of a right is a function of the strength of the relevant claim itself. It is independent of how many other people have a similar claim.

It could be replied that both of these objections assume that primary macro-allocation has to be illness-focused, rather than wellness-focused. If that were true, the right to health care would in fact not be a right to health care but a right to disease care.

The argument has some merit. However, we could accommodate if by beginning with the assumption that there is an average basic homeostatic status for individuals in society as determined by the general environment and the nature of the population. The primary macro-allocation of health care resources would then be designed to maintain that balance for the average individuals under such conditions.[19] It would include a calculation of the prevailing conditions and of the health care requirements that could reasonably be expected to arise. This would allow for flexibility in allocation as the health status base and health care needs change.

Equality versus Equity

However, not all people would have their health care needs met by this approach. Genetic, environmental and socio-economic factors produce inequalities that manifest themselves in different health status and health care needs. Social institutions that do not take this into account are egalitarian in nature, and treat everyone the same. However, by that very token such social institutions are unjust. Because they do not respond adequately to the increased requirements of those patients whose health-status is lower, they confirm this lower status and perpetuate an undeserved but correctable inequality. In effect, they punish the disadvantaged for being the victims of bad luck, and reward the advantaged for their undeserved stroke of good fortune.

Equity and justice therefore demand an approach that adjusts allocation to allow for the special needs that people have. In other words, equity and justice demand an approach to these problems that proceeds on the basis of equity rather than equality.

Secondary Macro-Allocation

This means that there is a need for a secondary macro-allocation. This allocation has to be geared to identifiable groups of people. More specifically, it has to be geared to identifiable groups whose needs are not met by the primary macro-allocation that accrues to all people. In a sense this is allocation on the basis of need. However, need is like a bottomless pit. It can swallow up a whole health care budget—sometimes even without reasonable expectation of positive results. Cancer funding is a good example. If cancer care and research were funded solely on the basis of need, where need is identified as the need for a cure, the amount of money would be staggering. Justice therefore demands that secondary macro-allocation involve some limitation and some balancing. We suggest the following as possible limiting conditions:

1. To the best of our understanding, the type of condition must be in principle correctable. (This is merely the principle of impossibility in action.)

However, the mere fact that people suffer from an unusual but identifiable condition does not mean that they automatically require special funds. For instance, the fact that some people suffer from baldness does not mean that special funds should be set aside for them and that they should receive treatment. It may be that baldness is a health condition. That does not, however, mean that it results in a lower-than-average health status.

2. The health status that is traceable to that condition must be lower than the average health status within the society as a whole.

The principle of equality and justice and the principle of relevant difference entail that it is unethical to treat persons differently unless there is an ethically relevant difference. The reason for secondary macro-allocation is that we assume that there is such a relevant difference.

However, just as no-one may be penalized for having a lower than average health status (and therefore a greater than average need), neither may anyone with a better than average status under equal primary macro-allocation be punished for that fact. In both cases we are dealing with a matter of happenstance.

Of course, it would be unrealistic if people who are in a privileged position as a result of primary macro-allocation were to expect society to increase that advantage still further through special support. However, the people who happen to find themselves in this privileged position may expect that primary macro-allocation remain at a level where it will maintain their average health status. If the funds available for ensuring average health status were lowered because of an increase in funding for secondary macro-allocation, this would threaten the health status of people who happened to be privileged by fate. This would be reverse discrimination. This sometimes happens when funds that would normally go to preventive programs or the delivery of normal health care are diverted into areas like cardiac by-pass surgery, transplantation and so on. Therefore, we would put the point like this:

> 3. The average health status of society (as achieved by primary macro-allocation) must not be adversely affected by the special, secondary macro-allocation.

There is an old saying that goes something like this: It is silly to throw good money after bad. In health care funding it is not only silly, it is also unethical. The fact that resources are limited means that what is not used effectively is misused. While it may be necessary to provide a greater-than-average allocation merely to retain the status quo for a particular disadvantaged group, that allocation must be effective. Therefore, if neither the improvement in the health status of this group nor even the retention of their status quo is traceable to this secondary allocation, then that allocation is pointless. It violates the principle of best action. Of course we cannot know beforehand whether the secondary funds that are allocated will be effective in this way. However, we can require that macro-allocation planning take this consideration into account:

> 4. The projected (reasonably-to-be-expected) health status of the recipients of preferential (secondary) macro-allocation must be at least as good as the one that existed prior to the allocation and the improvement/retention of the status must be traceable to the secondary allocation.

We are not suggesting that these considerations are the only ones that are appropriate for macro-allocation or that they exhaust what could be said on the subject. They are merely intended to give some idea of the mix of ethical and pragmatic variables that go into an acceptable macro-allocation policy. However, we would like to emphasize three points.

First, the criteria that we have suggested take both the average and the abnormal health care needs of people into account. However, the quantum level effect that we talked about earlier may entail that there will be health care needs that will not be met. As things stand, Huntington's Chorea, and Tay-Sachs for example will be implicated. In their case, only palliative care (and a certain amount of research) will be available.

Second, the criteria are sufficiently flexible to allow for shifts in macro-allocation in response to shifts in need patterns and also in the amount of the resources available.

Third, this approach is based on the conviction that there is no absolute and universally valid pattern of health care macro-allocation that holds for all societies. Variations in the health of a society and in the total environment in which that society is embedded play an important role in determining what a society is and what it is not ethically obligated to provide in terms of health care.

Fourth, while this approach recognizes the legitimacy of special needs, it suggests that adjustments to these needs cannot be open-ended. Ethical health care macro-allocation must distinguish what is possible and what can reasonably and fairly be expected.

Meso-Allocation

It sometimes happens that after a particular area of health care has been funded by macro-allocation, a conflict arises between the needs of some specific individual who falls under that rubric and a whole group of people who also fall under it.[20] Consider, for example, the following case:

> Alicia Morgenthau, a new-born infant, has been diagnosed as suffering from an irreversible heart condition which cannot be treated by medication or any other regimen. The only hope for her is a transplant. However, the cost of a transplant for someone in her position runs in the neighbourhood of $700,000, possibly going as high as $1.2 million if the follow-up treatment and incidental expenses are included. The province in which she lives has a transplantation budget of $15.5 million. The cost of a kidney transplant runs in the neighbourhood of $25—35,000[21]. If Alicia receives her transplant, 28 people will not receive a kidney. Some of them will die. Furthermore, the success-rate of paediatric heart transplants is very low. How should the resources within the transplant budget be allocated? [22]

Merit[23]

There are several ways of approaching this sort of problem. One way is to examine the merit of particular candidates by looking at their significance and status in society.[24] Whoever is in a position of responsibility, or whoever has made a substantial contribution to the welfare of society should get first chance at the resources.

Of course this would not work in the case of Alicia, and this would be one of the shortcomings of such an approach. Another problem would be that this approach makes two important assumptions. First, it assumes that everyone has had the same opportunity to contribute to society or of being in a position of authority or whatever. That assumption is highly questionable. Second, it is exceedingly difficult to assign a precise ethical weight to a particular level of contribution to the common good. The fact is that any attempt to develop a ranking scale will reflect socio-economic and/or political biases and nothing else. While in principle, therefore, this approach might yield a solution, in practice it will be unworkable.

First-Come, First-Served[25]

Another approach would be to proceed on a first-come first-served basis until the funds have run out. Therefore, if the needs of one person will the resources that could be used for many, that is just the luck of the draw.

This sort of approach would be workable from a pragmatic perspective in the case of Alicia Morgenthau. However, the problem is that it assumes that this type of lottery approach is in fact just and fair. This assumption has been seriously questioned.[26] Geographic location may have something to do with the ability to queue up.[27] There are other variables, like the ability to communicate[28] or the biases of the medical profession in identifying certain individuals as being in fact appropriate candidates for the relevant procedure. This is particularly obvious when one of the prospective candidates is someone who is mentally severely handicapped.[29] Furthermore, politicians would be committing political suicide if they followed this approach. Irate voters who were denied the necessary treatment because the resources had run out, or whose friends or next-of-kin found themselves in such a position, would raise such a furore such a policy would become politically untenable.

What often happens in such cases is that the conflict between the individual and the group is resolved on the basis of emotional appeal. The individual who is in need is paraded before the eyes of the public, with an appeal for special allocation. In this way, the resource limits that define (and cause) the problem are circumvented. This happens particularly in the case of transplant patients when organs are scarcer than usual, or in the case of cardiac patients who require surgery and cannot wait their turn in the long list of patients.

This approach has had great success in securing resources for individuals in specific cases. This is not surprising for it rests on what has been called the phenomenon of the identified victim.[30] It is psychologically easier to refuse resources to a group of persons whom we don't know as individuals, than to refuse the resources to someone we know. Presenting the identified victim to the public and appealing for help makes it very difficult for the public to refuse access to the needed resources. The anonymous group with whom this person stands in competition tugs much less strongly at our heartstrings.

However, it has recently been suggested this approach to meso-allocation is also flawed.[31] All it does is appeal to the public to extend the limits of the resources available while insisting that the specific individual who stands in competition with the group should have access to the newly extended resources. This is not to solve the problem of meso-allocation but to shift it to the area from which the new resources have to come.

Furthermore, it is to say that the particular individual on whose behalf the appeal is launched somehow should not be subject to the ranking procedures that determine access to the resources. However, to do so is to exempt this person from these criteria by definition. Ethically, such an approach cannot be defended.

Ability to Pay

Still another solution involves the introduction of a two-tier system. On one tier there are the people whose health care expenses will be defrayed by society. They have to queue up for the resources, meet certain criteria of eligibility and then wait their turn. On the other tier, access and eligibility are determined solely on the basis of the ability to pay. Those who can pay the price will get the resource. This sort of solution has been tried in Great Britain, and it is essentially the one that is in effect in the United States.[32] An example of this solution would be the following sort of situation.

> A young woman is admitted to a private clinic for a kidney transplant. Since she can pay for the kidney, she receives it. The kidney is rejected several weeks later, and after some time on dialysis, she again has a transplant at the private clinic. Again the kidney is rejected, and she goes on dialysis again. Since she comes from wealthy family, she has another kidney transplant—again defrayed by her family. In the meantime, at the public clinic there are lists of people waiting for their first kidney.[33]

This case illustrates some of the problems with the two-tier pay-as-you-go approach. In the first place, it assumes that the amount paid by private individuals really defrays the actual expenses of the health care services that they buy. However, the fact is that the various health sciences in general and medicine in particular are social goods. They have been developed using social research funds, and draw on knowledge gained in such diverse disciplines as chemistry, physics, mathematics, engineering and the like. The fees charged for the services do not reflect their true value. Therefore, a two-tier system would in effect subsidize the rich at the expense of the poor.

Furthermore, this solution is socially unjust. It assumes that everyone in society starts out from the same basis in socio-economic terms and has the same opportunities for acquiring the funds that are necessary to enter the second tier. This is false.

This approach is particularly unjust in situations involving access to human tissue, such as organs, blood and the like. It is ethically objectionable to buy and sell these things as though they were goods like all others. They are social resources. They are useful only in the medical and health care context. Outside of it, they are just so much tissue.

To put it in more concrete terms, in and by itself a liver or a heart, or even blood, is useless. What turns it into something useful and usable is the professional and social context in which they are to be used. This involves the medical teams, the bio-technical support services, the institutional services that led up to the establishment of clinics, and so on. It also includes a whole history of development and experimentation that involves people at every step.

General Considerations[34]

We could go on, but perhaps it will be more fruitful if we focus on some general considerations about meso-allocation. First, it is doubtful that meso-allocation dilemmas can be resolved by appealing to numbers: one against many. This would be possible if rights could be quantified and added. We could then say that the collective weight of the resulting sum outweighed the right of the individual person. However, rights cannot be quantified. Therefore, they cannot be calculated either. Which means that a balancing that depends on comparing the rights of the one against the many in calculative terms is fundamentally flawed.

Second, whatever the solution proposed, it must not recreate or exacerbate problems in different area. This happens when the allocation boundaries within one area are shifted in response to the phenomenon of the identified victim by taking funds from another area of health care. That is to pay Peter by robbing Paul.

Third, a solution that is bought at the price of violating the principle of equality and respect for persons is not an ethically acceptable solution. Therefore, even if a great improvement in the average health status of the group could be achieved by ignoring the needs of a specific individual and shunting the resources to the group instead, it would be indefensible.[35]

Finally, the point of health care allocation is not simply to produce the maximum amount of health status improvement possible under the circumstances. If that were the driving aim, there would be no allocation problems. Cost-effectiveness considerations would dictate allocation policy at all levels. Rather, the aim of allocation in general, and in this case of meso-allocation, is to balance competing rights. In meso-allocation it is the rights of the individual against those of the group.

The key word is here "balance." This means that the rights of the individual must be given due consideration. Which in turn means that such a right cannot be overruled by pointing to pragmatic results. The right of each individual has to be balanced against the right of every other member in the group with which it is in competition, taken one by one.[36] If the right is outranked at any point by another right, then of course the person who holds the initial right loses. However, when this is not the case, the person's right remains in effect. It does not matter how many others there may be whose lot could be improved; to improve it in this fashion would be unethical.

Therefore, despite inequities inherent in the first-come first-served approach, it is probably the appropriate road to follow, provided that certain conditions are met. We have already pointed out some of these in terms of equality of opportunity of access. The Hall Report and the Lalonde Report, as well as the Canada Health Act take some steps towards enshrining the principle of equality of opportunity into the Canadian health care system. Inequities remain, especially in terms of demographically identifiable variables. However, this does not mean that the approach itself has to be rejected.

Micro-Allocation

Allocation problems at the level of individuals are usually called micro-allocation issues. In a way, they are the most difficult of all. The reason is simple. At this level we are no longer dealing with abstract entities like populations and sub-groups, for example. We are dealing with the individuals who make up these groups. We are dealing directly with persons and on a one-on-one footing. The impact of a particular decision is here as immediate as it is apparent. Such immediacy carries great psychological weight.[37]

Another reason is that unlike allocations that involve groups, the impact of a decision cannot be lessened by shifting it to another area. There is no slack, no sub-choices that could spread the negative effect over a larger base.

Finally, it is at this level that the impact of macro-and meso-allocation becomes apparent. They set the stage, so to speak. Micro-allocation constitutes their focus. Therefore micro-allocation is the final point at which the ethics of the whole allocatory system must prove itself.

However, before going any further, there is something that we should make quite clear. Micro-allocation problems find their basis in the fact that resources are finite. This might give the impression that if macro-allocation decisions were made better, there would be no micro- and no meso-allocation problems. We suggested that is true up to a point, that an appropriate macro-allocation approach should allow for a minimum entitlement of health care services for everyone. However, this does not mean that society can allocate and actually set aside a certain amount of resources like beds or drugs or whatever for each person who would a potential health care consumer. Macro-allocation is based on statistical models. This means that there may be situations where the forecast is inaccurate, or where all potential users will need the facilities and personnel simultaneously. This is especially true about needing personnel. Even if everyone in society became a health care professional, there would still be the possibility that all would need health care services at the same time. We have witnessed such event in past centuries, when plagues swept the world. Therefore, selective allocation at the level of individual persons is an inescapable result of the finitude of society itself.

Furthermore, to set resources aside and hold them ready in anticipation of use would be incredibly wasteful. There are other areas of legitimate social endeavour which also have to be funded. The fact that a society has a rational and ethical allocation policy does not mean that there will be no micro-allocation problems. That is why competition for ward beds, surgery dates and even emergency room services at the micro-level does not necessarily mean that the macro-allocation policies were unacceptable. Competition even for the basic minimum due to everyone is an inescapable reality.

This does not mean that the right to fundamental primary allocation at the individual level is a sham. However, it does mean that allocation criteria at the micro-level must dovetail with the allocation-ethics of the macro-level.

Various criteria have been proposed. One is temporal priority: first come, first served.[38] We already suggested that this has a severe bias in favour of those who are geographically nearer to the centre of services. Even with the best transportation system available, those who live and work in outlying areas will be disadvantaged.[39] It would also favour those who are financially sufficiently well-off to be able to afford the time necessary to access the relevant services. It may not be true for these who cannot afford bay-sitters, or afford to take time off from work.

Another criterion focuses on ethical status. It contends that criminals or other deviants should take second place. As one commentator put it, " ... to assume that there was little to choose between Alexander Fleming and Adolf Hitler ... would be nonsense."[40]

The criterion has its attraction. However, it is not without problems. Pragmatically speaking, it would not resolve micro-allocation conflicts between people who have the same ethical status. Not only that, the clear difference between a Hitler and a Sir Alexander Fleming is not something that we encounter in the ordinary health care setting. The vast majority of people whom we encounter in allocation contexts are not all that distinct from each other.

Furthermore, this criterion assumes that all persons start ethically on the same footing when they are born, and that all people are wholly responsible for their acts. It may be that we do not want to abandon this assumption in the case of Hitler and Sir Alexander Fleming. However, in its generality it can be challenged. Not that there are criminal personalities. Rather, the environmental factors in which people grow up may have a very important influence on shaping their personality and therefore on how they will behave in later years. Therefore, unless we could guarantee in some way that these factors could be taken properly into account, this sort of approach would be unfair.

It would also be unfair in another assumption. It assumes that whoever is convicted as a criminal is in fact a criminal. This is not necessarily true. Miscarriages of justice have occurred. The quality of legal defense available to people plays an important role in this matter. The Canadian justice system assumes that only criminals will be convicted. This assumption is naive.

Reliance on the justice system also assumes that all criminals will be convicted. Again, this is not true. The fact that there are unsolved crimes, including murder, proves it. However, this means that only those who are caught and convicted will be discriminated against by this criterion, and this would violate procedural justice.

Finally, this criterion would turn health services into an instrument of social policy. Health care is concerned with health, not with the administration of criminal justice.

However, having said all that, there is some sense in which we can say that there are ethical differences in the conduct of our lives, and that these differences do have implications for us as right-holders. As we noted in the beginning chapters, rights arise among people by virtue of the context in which they stand to one another. To some extent, the context conditions the nature of the rights that arise.

Included in this context are certain presumptions. One of them is that people will act ethically towards each other and that they will respect each other's rights. The effectiveness with which someone can claim a right therefore depends in part on the degree to which these presuppositions are met. Therefore, in principle, ethical status is an acceptable criterion of discrimination on the micro-level. In practice, however, it is almost impossible to apply. There are rare exceptions. For instance, when it comes to competition between a confessed and convicted murderer and children. But as a general and especially a workable criterion, we should look for some other more easily applicable criterion.

There are other approaches to micro-allocation. For instance, age,[41] likelihood of successful intervention,[42] cost-effectiveness and cost-benefit[43] applied to individual cases,[44] dependence of others on the individual who needs the resources,[45] lottery,[46] life-expectancy as a result of treatment,[47] adverse effects on the individual[48] and so on. We cannot go into all of these here. Instead what we would like to do again is to make some suggestions that take several of the various proposals into account.

Possibility

The first criterion we would like to suggest is possibility. Ethically, the principle of impossibility states that one cannot have an obligation to do what cannot be done. As the law puts it, equity does not require the impossible. Therefore, if it is not possible to do anything for one of the patients, then clearly the other patients should receive the scarce resource.

For instance, suppose that two people are competing for by-pass surgery but one of them is dying of metasticized cancer of the lungs, whereas the other candidate is suffering from moderate obesity on top of the cardiac problem. The purpose of the by-pass operation is to save and extend the life of the patient. It is highly unlikely that it will have this effect in the case of the moribund cancer patient. In fact, given her condition, it is likely she will probably die on the operating table. Therefore, it is really impossible for this allocation to achieve what it is intended to achieve. Consequently she should not have the operation.

However, and there is always a "however," we have to be careful not to understand the notion of possibility too narrowly. It refers only to the expected and intended result of the particular intervention for which there is competition. Therefore although the by-pass surgery would be uncalled for, all of the other health care services that are of a palliative nature and that are appropriate to this sort of situation would definitely be mandated. In fact, not to provide them would be unethical.

Need

Once possibility has been established, need is an appropriate criterion. Need-driven demands take priority over those that are not need-driven. The case of kidney transplants illustrates this rather well. Usually patients on a waiting list for a transplant are allocated points on the basis of such things or quality of antigen match, waiting time for the transplant and sensitization.[49] However,

> If the transplant physician judges another patient more suitable for an available kidney, then he/she may overrule the choice of the point system. For example, a physician could allocate an available kidney to a patient with urgent medical need even if the patient did not have the highest point score.[50]

However, this notion of need has to be handled carefully. When we say that a demand is need-driven we mean that failure to respond to the demand in an appropriate way will lead to an irreparable deterioration in the health status of the individual. This may be clear in the case of a serious infectious disease or of diarrhoea in an infant which, if not treated, would lead to a serious deterioration of health status and possibly even death. These are different from the cleaning out of a stiff elbow joint or the surgical correction of a foot defect. However, it may not be so clear in other cases. For instance, how would one evaluate the psychological damage done to someone's psyche by having to wait a long time for corrective surgery on the foot, or on a deformed arm or nose?

Priority: Life-Saving versus Quality-Enhancing

The criterion of need does not always allow us to distinguish between competing claims. In both cases, failure to respond may result in irreparable harm. Fortunately, however, not all need-driven claims are the same. We can distinguish further between those needs that are life-preserving and those that are quality-enhancing. Quality-enhancing demands are those that would improve the quality of life of the individual if they were met—as for instance cosmetic surgeries like breast enhancement or the repositioning of ears, or orthopaedic surgery to correct an arch malformation, etc. Life-preserving demands are those like the removal of a duodenal atresia or the adminstration of an antibiotic.

Another way of arguing for this criterion is to appeal to the principle of priority. Rights have a presupposition structure. For example, the right to a certain quality of life presupposes for its exercise and fulfilment that the individual whose right it is, is in fact alive. The right to a certain quality of life, therefore, presupposes the right to life as an enabling condition. The right to life is therefore more fundamental. Therefore, if the two rights conflict, for example, the right to cosmetic surgery and the right to a life-saving appendectomy, then all other things being equal,[51] the latter takes priority.

Status: Child versus Adult

Furthermore, we can distinguish between the need-driven claims of children and the claims of all others. The need-driven demands of children take priority over the need-driven claims of all others. This is not reverse discrimination. The reason lies in the fact that society permits children to be borne knowing that children are unable to look out for themselves and knowing that they will have special needs. To bring someone into the world knowing that they have special needs and not to make special arrangements to meet those needs is to injure that person. Therefore, an ethical society commits itself to taking care of those needs. If it is not prepared to do that, it should not have children.[52] In the words of Paul Ramsey, "Utter helplessness demands utter protection." Therefore, all other things being equal, the need-driven claims of children take priority over those of adult members of society. The only exception would be when the survival and welfare af an adult person is necessary in order for the children to receive the relevant services.[53]

Origin: Auto- versus Hetero-Induced

In an article entitled "Patients' Ethical Obligation for their Health," R.C. Sider and C.D. Clements[54] argued that patients have a responsibility to try and maximize their chances for health. If the patients don't, then this would be an ethically relevant difference that serves to distinguish the weight of their claim from that of competing other patients. It is therefore appropriate to take this into account when it comes to micro-allocation. A similar point was made recently by The University of Western Ontario when it issued guidelines for liver transplantation that said that people who are alcoholics and the author of their own need should not have the same ranking for access to liver transplants as other people.

The point of these considerations is that we can then distinguish between needs that are auto-induced and needs that are hetero-induced. Auto-induced needs are the results, if not completely, at least to a large degree, of people's own actions. Implicated here are cases of lung-cancer and heart disease traceable to smoking, severe lacerations, fractures and contusions as a result of not wearing appropriate safety devices when in an automobile, and so on. Hetero-induced needs are needs that arise because of circumstances that are essentially outside of the control of the individual. They include genetically-based diseases like Huntington's Chorea or cystic fibrosis, infectious diseases like rubella, leprosy and malaria when contracted accidentally and despite appropriate precautions. Therefore, what these considerations suggest is that when all else fails, this distinction provides us with a criterion of ranking candidates.

The argument in favour of this criterion focuses on the nature of rights themselves. No right arises in isolation, but in a set of social conditions that determine their nature. One of these conditions is a universal condition for all rights: No-one should deliberately interfere with the legitimate rights of others or bring about conditions that will endanger the exercise of the legitimate rights of others. In auto-induced conditions involving conflict this universal condition is not met. What otherwise would be an effective right therefore becomes ineffective.

In principle, we would agree with this line of reasoning. All other things being equal, auto-induced needs should have a lower priority than hetero-induced needs.[55] Society's resources are limited. Therefore, there is a general duty to use the resources that are available wisely and prudently. Not to use them in this way is to increase the existing shortage, which will interfere with people's ability to receive the services they could otherwise obtain. Anyone who does not take care of their health and then uses the health services that are available puts others at risk. To do so violates the principle of best action and the principle of relevant difference.

Furthermore, it could be argued that if this difference between hetero- and auto-induced was not taken into account, then we would have to give everyone an equal chance.[56] This would mean that those who lived responsibly and did not decrease the amount of resources available by their actions would have no better access to those resources than those who lived irresponsibly and without concern for others. However, this would mean that in effect the responsible and considerate people would be punished for being responsible and considerate, and that irresponsible people would be rewarded. This would violate the principle of equality and justice.

These considerations strike us as persuasive, but not entirely so. It is sometimes difficult to determine whether a health care need is in fact auto-induced. We mentioned the alcoholic's need of a liver. There is beginning to be some evidence that alcoholism is at least in part genetically determined. We do not know how many other diseases this could be said of. We also do not know what weight to attach to a genetic predisposition for a certain disease or addiction and therefore to the need that is caused by it. We do not want to say that therefore this distinction between auto-induced and hetero-induced conditions should not be used at all. On the contrary, as we said, we are persuaded that it is appropriate to use it when all other things are equal. However, we would like to suggest that it should be used with extreme caution.

We would like to sound another note of caution. It concerns what are sometimes called dangerous professions. These are professions like mining, fishing, and logging, for example. They have a statistically higher accident rate and a higher rate of certain diseases than is normal in the population. No one is forced to become a fisherman, a miner or a logger. One could argue that the health care needs that such workers have are auto-induced and therefore fall under this criterion.

We would reject such a proposal, because these professions are socially approved. In fact, without mining, modern medicine would not be possible, and without fishing, it would be impossible for people to follow the cholesterol-reducing diets prescribed by physicians as conducive to a healthy lifestyle. We would therefore say that if a health care need is associated with a lifestyle or profession approved by society or necessary for the survival of society as we know it, then it should not fall under the rubric of auto-induced needs.

It is also important to keep in mind that society condones the use of certain products like alcohol and tobacco which have predictable health-impairing properties. It would therefore be inconsistent for society to permit such use on the one hand, and to accept auto-induced need as reducing the right of access to health care resources on the other.

Lots[57]

The criteria we have sketched will not resolve all micro-allocation conflicts. Sometimes all other things are indeed equal. A good example would be when we are faced with two children who have both been in the same accident and both require immediate attention, and there is no way that we can tell with any degree of certainty which one is a better risk. In situations like this, the only option is to draw lots. Lots assign an equal chance to everyone. That is why they are inappropriate when all other things are not equal. In these cases they discriminate against those who are disadvantaged in some way. However, when all other things are equal, the fact that they assign the same chance to everyone is appropriate. They allow for discrimination while retaining the equality of those concerned. We can put all of this together in the visual decision structure shown in Figure 9–1. The degree of effectiveness of a right is inversely proportional to its position on the ranking tree: the lower down, the more effective. We should also note that as it stands, the tree is incomplete. It ignores the relations that may hold on the right-hand side of the various levels.

FIGURE 9-1
Teleological System

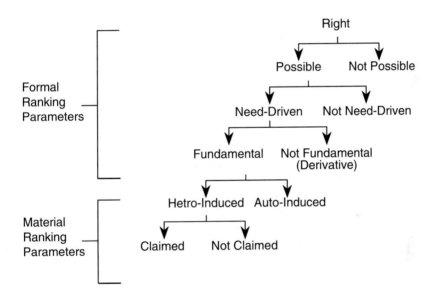

Success

When we began our discussion of macro-allocation we mentioned that success sometimes figures into allocation schemata. The argument is that we sometimes have to choose between giving scarce resources to people who will benefit greatly and people who will benefit only marginally from what we can offer. If we are going to be rational about it, we should really allocate scarce resources to those who will benefit the most.

These success-oriented schemata can be very scientific. They usually involve measuring the degree to which people can be helped. This measure is often expressed in terms of a cost/effectiveness ratio:[58] the ratio between the cost of the procedure or treatment for one group of people as opposed to the cost of treatment and returns for another treatment for another group of people.

One of the objections that traditionally has been raised against the success-oriented approach is that it is very value-laden. The notion depends on how effectiveness is defined. Effectiveness varies, depending on whether it is defined in terms of ability to work, life satisfaction, prolonged life, improvement over previous health status, or whatever. In recent years, some of the uncertainty and subjectivity has been removed by the introduction of the notion of QUALY's.[59] The term is an acronym for Quality Adjusted Life Years. QUALY is an attempt to assign a numerical value to an intervention by calculating the number of life years gained by the intervention compared with the quality of that life and the cost of the intervention itself.

One of the primary concerns with this sort of approach was that it is highly subjective in terms of quality-of-life determination. The use of standardized quality-of-life measures certainly removes a great deal of that subjectivity. However, this raises a special problem all its own. The instruments that are designed to give these numerical and objective data about quality-of-life do not and cannot capture the quality-of-life perception of the individual person. However, the quality instruments have to be standardized, otherwise the notion of a QUALY is useless. In other words, the notion of quality has to be statistical. Unfortunately, the individual person is not a statistical entity. Therefore quality-of-life is a highly subjective notion that may involve qualitative parameters not shared by anyone else. That is why we said that the concept cannot capture quality-of-life considerations on the micro-level. This of course means that the QUALY approach is here useless. In a sense, it would violate the principle of respect for persons.

But there is also another reason why we view QUALY's with suspicion. Our misgivings center on the very use of the concept itself. If we step back and look at the rationale for using the concept, we notice that it is based on the ethically rather dubious premise that producing a higher quality-of-life ratio over a greater number of years is more worthy of help than producing a lower ratio. When we translate this into more concrete terms, it means that a bigger aggregate bang is ethically better. However, in order to accept that premise we would have to abandon equality and respect for persons and accept the premise that we can calculate the ethical worth of people by evaluating the temporal segments of their lives in qualitative terms and summing the total. This would mean that we would have to abandon the premise that persons are beings of incommensurable value. We would have to abandon our conviction that rights cannot be defined in terms of outcomes, and that they cannot be expressed in arithmetic terms. We are not prepared to give up these premises. We are not prepared to say that a person's right to health care lapses because someone else can be helped more. Abraham Lincoln put it well: "You say your skin is whiter than his? Take care, that you do not become the slave of the next man you meet whose skin is lighter than yours."

Extent

What we have sketched has focused on access: Who shall have when not all can have? However, that is only part of the question. The other is, "How *long* shall someone have when not all can have?" In other words, we have not yet dealt with, the question of extent. This may be called the question of limit.

Contemporary discussions have not really addressed, let alone dealt with, the subject. The subject is important because the mere fact that a micro-allocation is appropriate at one point in time does not mean that its appropriateness, or for that matter its ethical defensibility, is settled for all time. We only have to look at people like Elaine Esposito or Karen Ann Quinlan, who for years were in a permanent vegetative coma, to see the point. The fact that it was appropriate to provide them with scarce resources on a micro-allocation basis in the beginning does not mean that we had an obligation to continue.

Our reasoning, therefore, could be summed up like this:

1. Each individual who has legitimate access to health care services is entitled, *prima facie,* to a basic allocation as determined in the primary macro-allocation.

2. Greater-than-average allocation is warranted if and only if the health status of the individual is correctably lower than the health status of the average member of society or otherwise falls into an allocation rubric covered by secondary macro-allocation.

3. However, greater-than-average allocation under any rubric is acceptable if and only if it does not lower (or is not reasonably expected to lower) the health status attained by other persons on a standard allocation within that rubric.

4. The special allocation must be (reasonably expected to be) effective in producing an improvement or at least retaining the status quo.

5. The special allocation must be reviewed at appropriate intervals.

The real thrust, of course, lies in point five. Each allocation at the micro-level has to be reviewed as and when the situation changes. This includes the diagnosis as well as the prognosis. If there is a scarcity of resources, then the allocation has to be reviewed in terms of the various micro-allocation criteria that we suggested. Otherwise, we would suggest that points one to five provide the beginnings of a schema.

Non-Validated and Experimental Therapies

We have tried to sketch the outline of an ethics of discrimination in the field of health care. What have tried to do is show that discrimination is not only appropriate but necessary, lest justice and fairness fail. We would like to conclude with a brief word about non-validated and experimental procedures.

Most non-validated and experimental therapies or treatment regimens are very expensive; particularly in such high profile areas as transplantation, artificial organ developments and therapies designed for those who are immuno-suppressed. People who benefit from such treatment have a special need.[60] Therefore, if we follow the schema above, their need should be approached from the perspective of secondary macro-allocation. This does not mean that the individual themselves and their group are invariably at a disadvantage. Their *prima facie* status will be the same as that of any other claimant. However, the health profile of society, its socio-economic position and its health care sophistication will become important considerations. Therefore, we cannot automatically presume that simply because these relevant treatments are possible *per se*, therefore they should be available as a matter of right. Not even the fact of feasibility as such will be ethically determining. Even here, what is central is the interplay of personal rights in the overall context of society as a whole.

Conclusion

Canadian society assumes that access, just and equitable access, to an appropriate level of health care is a matter of right. However, like any other right, this one also has limits. The limits lie in the finite nature of social resources and in the sheer inability to provide everyone with everything that they might have in an ideal world. This world is not ideal, at least not in that sense, and it never will be. This world has limits. And given that it has limits, we have to find some way to allocate in a just and equitable fashion the finite resources that are at our disposal. Any such allocation will disadvantage someone; but that is not really the issue. The issue is, whether the fact of comparative disadvantage amounts to unethical discrimination. It is all too easy to lose sight of that fact that what is experienced as a disadvantage, either at first hand or by considering the plight of others, may be strongly coloured by the psychology of our experience. The phenomenon of the identified victim is a powerful force in the politics of health resource allocation. However, it would ultimately be to everyone's disadvantage if a perception that has its roots in the psychology of experience were to govern a process that should really be determined by considerations of ethics.

ENDNOTES

[1] See F.T. Denton and B.G. Spencer, "Population Aging and the Economy: Some Issues in Resource Allocation" in J.E. Thornton and E.R. Winkler, *Ethics and Aging: The Right to Live and the Right to Die* (Vancouver: UBC Press, 1988) 98–123. For a somewhat contrary view, see Evans R., "Hang Together, or Hang Separately: Universal Health Care in the Year 2000," *Health Care for the Elderly in the Year 2000: Symposium Proceedings* (B.C. Ministry of Health: Victoria, 1986).

[2] This difficulty is inherent in the distribution of powers in the Canadian federal system, dating back to the British North-America Act of 1867.

[3] Quebec is an exception.

[4] See Canada Health Act Sections 7–20, especially s.20: " 20. (1) where a province fails to comply with the condition set out in section 18, there shall be deducted from the cash contribution to the province for a fiscal year an amount the Minister, on the basis of information provided in accordance with the regulations, determines to have been charged through extra-billing by medical practitioners or dentists in the province in that fiscal year or, where information is not provided in accordance with the regulations, an amount that the Minister estimates to have been charged."

[5] What follows is based on an invited seminar to the Treasury Board of the Province of British Columbia, 1987. A revised version of it was presented at the 8th Biennial Conference of the North-East Canadian-American Health Council (Danvers, Mass., April 26–28, 1990).

[6] See Thomas McKeown and C.R. Lowe, *An Introduction to Social Medicine* 2d ed. (Oxford: Blackwell, 1974); and Thomas McKeown, *The Role of Medicine: Dream, Mirage or Nemesis?* 2d ed. (Oxford: Blackwell, 1979).

[7] See Robert Veatch, "Who Should Pay for Smokers' Medical Care?" *Hastings Center Report*, 4 (Nov.1974), 8–9.

[8] Janet Storch, *Patients' Rights, Ethical and Legal Issues in Health Care and Nursing* (Toronto: McGraw-Hill, 1984), 122.

[9] Veatch, ref. note 7, 9.

[10] Gene Outka, "Social Justice and Equal Access to Health Care," reprinted in T.A. Mappes and J.S. Zembaty, *Biomedical Ethics* (New York and St. Louis: McGraw-Hill, 1981).

[11] Outka, ref. note 10, 530.

[12] Outka, ref. note 10, 535.

[13] Ottawa, Queen's Printer, 1964.

[14] Ottawa, Queen's Printer, 1974.

[15] Cost/benefit analysis assigns numerical coefficients to the costs for a given treatment modality and to the financial benefits to society of the outcomes, and then compares the different modalities relative to each other. For a good discussion, see Michael Drummond, "Guidelines for Health Technology Assessment: Economic Evaluation," in David Feeny, Gordon Guyatt and Peter Tugwell, eds., *Health Care Technology: Effectiveness, Efficiency and Public Policy* (Montreal: Institute for Research on Public Policy, 1986).

[16] Cost/effectiveness analysis compares numerical coefficients assigned to costs as opposed to the amounts of resources (money) saved for comparable forms of treatment. For several good discussions, see M.F. Drummond, *Principles of Economic Appraisal in Health Care*, (Oxford: Oxford Medical Publications, 1980); R. Sugden and A. Williams, *The Principles of Practical Cost-Benefit Analysis* (Oxford: Oxford University Press, 1978); H.E. Klarman, J.O. Francis, G.D. Rosenthal, "Cost-Effectiveness and Analysis Applied to the Treatment of Chronic Renal Disease," *Medical Care* 6 (1968) 48–54; Norman Daniels, *Just Health Care*, (Cambridge and London: Cambridge University Press, 1985).

[17] QUALY's or Quality Adjusted Life Years calculations assign numerical coefficients to quality-of-life evaluations and compare them to the cost involved in bringing about the extended life-span. See Feeny, ref. note 15, for several good discussions from an economic perspective.

[18] Drummond, ref. note 16.

[19] Average, because society cannot be expected to provide, as a matter of course, extra ordinary allocations in the first instance. No one has a right to be treated as unusual unless there is a case for it (principle of relevant difference).

[20] In technical terms, this is called a horizontal one-many allocation dilemma.

[21] These figures were offered by the British Columbia Ministry of Health in response to questions from the author.

[22] Based on the case of Baby M.

[23] See Rescher, full ref. in note 24, below.

[24] For a discussion of this and other proposals, see Nicholas Rescher, "The Allocation of Exotic Medical Lifesaving Therapy," *Ethics* 79: 3 (April 1969) 174–186. Although somewhat dated, this is a classic discussion.

[25] See Paul Ramsey, *The Patient as Person* (New Haven and London: Yale Univ. Press, 1970); see Rachels, ref. note 46.

[26] See Daniels, ref. note 16 above.

[27] See President's Commission for the Study of Ethical Problems in Medicine and Biomedical and Behavioral Research, *Securing Access to Health Care* (Washington, D.C.: U.S. Government Printing Office, 1983) 3 vols., vol 1 chapters 1 and 2.

[28] Those who have a language barrier will not be able to access the queue easily. This is particularly important in the multicultural context of Canadian society.

[29] See Diana Crane, *The Sanctity of Social Life: Physicians' Treatment of Critically Ill Patients* (New York: Russell Sage Foundation, 1975) Part I, chapters 3 to 5, with respect to treatment options considered appropriate for mentally handicapped.

[30] Thomas Schelling, "The Life You Save May be Your Own," *Problems in Public Expenditure Analysis* edited by S.B. Chase, Jr. (Washington, D.C.: The Brookings Institute, 1966) 127–166.

[31] See E.H.W. Kluge, "Designated Organ Donation: Private Choice in Social Context," *Hastings Center Report* September/October 1989, 10–15 for similar considerations.

[32] See President's Commission, *Securing Access*, vol. I, ref. note 27.

[33] This case is based on a series of cases from St. ... Hospital in London, England.

[34] We have not discussed allocation on the basis of age, since it is almost universally recognized that age *per se* is an ethically indefensible criterion of allocation. For more on this, see Thornton and Winkler, *Ethics and Aging*, and Report of the Council on Ethical and Judicial Affairs of the American Medical Association, *Ethical Implications of Age-Based Rationing of Health Care* (Chicago, Ill.: American Medical Association, 1988) I–88.

[35] With due alteration of detail, a similar situation holds at the macro-level. The answer there is analogous to the one sketched here.

[36] For a judicial recognition of this and a rejection of a utilitarian approach to individual rights, see the comments of Mr. Justice Dickson in *R. vs Perka et al.* (1982), 69 C.C.C. (2d) 405 (B.C.C.A.).

[37] This is sometimes called the problem of the identified versus the general victim.

[38] See Elizabeth Anscombe, "Who Is Wronged?" *The Oxford Review* 5 (1967) 16–17.

[39] Since farmers and other primary production workers are affected, and since these are essential to the survival of society itself, their position cannot be dismissed as being a predictable outcome of a deliberate choice. Society here has a special obligation. Professional mountaineers, however, would differ radically. Compare *Securing Access*, vol. I. (ref. note 27).

[40] See F.M. Parsons, "Selection of Patients for Haemodialysis," *British Medical Journal*. (March 11, 1967 622–624). Rescher, (see note 24 above) seems to involve something like this in what he calls the "retrospective service" factor.

[41] This is used in the U.K. in the forms of guidelines for access to transplantation.

[42] Rescher, (see note 24 above).

[43] This is reflected in David Feeny, Gordon Guyatt and Peter Tugwell, eds., *Health Care Technology: Effectiveness, Efficiency and Public Policy*, (Montreal: Institute for Research on Public Policy, 1986); and Parsons, note 40 above, 623, who maintains that in selecting patients "gainful employment in a well-chosen occupation is necessary to achieve the best results [since] only the minority wish to live on charity."

[44] Robert Young, "Some Criteria for Making Decisions Concerning the Distribution of Scarce Medical Resources," *Theory and Decision* 6 (1975) 439–455.

[45] Young, ref. note 44 above.

[46] Paul Ramsey, *The Patient as Persons* (New Haven and London: Yale University Press, 1970) 252–259; James F. Rachels, "Who Shall Live when Not All Can Live?" *Soundings: An Interdisciplinary Journal* 53 (Winter, 1970) 339–355.

[47] Nicholas Rescher, "The Allocation of Exotic Medical Lifesaving Therapy," *Ethics* 79 (1969) 173–180.

[48] See Feeny, Guyatt and Tugwell, ref. in note 43 above, 190.

[49] P. Singer, "A Review of Public Policies to Procure and Distribute Kidneys for Transplantation," *Archives of Internal Medicine* 150: 3 (March 1990) 523–527, 525–6.

[50] Singer, ref. note 49 above, 526.

[51] We are here assuming the proposed cosmetic surgery is not intended to correct a suicidal tendency that derives from hideous disfigurement, etc.

[52] The reason for this will be discussed in more detail in Chapter 12 when we consider the right to have children and corresponding duties.

[53] A version of this principle was explicitly stated in the U.S. case of *U.S. vs. Holmes* (1842), 1 Wall Jr. 1, where the court asserted the position that in life-boat situations some of the crew might take priority over some of the passengers if the survival of the passengers depended on there being some crew members to man the lifeboats.

[54] *Journal of Medical Ethics* 10: 142. (1984); See also Veatch, ref. in the bibliography to this chapter.

[55] We presume, of course, reasonable care having been taken by the individuals in the performance of their jobs, etc.

[56] All other things being equal, of course. However, that may not always be true.

[57] See pp. 218 for a variation on this in terms of first-come, first-served. The first-come, first-served approach differs from a general lottery approach because the socio-economic and demographic variables that determine access to a health care facility are inherently discriminatory.

[58] See Feeny, Guyatt and Tugwell, ref. note 59 below.

[59] See Kathryn Bennett and David Feeny, "Clinical And Economic Evaluation of Therapeutic Technologies: The Case of Neonatal Intensive Care Programs," in D. Feeny, G. Guyatt and P. Tugwell, eds., *Health Care Technology: Effectiveness, Efficiency and Public Policy* (Montreal: Institute for Research on Public Policy, 1986) 199–223.

[60] See Benjamin Freedman, and others, ref. in the biblography to this chapter.

SUGGESTED READINGS

- Bell, Nora K. "The Scarcity of Medical Resources: Are There Rights to Health Care? " *Journal of Medicine and Philosophy* 4: 2(1979) 158–169.

  Bell's article is one of the earliest articles in the U.S. advocating a position opposed to that of Sade. However, she does not go as far as Lalonde, and therefore provides an interesting contrast to the latter's position.

- Daniels, Norman. *Just Health Care.* (Cambridge and London: Cambridge University Press, 1985, 115–139.

- Drummond, Michael. "Guidelines for Health Technology Assessment: Economic Evaluation," in D.Feeny, Gordon Guyatt and Peter Tugwell, eds., *Health Care Technology: Effectiveness, Efficiency and Public Policy.* Montreal: Institute for Research on Public Policy, 1986, 107–128.

  Drummond, a prominent Canadian health care economist, looks at the problem of allocation of resources from the perspective of quality control and technology assessment. This selection complements that by Evans in that it deals with the question of what resources should be mad available under what conditions, whereas Evans focuses on the question of who should have the resources.

- Evans, Robert. "Hang Together, or Hang Separately: Universal Health Care in the Year 2000," from *Health Care For the Elderly in the Year 2000: Symposium Proceedings*. Victoria: B.C. Ministry of Health, 1986.

  The percentage of elderly in Canada is increasing. This presents allocation problems, because it appears that the elderly consume a disproportionate amount of health care resources in the last years of their life. This article is a look by one of the foremost Canadian health care economists at the issues of resource allocation for the elderly. Evans contends that properly managed, there need not be an allocation problem.

- Freedman, Benjamin and the McGill/Boston Research Group. "Nonvalidated Therapies and HIV Disease," *Hastings Center Report* 19: 3 (June 1989)14–20.

  Although this article focuses on access to treatment for HIV disease, it deals with the much more general issue under what circumstances scarce resources should be used to provide therapies that have not [yet] been shown to be effective in Drummond's sense.

- Ingelfinger, Franz. "Haves and Have-Nots in the World of Disease," *The New England Journal of Medicine* 287(Dec.7, 1972) 1198–1199.

  This is one of the earlier articles from the U.S. context dealing with the effects of a two-tier health care system. The perspective is that of a physician.

- Kluge, Eike-Henner W. "The Calculus of Discrimination: Discriminatory Resource Allocation for an Aging Population," from Thornton and Winkler, full ref. in note 34, 84–97.

  Kluge addresses the question of criteria of allocation for special groups. Although focused on the aged, the issue itself is a very general one.

- Lalonde, Marc. "The Health Field Concept and Strategies for the Future," from Marc Lalonde, *A New Perspective on the Health of Canadians*. Ottawa: Information Canada, 1974, 26–37, 55–72.

  This selection is from the position paper of the Liberal Government on the delivery of health care for Canada. It was a modification of the proposals of Mr. Justice E. Hall in the Hall Report ten years earlier. While it still accepted the idea of a right to health care, it limited it to the notion of a universal right of equitable opportunity of access to health care.

- President's Commission for the Study of Ethical Problems in Medicine and Biomedical and Behavioral Research. *Securing Access to Health Care*. Washington: U.S. Government Printing Office, 1983, vol.1–3.

  This three-volume study by the President's Commission constitutes a turning point in U.S. government perception on the right to health care, in that it is the beginning of a development in the direction of the Canadian system: a development that is still going on. The last two volumes contain articles by most of the prominent health care economist and ethicists concerned with the theory and practice of selective allocation of resources in health care.

- Sade, Robert M. "Medical Care as a Right: A Refutation," *New England Journal of Medicine* 285: 23 (Dec.2, 1971) 1288–92.

    Sade, a physician, rejects the idea of a natural right to health care. He points out what he considers to be some unacceptable consequences if such a right were to be granted as a matter of social policy. He is especially concerned about the impact this would have on the position of physicians as professionals and on the physician/patient relationship.

- Veatch, R.M. "Voluntary Risk to Health: The Ethical Issues," *Journal of the American Medical Association* 243 (Jan.4, 1980) 50–55.

    Veatch, one of the most prominent contemporary ethicists in the U.S., addresses the question of the relationship between the right to health care and the responsibility of individual health care consumers for their own health.

10

The Ethics of Deliberate Death: Euthanasia

The aim of this chapter is to clarify the notion of deliberate death with particular focus on euthanasia. Having read this chapter, you should be aware of the distinctions that are sometimes drawn between active and passive euthanasia, have formulated a perspective on the ethical tenability of these distinctions; and in general terms be able to present and defend a position on the subject of deliberate death.

The following questions should be kept in mind:

1. What is the problem of euthanasia? How does a "living" will fit into this?
2. Is there a difference between active and passive euthanasia? Can you give a brief evaluation of the ethical tenability of the distinction?
3. What is the difference between direct and indirect euthanasia, and how could the distinction be defended from an ethical perspective?
4. What is meant by the distinction between ordinary and extraordinary means of saving/sustaining life? Is there ever a use for the distinction?
5. Is it ethically acceptable to let "nature take its course?" Does the answer depend on whether you accept a deontological ethical framework or a utilitarian framework?
6. Is there a place for the notion of quality of life in decisions surrounding the question of deliberate death?
7. Sketch and evaluate several arguments in favour of (against) euthanasia. Which do you accept? Why? Defend your position in terms of the general ethical framework you adopt generally.

Introduction

Is it ever ethically acceptable for a physician to bring about the death of a patient deliberately?

The immediate reaction is to answer no. It is never an option for the physician. The nature and tradition of medicine, after all, is to save life, not to take it. Nor is this tradition new, something that has entered the profession only in recent times. The Hippocratic Oath contains an injunction against deliberately causing the death of a patient,[1] and the prohibition is repeated in every other medical code of ethics since then. *The Code of Ethics of the Canadian Medical Association* expresses it in the following way: "Consider first the well-being of the patient."[2] This position is usually interpreted as meaning that the active and deliberate termination of the life of a patient is ethically unacceptable. Nor is the Canadian Medical Association alone in holding this position. The Royal College of Physicians and Surgeons has also rejected the concept of active euthanasia, and most Canadian medical commentators agree that, at the very least, it is illegal.[3] In the United States, as early as 1973, the House of Delegates of the American Medical Association adopted the following statement:

> The intentional termination of the life of one human being by another—mercy killing—is contrary to that for which the medical profession stands ... [4]

The AMA has reiterated this position on various occasions.[5]

Organized Canadian medicine is therefore not alone in adopting this prohibitive stance. Furthermore, quite aside from any professional considerations, it seems obvious that deliberately bringing about the death of a human being is murder. The *Criminal Code of Canada* leaves little doubt on that score. Section 222 reads as follows:

> 222. (1) A person commits homicide when, directly or indirectly by any means, he causes the death of a human being.
> (2) Homicide is culpable or not culpable.
> (3) Culpable homicide is murder or manslaughter or infanticide.
> 224. Where a person, by an act or omission, does anything that results in the death of a human being, he causes the death of that human being notwithstanding the death of that human being might have been prevented by resorting to proper means.

Furthermore, neither that fact that a person has consented to or even requested that he or she be killed, or that he or she be allowed to die, would exonerate the physician (or for that matter, anyone else). For, as the *Criminal Code* puts it,

> No person is entitled to consent to have death inflicted upon him, and such consent does not affect the criminal responsibilities of any person by whom death may be inflicted upon the person by whom consent is given.[6]

It would therefore seem that the physician may never be an agent of deliberate death.

Some Considerations

The reality of medical practice, however, is rarely as simple and as neat as tradition and the law would have us believe. For instance, what about abortion? Abortion is countenanced as acceptable both by the *Criminal Code* as well as the medical profession. Yet clearly, whatever else may be true about it, and we shall deal with the subject a bit more fully later, abortion is the deliberate taking of a human life. Or, what about situations where both physician and patient agree that it is better that all life-saving and/or sustaining efforts cease and the patient be allowed to die? That happens not infrequently. Isn't there an ethical difference between this and actively bringing about the patient's death? Surely there is a difference between the following two cases:

> (a) J.B. had been diagnosed as having AIDS some three years ago, and right from the very beginning, the disease had taken a very rapid course. Opportunistic infection followed opportunistic infection and beset J.B.—until finally he had contracted Kaposi's sarcoma. J.B. was tired of fighting what he knew, or at least what he believed, was a final and irrevocable death sentence. He had made peace with his circle of friends, and come to terms with his own increasing deterioration. As he put it to them, and to his physician, appearance and style had always meant a great deal to him. He would rather die while he still was *compos mentis* and had at least the semblance of the appearance that he had when he was healthy than battle the disease still further and ultimately die an unrecognizable and demented wreck. He therefore asked his physician to desist from further efforts, to simply keep him comfortable—and to let him die.

> (b) M.Q., a former comptroller for a large oil company, suffered from Alzheimer's disease, a progressive and irreversible neurological disorder of unknown etiology involving among other things severe impairment of the cognitive functions, memory and other thought processes due to loss of brain cells. M.Q. had lucid periods. During those periods she stated very emphatically and very clearly to her physician and to her next-of-kin that she did not wish the disease to run its full course in her, but that when it seemed certain that she had reached such a state of cognitive deficit that she would probably not function at any appreciably coherent and sapient cognitive level, she be given an injection and allowed to die. As she put it, she simply did not consider such a life worthy of the term "human"; she found it degrading and humiliating, and would rather be dead.[7]

The two cases are of course quite different. In the first, the physician is not being asked to be the direct and active agent of death. Instead, the request is to refrain from any further action that might prolong the length of a process that in many ways could be compared to a protracted way of dying. This sort of stance is clearly allowed for by clause 18 of the *Code of Ethics of the Canadian Medical Association:* An ethical physician "will allow death to occur with dignity and comfort when death of the body appears to be inevitable."

Furthermore, if J.B. is competent, the ethics of informed consent require that his wishes be honoured by the physician. These ethical considerations even have legal bite—as the old Alberta case of *Mulloy vs. HopSang*[8] and the more recent Ontario case of *Malette vs. Shulman*[9] illustrate only too well.

The second case, however, appears to be fundamentally different. Here the physician is not being asked to allow nature to take its course. Instead, she is asked to become the immediate and active agent of death. This, however, is murder by any definition, and therefore is ruled out absolutely.

The difference between the two sorts of cases, therefore, seems clear. It is one thing to stand back passively at the request of a competent patient and allow death to occur; it is another thing entirely actively to bring about that death.

However, this distinction has also been challenged. For instance, it has also been argued that to see the two as different is to fall prey to an illusion. The difference between an active and a passive stance, so it is said, is merely one of perspective. Ultimately it has not ethical but only psychological significance.[10] Furthermore, some Canadian physicians have suggested that irrespective of what one may think about the cogency of the active-passive distinction, the physicians do have a duty to honour the request of their competent patients, even in situations like that illustrated by case (b). As Dr. Gifford-Jones put it in a recent article entitled, "It's Time to Legalize Euthanasia," in which he compared the Dutch permissiveness of active euthanasia as practised by physicians and the Canadian medical perspective:

> I'm ... sure Canadian physicians will find a host of moral, ethical and religious reasons to damn such active euthanasia. Some would agree with it in the privacy of the doctors' lounge. But publicly they will not have the courage to say so.
>
> Current attitudes on ethical issues in this country worry me and they should concern others who believe in personal privacy and freedom of choice. I'm tired of listening to moralists who believe they have a profound understanding that the rest of us don't. And that their moral code, having the stamp of the Almighty, is beyond reproach.
>
> It's time to say, "You have the right to die any way you wish, and I demand the same unrestricted freedom."[11]

Dr. Gifford-Jones is not alone in holding this position, even when we turn to the public. A recent Gallup poll across Canada shows that 77% of Canadian answered positively to the question,

> When a person has an incurable disease that causes suffering, do you think that competent doctors should be allowed by law to end the patient's life through mercy killing if the patient has made a formal request in writing?[12]

The same opinion is expressed, albeit in a somewhat more mitigated form, by 10 of 12 authors of an article entitled "The Physician's Responsibility toward Hopelessly Ill Patients: A Second Look," which appeared recently in a 1989 issue of *The New England Journal of Medicine*.[13] In that article the authors maintain that while appropriate palliative care should always be the treatment of choice, there may be occasions where the physician should assist the patient in committing suicide with appropriate medication. While the physicians should not be an active participant, he or she should definitely not refuse appropriate help. That position is also shared by a judge in California, who was involved as a concurring judge in the Bovia case. He argued that a patient has the right to enlist the help of a physician to make death as swift and painless as possible.[14]

In the eyes of Dr. Gifford-Jones and those who think like him, the fact that a competent patient has made an informed request would exculpate the physician from whatever blame would otherwise attach to the relevant act. Dutch physicians apparently feel likewise. Although the Netherlands has not officially legalized active euthanasia under such circumstances, the authorities have gradually adopted a relaxed attitude towards physician involvement in the area, so that at present approximately 5,000 people a year die in Dutch hospitals under these circumstances.[15] In fact, those who hold this position go further. They maintain that a request by a competent patient imposes a duty on the physician to perform the required act—the letter of the law and the clauses of the CMA Code of Ethics notwithstanding.

In fact, the argument has been carried still further. It has been argued that incompetent patients must not be treated differently from the way in which competent patients are treated. That would amount to discrimination on the basis of handicap: something that is not only ethically indefensible, but also is prohibited by Section X of the *Charter of Rights and Freedoms*. Therefore, with due alteration of detail the option of deliberate death should be open to the incompetent as well: for example: to radically defective neonates, the mentally severely retarded, and brain-damaged patients.[16] Of course, incompetent persons cannot make decisions for themselves. Surrogate decision-makers have to be appointed to exercise their right of decision-making for them. However, it would be unethical to limit the choices open to these surrogate decision-makers in a way in which they are not limited for competent persons. To do so would make a mockery of the notion of surrogacy itself. The option of deliberate death must be an option that the surrogate decision-makers may seriously consider as and when it becomes appropriate. There must not be any preconceived position that deliberate death may not be an option. The principle of equality demands it.

Finally, it has also been suggested that the prohibition against actively taking a human life is not really a fundamental value in our society. It is not accepted fully either by the medical profession or the law. After all, as we have already mentioned, physicians do perform abortions, and doing so is not thought unethical by the profession. The position statement on abortion by the Canadian Medical Association makes this very clear.[17] It is ethically permissible for a physician to perform an abortion, which is defined as the deliberate termination of a human pregnancy prior to 20 weeks gestation, or up until that time has been reached.

As to the law, even though the Sections of the *Criminal Code* which had controlled abortion have been struck down by the Supreme Court of Canada in the case of *Morgentaler vs. the Queen*,[18] these sections were not struck down because the Supreme Court thought that killing human fetuses was unacceptable. On the contrary; the acceptability of killing fetuses was never really questioned in the majority judgement. Instead, the main reason for striking down these sections was that they contained provisions which prevented Canadian women in general from having equal access to abortion itself.[19] In other words, the Sections were struck down not to prevent abortions but to equalize their availability. If we had to identify an ethical reason for striking them down we would have to say that it was the principle of equality and justice as applied to Canadian women, not some concern over human life.

The issue of deliberate death, therefore, is not quite as decided or even as clear as it may have seemed at the outset. All of this could be ignored and dismissed as theoretical logic-chopping were it not for the fact that, sooner or later, most physicians come face-to-face with the issue of deliberate death in their practice. This may happen when they contemplate allowing death to occur, or in situations where the patient requests death, or in situations that involve accelerating death in some deliberate fashion. None of this is any longer unusual.[20] It therefore seems appropriate to discuss the issue of deliberate death more fully. However, we shall not address the topic in its full ramifications. Instead, our focus will be euthanasia alone. We shall deal with abortion later.

Nor shall we consider infanticide as a separate issue. As will become clear from what follows, infanticide is a special name given to the deliberate killing of neonates. In its usual sense, it is nothing more than euthanasia in the paediatric context. However, this context is importantly different from the usual sort of situation in which the issue of euthanasia is raised. In the usual setting the person who is euthanatized is someone who has been competent, who has had the ability to form preferences, likes and dislikes; to acquire values and to live according to them. None of this is the case with neonates. Neonates are like congenitally incompetent persons in that they have never been competent. They have never had the opportunity to form, let alone express, preferences in any sapient cognitive fashion. (In some cases they also don't have the capacity.) Therefore, (in the case of infanticide) the usual arguments that are based on an assumption of prior autonomy do not apply. The subject of infanticide is so difficult that it deserves separate discussion, which we have provided elsewhere.[21] Here we can only indicate some general guidelines. As we said in our introductory discussion at the beginning of this book, ethical rules and principles must be the same for all persons. Therefore, to treat infants differently, merely because they are infants, would violate the principle of equality, and discriminate against infant persons solely because of their age. Whatever conclusion we reach with respect to non-paediatric persons must be applicable to infants as well—with the alteration of detail that is required because of the inherently non-competent nature of the neonates. Our previous discussion of proxy decision-making in Chapter 6 will give some indication of how such an adjustment should proceed.

We shall also not consider suicide separately or to any great extent. Suicide is not a crime.[22] More important than that, the principle of autonomy entails that unless there is a psychiatric or other relevant condition that interferes with competence and autonomy, every person has the right to do with his or her life as he or she pleases—including the right to end it. But we shall say more about that presently.

Euthanasia

The word "euthanasia" is of Greek origin. Originally it signified a good, easy or honourable death.[23] In the last few decades, however, it has come to be used with a variety of different meanings. For instance, it has been used to describe a "quick and easy death,"[24] the "failure to supply ordinary means" to save or sustain human life,"[25] as well as simply what has been called "mercy killing,"[26] to mention but a few of the terms associated with it.

Instead of debating the historical accuracy of these definitions or the acceptability of a particular usage, let us agree that for present purposes we shall simply use the term to mean the bringing about of the painless death of a person suffering from an incurable and distressing condition or disease.[27] Nothing is said in this definition about imminent death or life-threatening situations. This may seem astonishing; but, the reasons for this omission will become clear as we continue.

Ordinary versus Extraordinary

Let us begin our discussion with the distinction between what are called ordinary and extraordinary means respectively. Such a distinction is not entirely new. It underlies the traditional contention that even from a medical standpoint it is not always in the patient's best interest to save and/or sustain his life. The quality of the life that may be saved may be so low, the type of existence so filled with nausea, pain and general suffering, and the lack of human potential and interaction so great that even when weighed in the balance of best interest, continued life is found wanting.[28] However, the distinction between ordinary and extraordinary means, attained to international prominence when in 1957, Pope Pius XII, in an address to an international congress of anaesthesiologist, asserted:

> Natural reason and Christian morals say that man (and whoever is entrusted with the task of taking care of his fellow man) has the right and duty in the case of serious illness to take the necessary treatment for the preservation of life and health ... But morally, one is held to use only ordinary means—according to the circumstances of persons, places, times and cultures—that is to say, means that do not involve any grave burdens for oneself or another. A more strict obligation would be too burdensome for most men and would render the attainment of a higher, more important good too difficult.[29]

The same position was reiterated in 1980 by the Sacred Congregation for Doctrine of Faith:

> It is ... permissable to make do with the normal means that medicine can offer. Therefore, one cannot impose on anyone the obligation of having recourse to a technique which is already in use but which carries a risk or is burdensome. Such a refusal ... should be considered as an acceptance of the human condition or a

wish to avoid the application of a medical procedure disproportionate to the results that can be expected, or a desire not to impose excessive expense on the family or the community.[30]

Since then, in one form or another, the distinction has entered almost every discussion of deliberate death. Its primary use has been to draw a line between acceptable and unacceptable forms of permissible death.

Despite its widespread usage, the distinction has met with some opposition. For instance, it has been suggested that both the definition itself as well as the reasoning surrounding it are nonsensical and useless, because one simply cannot distinguish between medical procedures and regimens in this fashion. Whether a particular practice is ordinary or not is not something that is inherent in the technique or procedure itself. Instead, it depends on the context in which it is practised or proposed. So, for example, an appendectomy under primitive conditions, in a yurt in Outer Mongolia perhaps, would definitely have be considered extraordinary treatment, whereas in a well-equipped Parisian hospital it would be quite ordinary. Likewise, a corneal transplant would be ordinary for an otherwise healthy nine-year-old child, whereas the same procedure for a nonagenarian suffering from the last stages of Parkinson's disease would be an extraordinary procedure; and so on. In other words, it has been argued that the very relativity of the ordinary-extraordinary distinction makes it ethically useless.[31] It lacks sufficient provision to be applicable in an objective fashion.

However, such a critique is short-sighted. In fact, it commits what could be called the fallacy of isolation. That is to say, it makes the mistake of trying to evaluate the ethical nature of a decision, or course of action, independently of the context in which that decision or action takes place. This is a mistake because not only the ethical status of the act, but indeed its very nature as an act, is always context-dependent.

An example will make this clear. The act of injecting a narcotic analgesic into a patient is an assault when done against the wishes of a competent patient even though he or she may be in excruciating agony. On the other hand, it is an act of good health care and acceptable palliative practice when it is done with the patient's informed consent. Or, to take another example, the act of amputating a gangrenous right hand is good medicine when it is performed with the consent of the patient; but it is assault and battery when it is done against his expressed wishes—as Dr Mulloy found out to his regret in the Alberta Court of Appeals case of *Mulloy vs. HopSang*[32].

Or, to vary the example, giving a placebo to satisfy a "difficult" patient is an act of deception and ethically reprehensible; but the very same act, namely giving a placebo, is ethically acceptable when it is done in the course of a double-blind experiment[33] to which the patient has competently, voluntarily and informedly agreed. In other words, the fact of the matter is that the same material action may now be called ordinary and now extraordinary, depending on the circumstances. However, this is not a shortcoming of the distinction but a strength. In fact, the distinction would be flawed if it were otherwise, because things do differ in this way.

Therefore, if there is any ethical difficulty with the ordinary/extraordinary distinction, it does not lie here. If it lies anywhere, it lies in the assumption that no one has an obligation to go beyond what is ordinary. The problem with this, however, is not simply that it is false in its generality, but that even when it is true, it is not clear what it means in practical terms.

Perhaps we can clarify this by the following example. Suppose that Dr. K. has a patient who is pregnant and who wants an abortion. Let us also suppose that Dr. K. is a confirmed Roman Catholic who believes in the sanctity of all human life. Dr. K. would therefore not want to perform an abortion, and would normally refer the woman to a colleague who would help her in that matter. Dr. K. would ordinarily be supported and justified in her decision by clauses 12 and 16 of the *Code of Ethics of the Canadian Medical Association*.[34] However, Dr. K. practises in a small rural community several hundred miles distant from the nearest other centre where there is another physician. For Dr. K. to suggest that the young woman go there to obtain an abortion would not only present some considerable hardship to the latter, but would also run a clear risk of having her condition and the fact of her abortion become known in the community, with devastating results for the future of the woman. The young woman is aware of the very real impact on her life that such a scandal would have and threatens suicide if Dr. K. does not perform the abortion.

Under such circumstances, so it could be argued, Dr. K.'s duty is not confined within the limits of the ordinary. That is, the scope of her obligations is not simply to refer the young woman to her conseure in the nearest urban centre. Clearly, that would not solve the problem. Instead, the nature of the physician-patient relationship, and particularly of the physician-patient relationship in rural areas, requires that Dr. K. go outside the bounds of what ordinary medical practice requires.

That is to say, Dr. K. here has an obligation to go beyond the ordinary and make some arrangements for the young woman to have an abortion, and to have it in such a way that her life not be blighted and, certainly, that the likelihood of suicide be minimized. This may mean that Dr. K. has to arrange for a replacement who will come in on a *locum* and do the abortion. It may even mean that Dr. K. will have no choice but to do the abortion herself. But whatever actions Dr. K. will take, they cannot be confined to what is ordinarily expected of physicians.

What is ordinarily expected of physicians, or, for that matter, what is ordinarily expected of any person in society, is merely the basic level of obligation: a level that holds without consideration of the conditions that obtain. In the language of the first few chapters, it is a basic *prima facie* level of obligation. The actual obligations are determined by the circumstances as and when they arise; and they may go far beyond the level of what is ordinary without, for all that, ceasing to be obligatory. Anything else would be tantamount to saying that the statistical norm determines the scope of ethics. It would elevate statistical normalcy to the level of an ethical absolute. And that would be a mistake. The proper approach is to realize that the moral status of an action is always context-dependent: dependent, as it were, on the "time and the circumstances," which are individual variables. But then, the principle of relevant difference entails no less.

Furthermore, to say that no-one has a duty to do what is extraordinary is really not to say very much unless the difference between what is ordinary and what is extraordinary is defined in some way. The obvious way of doing this, of course, is to draw the distinction in terms of what is statistically normal and what is not.

However this distinction, even though it may appear to be quite clear and definite, actually isn't. Because the next question becomes, "Statistically normal for whom? "—and here there are several possible answers: statistically normal for patients in general; for patients of the specific sort of this particular patient; for physicians in general; for physicians like this particular physician under these sorts of circumstances; and so on. There is a crucial ambiguity here, and unless this ambiguity is resolved, the general claim makes little sense. Once this is pointed out, however, the attractiveness of the initial claim about duties being limited by what is ordinary disappears.

How does all this impact on the issue of euthanasia? It shows two things. First, it shows that the distinction between ordinary and extraordinary means is not absolute but context-dependent. Second, it shows that the distinction itself has nothing whatever to do with whether a particular act or omission constitutes euthanasia. Euthanasia is the bringing about of a painless death. Whether that painless death is brought about by ordinary or extraordinary means does not change the fact that such a death was brought about. The real question, the important question, is not, "Were the means that were (or were not) employed ordinary or extraordinary? " but rather, "Was it ethically acceptable to bring about that death at all? "

Active versus Passive Euthanasia

So far, we have talked about euthanasia by using such phrases as "bringing about the death of a person," "allowing death to occur," and the like. We have used these phrases interchangeably, as though they were logically equivalent in meaning. However, there is a very strong current of thought that maintains that this is not correct. The proponents of this view contend that to bring about the death of a person by allowing it to occur is one thing, particularly when the patient has requested it; but that to actively do something, perhaps to give an injection, is something else entirely.

So, for example, the Law Reform Commission of Canada, in its Working Paper 28, *Euthanasia, Aiding Suicide and Cessation of Treatment*,[35] stated that no matter how it is construed, deliberately bringing about the death of a person is murder in the eyes of the law,—a position it reiterated in its report to parliament one year later.[36]

Likewise, the Canadian Medical Association has gone on record as rejecting active euthanasia, while admitting that an ethical physician[37] "will allow death to occur with dignity and comfort when death of the body appears to be inevitable."

In its policy paper on resuscitation the CMA maintains very clearly that to bring death about deliberately is unacceptable to the ethics of the profession.

In adopting this stance, the CMA is in close agreement with medico-ethical commentators from other countries, as for example Sade and Redfern, who have argued that:

> Passive euthanasia is not an act of killing, it is death suffered by incurable disease, without suffering ... Active termination of life [on the other hand] ... is an act of killing, and no humanitarian rationalization can make it morally defensible ... There is a profound moral difference between allowing a patient to die of his disease in comfort and taking active measures to end his life.[38]

or J.R. Connery, who has maintained that:

> Obviously there is a clear difference between turning off a respirator and injecting a bubble into a patient's vein. The latter is the real cause of death. The respirator does no more than prevent natural causes of death from taking their effect.[39]

Closer to home, the Canadian philosopher Douglas Walton[40] has supported this stance and has argued that:

> ... there is a difference, sometimes, in our readiness to allocate responsibility according to whether an action is positive or omissive.

He has gone on to defend his position by the following train of reasoning:

> ... to make something happen is to ensure that outcome, virtually to force that outcome or nature (or other agents), by in effect blocking off all outcomes that do not contain the state of affairs brought about ... Metaphorically speaking, "Nature is left no alternative" ... But to let something happen is to leave open alternatives from a viewpoint of the agent himself, even if Nature or Society should carry through the outcome enabled by the agent anyway ... At bottom, I feel that we tend to think passive euthanasia less culpable because we conceive Nature as the dominant agent in these cases—the physician merely lets happen what Nature inevitably brings about.[41]

It would seem, therefore, that the distinction between active and passive euthanasia is well-founded and generally accepted.[42]

However, although there is widespread agreement with this distinction, it is by no means universal. For instance, the noted U.S. ethicist James Rachels has argued that:

> Fixing the cause of death may be very important from a legal point of view, for it may determine whether criminal charges are brought against the doctor. But I do not think that this notion can be used to show a moral difference between active and passive euthanasia. The reason why it is considered bad to be the cause of someone's death is that death is regarded as an evil—and so it is. However, if it has been decided that euthanasia—even passive euthanasia—is desirable in a given case, it has also been decided that in this instance death is no greater an evil than

the patient's continued existence. And if this is true, the usual reason for not wanting to be the cause of someone's death simply do not apply.[43]

and as we had occasion to observe above,[44] even some well-known Canadian physicians reject this distinction between active and passive euthanasia as being ethically irrelevant. They have maintained that there is no ethically relevant difference between doing something—say, giving an injection—and merely letting the patient die. And as to actions like unplugging a respirator or switching off a life-support system—or for that matter, failing to give antibiotics, or withholding fluids or nutrition—they all fall into the same category. One and all, they bring about death, and physicians ought not to hide that fact from themselves.

Ironically enough, this very stance can also be supported from the writings of Law Reform Commission itself. In its Working Paper 33, *Homicide*,[45] the commission states:

> 4. Everyone commits intentional homicide in the second degree who kills another meaning to kill a person other than himself (*or knowing for virtually certain that his conduct will do so*).

where the words in italics clearly apply to omissions. More explicitly still, the Commission characterizes omissions as follows:

> ... a person who creates or is control of a danger should have a duty to take reasonable steps to prevents harm to others therefrom.[46]

It also maintains that

> ... all persons have a duty to take reasonable steps to carry put any undertaking, gratuitous or otherwise, whose non-performance will cause serious danger to life.[47]

and explicitly suggests that

> ... the criminal law should recognize a general duty to give reasonable aid and assistance to anyone in instant and overwhelming danger ...

> ... the special Part [of the *Criminal Code* should] provide that everyone commits a crime who fails to take reasonable steps to assist another person whom he sees in instant and overwhelming danger unless he is incapable of doing so without serious risk to himself or another or there is some other valid reason for not giving assistance.[48]

In this, so one might argue, the Law Reform Commission is only expressing what those who reject the active-passive distinction have been saying all along: While the distinction may be psychologically comforting, ethically (and perhaps legally as well) it makes no sense.[49]

Furthermore, those who reject the distinction can also point to the Quebec *Charter of Human Rights and Freedoms*. In Section 2 that Charter states that every human being whose life is in danger has the right to assistance, and that everyone who is in a position to come to that person's assistance has an *obligation* to do so unless there is some overwhelming and legitimate reason to the contrary.[50] That clause, so it could be argued, would be indefensible were it not for the fact that, as

Jonathan Bennett has stated so clearly, "Sometimes cases of letting-die are also cases of killing."[51] And so far from remaining merely an expression of a moral expression, the Quebec stance has found pragmatic recognition in the 1980 case of *R. vs. Fortier*[52].

Causality

Which of these conflicting positions is correct? Is active euthanasia really ethically different from passive euthanasia, or are the two morally the same?[53]

Let us begin our discussion by noting that putting the question in such simplistic terms is really deceptive. It suggests that the issue can be resolved by giving only a single answer. In actuality, the issue is much more complex. There are two central points that are here at issue. The first centres in the *notion of causality*. It may be put like this: "Can a failure to act itself bring about a certain outcome? " The second question centres in the *issue of responsibility*. It is captured more aptly by the following question: "Is the deliberate bringing about of an otherwise preventible death always ethically objectionable? "

The answer to the first question is clear. There is more than one way in which one can be the cause of a particular state of affairs. One can be the cause of that state of affairs by actually doing something—as when a physician accidentally gives a patient a drug such as penicillin to which the patient is allergic and the patient then dies of an induced allergy reaction.

On the other hand, one can also be the cause of a state of affairs by not doing something—as when a physician simply stands by and watches a patient who has gone into fibrillations die without lifting a finger. In both instances, the ethically relevant fact is that the physician was in a position to do something in order to affect the chain of events. In the first case, the physician did do something: She gave the drug; and by that action she altered the chain of events in such a way that a state of affairs which would not have come about had she not acted, did in fact come about.[54]

In a very clear and obvious sense, the physician here was the determinant of that state of affairs. But this holds equally true in the second case, even though the physician did not act but simply stood by. The fact of the matter is that she was in a position to interfere in the situation by taking appropriate steps, but she did not do so. That fact—the very fact of non-intervention—led to a state of affairs that was other than the one that would have existed had she intervened. Therefore, her non-intervention, her lack of action, determined the result, namely death.

This conclusion is important and is worth repeating. Whether someone is physically active or passive has nothing to do with whether that individual is the determinant of a particular outcome. An outcome or a state of affairs may be brought about in either of two ways: by what is sometimes called positive action: i.e., by exerting oneself and thus affecting the causal flow events to ensure (or attempt to ensure) that it follows a certain direction; or by failing to act—by failing to exert oneself precisely in order to ensure that the establish course of events continue and thereby a certain outcome be reached.

FIGURE 10-1
Multiple Effects

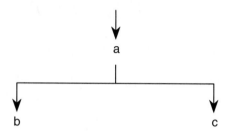

FIGURE 10-2
Multiple Causes

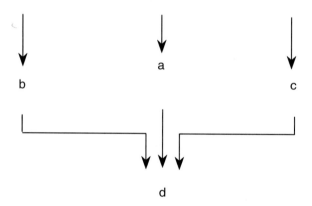

These considerations are represented in figures 10-1 and 10-2.

In Figure 10-1, (a) is a causal determinative (gives rise to) of both (b) and (c), which exist precisely because of that causal determination. In Figure 10-2, (d) is in the state in which it is (or even simply exists) because of (a) and (b) as well as (c).

A practical illustration of the sort of thing represented by Figure 10-1 would be the 1935 Alberta Court of Appeals case of *Mulloy vs. HopSang*. That case centred around the question of whether the physician, Dr.Mulloy, should have amputated the gangrenous hand of Mr. HopSang against the latter's express wishes. Mr. HopSang would not have been without a hand (b)—or, for that matter, alive (c)—if the amputation (a) had not taken place: i.e., if Dr. Mulloy had not amputated.

The relationship in Figure 10-2, on the other hand, could be illustrated by the case of a heart-transplant for Infant M. Her heart would not have been replaced (d) unless there had been some involvement by her family physician (a), by a team of surgeons (b), and others had not contributed further efforts (c) (financing, tissue-matching, size-matching, etc.) as contributory factors.

In reality, of course, causal situations are rarely as simple as the ones we have just considered. Usually the range of actions that are possible for all participants in a causal drama are much wider than our diagram would suggest. For example, the gangrene could have been treated differently—or run a different course; the heart surgeon, the transplant candidate, the team—all these could have behaved in a different fashion; other medical social and material factors could have intervened; and so on. And given the laws of nature as general factors that affect all aspects of every causal chain, each part of the whole process could have been in some other state. Therefore, Figure 10-3 is a much better representation of various possibilities that are open at any given point in time. Where the option, 1 to n+1 represent the possibilities open to the object, depending on what is done.

FIGURE 10-3
Possible Outcomes

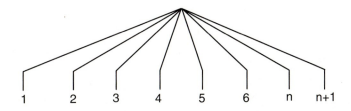

Depending on what is done—or not done. Because, clearly, the amputation might not have taken place because Dr. Mulloy had the flu. More drastically, perhaps, the operation might not have taken place if the relevant surgical technique had not been developed—had been unavailable. If any of these possibilities had been realized, a different outcome, a different future, would have come about. Therefore, if an act is defined as the determination of an outcome from among all those that are possible (Figure 10-3), either directly or in combination (Figures 10-1 and 10-2), then the question of how that outcome is materially achieved, that is to say, what material means are used to bring it about, is really irrelevant.

Ethical Responsibility

What all of this shows is that physical, overt or positive action is not necessary in order to be the causal determinant (cause) of a particular outcome. The very failure to act may function as a causal determination. Which brings us to the second question: responsibility. Some, for example Walton,[55] have said that even when we admit that the physician who passively stands by and lets a death occur is the determinant of that death, that physician will not be guilty of murder.[56] The reason is that by standing passively by, the physician is merely letting nature take its course. It is nature as the dominant agent that bears the responsibility for the death: "We conceive of Nature as the dominant agent in these cases—the physician merely lets happen what Nature inevitably brings about."[57]

But the question that we have to ask ourselves here is, whether this involvement of Nature really makes any difference, ethically speaking, that is. Because what we have to keep in mind is that *any* causal situation, even one that involves a voluntary agent, requires the complicity of Nature. An injection of morphine, for example, or of penicillin will not work unless there are laws of nature. But neither will pulling the plug lead to the death of the patient unless the standard and familiar laws of nature hold sway. And they do. No-one and nothing can violate the laws of nature. Furthermore they are always present, whether the stance we adopt is active or passive. So pointing to the fact that Nature is dominant does not settle the issue of responsibility. Nature is always the dominant cause. That dominance is inherent in inescapable operation of the laws of Nature themselves. Without this dominance, medicine itself would be impossible.

The real question, therefore, is not one of dominance or even causality but of control. Moral responsibility is only assigned on the assumption that we have the power to be causally determinative. It is unethical to praise or blame someone for something over which he or she had no control. Therefore, in any given instance, the first question we have to ask is whether the voluntary agent, which is to say the physician, is in a position to direct the way in which the train of events will go. If the answer to that question is affirmative, it then becomes important to ask whether he or she should in fact direct it differently. It is at that point and at that point only that it becomes appropriate even to consider praise or condemnation.

To this we have to add one further observation. The picture of certain possibilities as being left open by a passive non-active stance and of the future as being left uncertain when we do not act in any positive fashion is really quite illusory. Responsible medical decision-making does not occur in a vacuum, but in the context and against the backdrop of the physician's knowledge and training. That knowledge and that training allow the physician to form an opinion—an informed opinion—about status of the patient.

Therefore, when the physician decides to "let nature take its course," that decision is not made in isolation. It is made in the understanding that *because* the condition of the patient is what it is, *because* the history and nature of the disease or condition is such and so, and *because* the medico-social circumstances are what they are, *therefore* death is expected to occur if treatment is suspended. To put it bluntly, the physician who makes such a decision expects that only a miracle could alter the chain of events which foreseeably will lead to death. However, this is the very same understanding that underlies positive interference. When a physician acts positively, he or she expects that, except for a miracle, the laws of nature, together with his or her causal determination, will yield a fatal denouement.

Therefore, in each case there is the clear expectation of a fatal outcome. This expectation may be unstated; nevertheless it is there. In each instance the physician operates on the assumption that the laws of nature will proceed in their usual course and that the disease or condition will proceed in its usual fashion. There may be an awareness of the possibility that something else—some unforeseen or undiagnosed parameter—will intervene and change the course of events. The physician may even hope that this will happen. However, that is not what he or she *expects* will happen. If he or she did have this expectation, he or she would be remiss as a physician in not doing what was possible in order to bring it about.

Therefore the decision to let nature take its course is made in a climate of relative diagnostic and prognostic certainty. Otherwise the physician could not even talk meaningfully about letting nature take its course. After all, what course is nature here expected to take?

The answer, of course, is the expected course: the one which in all probability will lead to death. Things would be otherwise if physicians approached the future not as governed by the laws of nature but rather like a series of unpredictable, random or chaotic events. That sort of perspective, however, could not be reconciled with what is called scientific medicine.

Direct versus Indirect Euthanasia

The critics who reject the active-passive distinction, therefore, appear to be correct. The distinction is ethically irrelevant. Adopting a passive stance will provide no guarantee that whoever adopts that stance is free of responsibility for the resultant death. The same thing is true for the so-called direct-indirect distinction. To illustrate it, let us consider the following case:

> Aristotle J. has had a severe stroke, and has been brought to the emergency department of Our Lady of the Sorrows Hospital. He is being maintained on a respirator, but it is clear to the emergency room physician and the rest of the staff that he will not recover to any level of sapient cognitive awareness. The next-of-kin have been made aware of the current status of Mr. J. After consultation with the attending physician and the chaplain they decide that continuing treatment would

be pointless. They therefore authorize the physician to cease all efforts. The physician has some qualms about doing so, because on one level she feels that to turn it off is to kill the patient. However, after some reflection she decides that she would not be the primary and direct cause of Mr. J.'s death. Her causal involvement would be indirect only, since the direct causal agent would be the disease process that has brought Mr. J. to this state. She therefore turns off the respirator, confident in the opinion that no real responsibility for Mr. J.'s death falls on her.

This sort of reasoning is not all that rare in the medical setting; and like the active-passive distinction, it has tremendous psychological appeal. For all that, however, it is ethically quite dubious.

A full discussion of what is wrong with it would take us too far afield. Suffice it to say that as we pointed out a moment ago, and as should be clear from the example itself, medical decisions are not made in isolation. They are made in a particular context on the basis of certain pieces of information and with certain expectations. In the case above, the context is one where the patient requires assistance in staying biologically alive. This is known to the medical staff. There is also the expectation that if the respirator is turned off Mr. J. will be unable to breathe on his own. Under such circumstances, turning off the respirator is the deliberate initiation of a chain of events that foreseeably and predictably will lead to the death of Mr. J.—the foreseeable and predictable nature of the chain of events is what is here important. Deliberately to initiate a course of events, knowing full well that it will have a specific outcome if certain other elements are present—and knowing also that these other elements are in fact present—is to assume responsibility for that outcome. That is here the case.

If we look at figure 10-4 we see that, in more general terms, indirect causality involves several parameters either cooperating together, as in (a), or acting sequentially, as in (b), to bring about the final outcome E. However, in neither case does the complexity of the causal framework remove responsibility from the physician. *If* the physician was acting as a voluntary and competent agent; *if* he or she could reasonably have been expected to know that the relevant contributing causal factors would be present; and *if* he or she should have known that this particular causal chain would have this outcome, *then* he or she cannot claim reduced moral responsibility by pointing to the complexity of the causal structure or the causal distance between his or her action and the ultimate result. Moral responsibility, as we saw, attaches to acts. Acts, in turn, are defined in terms of contexts in which they are embedded. In the present sort of instance that includes both knowledge of the fatal denouement as well as the decision to opt for that alternative anyway. The full weight of moral responsibility therefore descends upon the physician.

The Morality of Euthanasia

What the discussion so far has shown is that the question whether euthanasia is morally defensible cannot be settled by looking at the material nature of the act itself.

FIGURE 10-4
Complex Causation

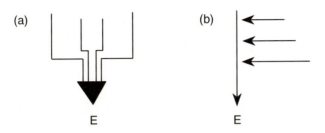

As in all other cases, the act has to be looked at in its own context. The question that we have to ask is, Are there contexts in which euthanasia is ethically defensible?

There are all sorts of arguments to show that there are not. Some are based on a particular perspective about the ethical relevance of the concept of a person; others are life-oriented; still others centre around a certain understanding of the nature of the medical profession; and then there are those having a pragmatic orientation. On the other hand, there is also no shortage of arguments to the contrary. There are arguments that derive from the concept of autonomy, from the duty to alleviate pain and suffering, and from equality and justice, to mention but a few. Obviously we cannot consider all of them here. What we can and shall do, however, is to sketch a representative few, look at them briefly and then outline what we take to be an acceptable position mandated by the ethical principles that underlie our discussion so far.

Life-Centred Arguments

Life-centred arguments fall into two general rubrics: those that take their cue from the principle that all life must be respected, and those that start from the principle that it is essentially only human life that has such a special status.

The first sort of position is well represented in the Buddhistic tradition. In the West, it's most prominent proponent was probably Albert Schweitzer. Schweitzer maintained that all life is sacred, not merely in a religious sense, but also in the sense that it has intrinsic or absolute value.[58] Any destruction of it, therefore—so he reasoned—if deliberate and avoidable, is anathema. As he put it,

> The ethics of respect for life does not recognize any relative ethics. It admits as good only the preservation and advancement of life. All destruction and harming of life, no matter what the circumstances under which it may occur, it designates as evil.[59]

The obvious reply to this, however, is, How could such an ethics be livable without contradiction? Taken as it stands, it would make us ethically guilty every time we ate, took a breath, or took a step. Indeed, on this token the very practice of medicine itself would be fraught with guilt. On the other hand not to engage in such activities would also result in death: namely our own. Surely, so it could be argued, the inevitability of guilt no matter which way we turn amounts to a *reductio ad absurdum* of this perspective.

Of course, not everyone who accepts the principle of respect for life has gone quite this far. Some have argued that the principle does not entail that we may not take life under any circumstances whatever. Instead, it demands that we should have respect for it; and that respect means just that. We should have good and overwhelming reasons for taking life if and when we do so. We should not treat it irresponsibly. The point remains, however, that an obligation of respect for life does not entail an absolute prohibition against taking it.

This approach would allow medical practice to proceed with its antiseptic and antibiotic regimens, research projects and the like. But by that very token it would also allow the taking of life under certain circumstances. And since the principle applies to all life and does not out single human life as special, it also allows taking human life under certain circumstances. All of which means that in principle it would not rule out euthanasia.

Which brings us to the second line of reasoning: the line which maintains that only human life has a privileged position. This sort of approach has sometimes been associated with the name Kant. There is some debate whether Kant actually held this position, but in the end it doesn't really matter. The point is that this position bases itself on the assumption that human life, as distinct from all other life, has intrinsic value; and that because it has intrinsic value, no one may take a human life, whether that be the person whose life it is, or anyone else.

> If, in order to escape from some burdensome circumstances, we were to kill someone or he asked to be destroyed, we—and he as well—would be using a person merely as a means to maintaining a tolerable condition to the end of life. Man, however, is not a thing, and therefore not something that may be used merely as a means, but in all acts must forever be considered an end in itself.[60]

But that approach, too, has been challenged. Ironically enough, in the first instance, by those who hold the position that we have just discussed. They maintain that singling out human life as special and alone as worthy of particular protection has no ethical foundation. It is simply ethical speciesm.[61]

Secondly, this whole position hinges on the premise that only human life has intrinsic value. The obvious question is, "How is that premise established?" And even if that premise were somehow shown to be true, the position would still be based on faulty logical reasoning. It does not follow from the fact that something has intrinsic value that therefore it should not be destroyed—or killed. What does follow is that its destruction should not be undertaken lightly—but that is an entirely different matter.

Furthermore, even if assumptions underlying this position were to be accepted, the conclusion that it is trying to advance would still not follow. One could always reply that it is precisely because human life has intrinsic value, and precisely because the human person is an end-in-itself that under certain circumstances it is not only permissible but even obligatory to take it, for instance, when the life in question is fraught with torture, is degrading to the individual, and so on. Not to end such a life would be to show disrespect for it, because it would be to degrade precisely that which makes it different from all other types of life, and which gives it its intrinsic value: its personal human nature. Bringing about an end to such an existence would be mandated, rather than prohibited. Anything else would be degrading.

Self-Realization

Another common argument against euthanasia bases itself on the claim that everyone has an obligation develop his or her potentials. These potentials involve not only intellectual capabilities but also personal ones: perseverance, humility, and so on.[62] Therefore, to end a life that affords the possibility to realize these potentials is to fail to rise to the challenge of what can make us human in the fullest possible sense.

This line of reasoning is sometimes heightened by an appeal to religious premises, such as revelation. Still, whether buttressed in this way or not, there is something very medieval about it. It suggests a trial by ordeal in order to attain an elevated plateau of personal goodness. It is reminiscent of the sort of perspective that we encounter in writings like *The Pilgrim's Progress*. We shall not analyze it in detail. However, it should be noted that this perspective is not without its opposition. It is sometimes argued that not only is there is a duty of self-realization, but also that this duty can be fulfilled only by clinging to life no matter what.

However, to this we could make the following reply: If the quality of life that lies in store for someone or that someone currently experiences makes it impossible for that person to enjoy socialization, cognitive sapient awareness, and emotional interaction with others, then to talk about self-realization is absurd. If the individual is still sapient at all, his or her energies will be devoted solely to staying alive. There will be no energy left for anything else. As to the possibility that others—onlookers, participants in the drama, and so on—might benefit and realize personal potentials they would otherwise not have realized, that would be to degrade the individual to the status of a tool for the benefit of others. However, if the sole purpose for keeping someone alive is that through this others may achieve their humanity, then something has gone drastically wrong. In principle, such a perspective would allow any kind of action so long as others benefitted as persons. Ethically, this is disturbing.

Ironically enough, this very stance would also allow euthanasia in those cases where the sufferer's circumstances no longer offer the possibility of self-improvement, either for himself or others.

Professional Obligation

There are many anti-euthanasia arguments that centre not on the health care recipient or the onlooker, but in the health care provider: the physician. Their focus is the claim that no physician can ever have an obligation (or indeed can be allowed) to participate in euthanasia. The very nature of the profession rules it out.[63] From the earliest time, the physician's profession has been characterized by the obligation to save and/or maintain life, not to end it. This obligation was first expressed clearly in the Hippocratic Oath:

> I will use treatment to help the sick according to my ability and judgement, but never with a view to injury and wrong-doing. Neither will I administer a poison to anybody when asked to do so, nor will I suggest such a course.

Every code of medical ethics after it has embraced a similar prohibition.

But like any other tradition, not even this one has gone unchallenged.[64] For instance, it has been argued that this sort of perspective bespeaks a very narrow, and mistaken, view of the nature of the health care professions. Their obligation is not, as suggested, to save and/or sustain life at all costs but to provide the best services possible within the domain of health care practice consonant with informed consent. Anything else would violate the principle of autonomy. Therefore, when such consent is lacking or withdrawn, the professional has no mandate to continue. A passive stance, therefore, when voluntarily requested by the patient, is not merely ethically acceptable but is, in fact, a duty.

Furthermore, there are cases where there is no more hope of cure or improvement, even of stabilization, for the patient; cases where only a palliative approach remains as a reasonable option. In such cases it may happen that the medications necessary to produce a proper palliative effect also shorten the life-expectancy of the patient who receives them. In some cases, they may even hasten death dramatically. Strictly speaking, the physician who embarks on such palliative actions thereby becomes an agent of death. After all, strictly speaking, death could be staved off a little longer if the physician employed the means that are available to sustain life. However, the fact that this may occur does not mean that the conscientious physician may not engage in appropriate palliative care under such circumstances, even when an accelerated death may be the outcome. This is clearly recognized by the Canadian Medical Association, which states that

> Palliative care to alleviate the mental and physical discomfort of the patient should be provided at all times ... [An ethical physician] will allow death to occur with dignity and comfort when death of the body appears to be inevitable.[65]

In the eyes of the CMA, there is no duty to prolong the dying process. The physician has an obligation of respect towards the patient: an obligation that follows from the principle of autonomy and respect for persons itself. To leave a patient in agony and suffering, or a state which is degrading, demeaning or otherwise an affront to human dignity would be to respect life as such, but it would also denigrate the person whose life it is. It would be to use the person for the sake of biological life itself. Therefore, unless the patient or the appropriate surrogate decision-maker has explicitly indicated the contrary, the obligation of the physician here is to use such means as preserve the quality of life of the patient insofar as that is possible, the life-shortening side-effects of these means notwithstanding. This position has also been accepted by other health care professionals, such as the Canadian Nurses Association.

The same conclusion, that palliative treatment is ethically acceptable even though it may shorten the life of the patient, is sometimes defended on a different basis: by arguing, for example, that in these sorts of cases only the good palliative effect is intended and not the negative outcome—the hastening of the death;[66] or by arguing that all shortening of life is indirect, not active euthanasia.[67]

However, when all is said and done, such arguments are really only psychological ploys. They may allow whoever uses this sort of reasoning to hide from him- or herself the fact that such palliative actions do involve a knowing and deliberate shortening of life. The standard distinction between consequences that are desired and consequences that are foreseen and not desired is here appropriate. In the sorts of cases we are here dealing with, the physician cannot will or intend the good (palliative) effect alone without at the same time foreseeing the negative outcome. Therefore, by intending the good effect, *while foreseeing the negative outcome which is an integral and ineluctable part of the scenario,* the physician is also willing that negative outcome. To try to separate the two would require an impossibly tortuous feat of self-deception and selective memory. What the physician does is to will the good effect *despite* the fact that it will hasten the patient's death.

The point to keep in mind in all of this is that being a determinant of death is not necessarily ethically reprehensible. It all depends on the circumstances. Once that is recognized, there is no need to hide behind psychological manoeuvres in order to come to terms with that fact.

Pragmatic Arguments

Of course, not all arguments against euthanasia are grounded in ethical considerations. There are several that have a pragmatic social orientation. The first bases itself on the *difficulty of legislation,* the second is the so-called *wedge or slippery slope argument,* and the third may be called the *argument from brutalization.*

The argument from difficulty of legislation has a very simple message: euthanasia, whether active or passive, is the deliberate taking of human life. In a word, it is homicide. Consequently it would be far too dangerous to legalize it without spelling out very clearly what the conditions are under which it would be permissible. And that, to put it simply, can't be done. The British Medical Association had a select panel look into the matter, and its conclusion was this:

> After careful consideration the panel is convinced that it would be impossible to provide adequate safeguards in any euthanasia legislation.[68]

Who, so the panel's reasoning seems to be, would have the ultimate decision-making power in such cases? The attending physician? A group of physicians, or an ethics committee? The family, or society as a whole? None of these alternatives will guarantee against religious, social and even professional bias; and all of them are, to some degree, subject to the personal and economic factors that stand in the wings. Under what conditions should euthanasia be permissible? Using what criteria? Within what limits? And the problem would not be solved by what has been called a *living will.* That is to say, by giving legal recognition to the right of the individual, while competent, to state formally that under certain circumstances he or she should be allowed or even made to die. If it is impossible at the legislative level to spell out precisely the circumstances under which deliberate death is to be permissible, that difficulty is not removed be transferring the issue from the legislative level to that of the individual person.[69]

The slippery slope argument does not question the possibility of drafting carefully and appropriately circumscribed legislation. Instead, its fear is that once deliberate death has been legally sanctioned in any context, no matter how carefully circumscribed, it is only a small step to its use as a tool to kill unwanted population. As J. Gould put it:[69]

> ... once the principle of the sanctity of human life is abandoned, or the propaganda accepted that to uphold it is old-fashioned, prejudicial or superficial, the way is open to the raising of—and satisfaction of—a demand for euthanasia for the severely crippled, the aged, and ultimately for all who are a burden on community services and the public purse.[70]

and as Yale Kamisar said in his classic article on the subject,.

> It is true that the "wedge" objection can always be advanced, the horrors can always be paraded. But it is less true that on some occasions the objection is much more valid that it is on others. One reason why the parade of horrors cannot be too lightly dismissed in some particular instances is that Miss Voluntary Euthanasia is not likely to be going it alone for very long. Many of her admirers ... would be neither surprised nor distressed to see her joined by Miss Euthanatize the Congenital Idiot and Miss Euthanatize the Permanently Insane and Miss Euthanatize the Senile Dementia ...[71]

> Another reason why the "parade of horrors" argument cannot be dismissed in this particular instance ... is that the parade *has* taken place in our time and the order of procession has been headed by killing the "incurable" and "useless." ... The apparent innocuousness of Germany's "small beginnings" is perhaps best shown by the fact that German Jews were at first excluded from the programme. For it was originally conceived that the blessing of euthanasia should be granted only to (true) Germans.

The message of the argument from brutalization is simple: legally sanctioning euthanasia will also lead to a general erosion of sensitivity, to a brutalization of public sentiment in the face of suffering. Suffering is not something to be valued in itself, or even encouraged. It is something that deserves our compassion. The suffering of fellow human being should evoke a helping response. Once euthanasia is legislatively permitted for those who are suffering, the stage is set for replacing compassion with—termination. Focus on the *person* of the individual will be replaced by a focus on the *condition* of the individual. Our response to human suffering will become the response to an object that no longer meets our expectations. The value of human life will become measured in quality-adjusted life units. It will be only a short step from this to the position that human life must be evaluated in terms of social utility.[72]

Clearly, these arguments raise serious considerations. It would be foolish to deny either the fact that euthanasia legislation has been misused in the past or that it might not be misused in the future. However, as with any fear, we must always ask ourselves whether it is misplaced or appropriate. In this case, the fear is based on an the fact that such misuse has occurred. However, when evaluating this kind of reasoning we should keep in mind that this misuse was set in a certain historical context, and that it took place in a legal tradition entirely different from ours. We should therefore ask ourselves whether enough of an analogy really remains to make the argument cogent.

Furthermore, the fear of misuse and abuse of euthanasia legislation if it were passed is something that can be raised in any area of legislation. Any law may be misused, broken or ignored. Euthanasia legislation would be no different from laws mandating incarceration, the death penalty or giving powers of professional discretion to physicians. The real danger lies not in the law itself, but in the people who use it. The crucial question is, how the relevant law would be interpreted and applied. So what this argument really says is that people cannot be trusted to use in an appropriate fashion the laws they themselves have made. Not only is that a sad commentary on our faith in our fellow human beings, it also means that even if we have laws that prohibit euthanasia, we should expect them to be broken. In this context it might be appropriate to remember the words of David Hume. Although they were intended for a different context, they do have relevance here:

> There is no method of reasoning more common, and yet none more blameable, than ... to endeavour to refute any hypothesis by pretext of its dangerous consequences ... When an opinion leads to absurdity, 'tis certainly false; but 'tis not certain an opinion is false because 'tis of dangerous consequences.[73]

As to the fear that permitting euthanasia in one context, no matter how carefully circumscribed, marks the beginning of a slide down a slippery slope, this is an argument from analogy. Such arguments are only as strong as the comparison on which they are based. The comparison that is drawn is always to Nazi Germany. Why not to Uruguay, which for decades has had legislative recognition of even active euthanasia under certain circumstances; or to Switzerland, which recognizes extenuating circumstances. Most notably perhaps the Netherlands, which is actively exploring the possibility of such legislation. These countries do not seem to feel that the dangers of the slippery slope are unavoidable. Furthermore, as Gerald Winslow recently stated,

> Such arguments tend to be tiresome and abused. They may also be offensive, with their intimations that ... people ... are so inept that they cannot (or will not) establish safeguards against such a slide.[74]

Finally, the argument from brutalization. It is not at all clear that the opposite conclusion is not more appropriate; that being saved and/ or maintained at all cost, betubed, sedated, glucosed, aerated and wired for pace-making and monitoring devices of all sorts without reasonable expectation of improvement, either in agony or so full of narcotics and analgesics as to be non-cognitive in any real sense, vegetating until the final systemic collapse occurs—it is not clear that this is not more brutalizing than making for "a fair and easy passage."[75] To force a congenitally and severely deformed and defective neonate to live by dint of technology and professional determination; to save and/or sustain a radical burns victim with no reasonable hope of recovery, or someone with incurably metasticized cancer, and so on, is less humane and less respective of human dignity than allowing an earlier but easier death.

Arguments in Favour

The matter could be pressed further. However, sooner or later the issue has to be faced squarely: can euthanasia be justified within the framework of a deontological medical ethics? If it can, then it cannot be in contravention of a properly formulated code of medical ethics.

Such a code, after all, derives its moral legitimacy from the general ethical system as a whole. Nor could pragmatic difficulties then be considered telling. Their only point would be to indicate particular situations under which the general conditions that permit euthanasia do not hold. And as to psychological and social problems, unless they could be shown to have ethical relevance, they would merely indicate that an educational effort is called for.

The fact that legitimating euthanasia would oppose current opinion, even if it were true, can not be considered an argument either. Slavery, the disenfranchisement of women, the legal prohibition of alcohol and abortion, the mistreatment of Japanese Canadians, all these have been sanctioned by public opinion; so the record on that score is not too great. But as a matter of fact, current public opinion does not reject the legalization of euthanasia. Recent Gallup polls indicate that an overwhelming majority of Canadians favour legal recognition of euthanasia under carefully controlled circumstances.[76] Of course this does not show that it is ethically acceptable; but it does suggest that the subject should be considered seriously.

As to the claim that euthanasia would contravene medical tradition: It would not be the first time that this has happened. The whole ethics of informed consent has developed in opposition to entrenched medical tradition. Perhaps medical tradition is mistaken in this instance as well.

So the question has to be faced squarely and on its own terms: Is euthanasia ethically acceptable within a deontological framework? It seems to us that the answer is yes.[77] To put this into context, let us consider the following case:

> Arthur Q. had been admitted to hospital with a diagnosis of cancer of the lung. A lobectomy had been recommended and he had agreed to it. In fact, he had been a most cooperative patient. He followed the prescribed regimen faithfully, and it looked as though the surgery had been successful. Three months later a checkup revealed that not all had gone as hoped. The cancer had metastasized into the liver, and several other metastases were noted. The other lung also was affected. Considered opinion was that the best that could be done for Arthur Q. was to give him palliative care. Arthur Q. accepted this. When the pain became too great and he could no longer eat, he was hospitalized. He grew steadily weaker—and the pain control regimen had to be increased steadily. After several weeks in hospital, he conferred with his attending physician and his nurses and told them that he did not want any more visits from his grandchildren and his next-of-kin. He had fought the good fight, and he felt that he now deserved to die. He had informed his family of his decision. While they had difficulty facing it, they respected it as his right. Arthur Q. was a proud man. He was a veteran—a World War II Spitfire pilot, decorated and a war hero. He wanted to die while he still had a shred of dignity left. He had no firearm—and in any case he was convinced that if he were to kill himself by such means, his family and above all his grandchildren would be deeply shocked. He therefore asked the physician to give him something that would allow him to die painlessly, peacefully and in his sleep.

The principle of autonomy and respect for persons entails that Arthur Q. may voluntarily forego any life saving or sustaining intervention. Furthermore, as a competent person he has the right to decide on the deliberate termination of his life, whether that be by active or passive means. Ordinarily this would not impose an obligation on the attending medical staff beyond the duty to refrain from life-sustaining interventions. If such a discontinuation were acceptable to Arthur Q., then that would be appropriate.

Of course, the physician who acted in this way would still be engaged in euthanasia. As our previous analysis has shown, the passive nature of the medical stance would not alter that fact that it would still be the deliberate and conscious determination of a chain of events that foreseeably will lead to the patient's death.

But let us ignore that. Instead, let us concentrate on the fact that Arthur Q. does not want to die in this way. Arthur Q. does not want to die in what he considers an undignified fashion: through starvation, incontinent, under the effects of increasing pain medication, and *non compos mentis*. He wants to die with dignity: painlessly, peacefully and in his sleep. If he had access to some means of killing himself in this way, in a way that would not shock his family and preserve his dignity, he would do it; but he doesn't.

The law of the land has denied him access to the means that would give him a dignified and easy death. These means and their use have been placed into the hands of the physicians. By law, physicians have become the gatekeepers. The principles of autonomy and justice therefore require from physicians that they provide or use these means when a competent patient asks for them under appropriate circumstances; and the principles also demand that the law allow this. Otherwise the law will have turned the right to life into a duty.

The profession of medicine, having accepted the role of gatekeeper and having accepted the privilege of service monopoly, must find some way to provide Arthur Q. with the means of ending his life. Otherwise it will be party to a fundamental violation of the principle of autonomy. This does not necessarily mean that Arthur Q.'s attending physician must end Arthur Q.'s life; nor does it necessarily entail that any other physician has that obligation. It may entail this if, for example, Arthur Q. were a quadripalegic or otherwise seriously incapacitated or incapable of performing the appropriate act. But this is not the case here.

What it means is that the medical profession must find some way of fulfilling Arthur Q.'s legitimate request in a way that preserves his dignity. This may involve providing him with some medication which he may self-administer, so long as he is able to do so. However, when he is unable to do so, the medical profession has a clear duty to bring about his death.

But suppose we alter the situation slightly. Suppose we say that Arthur Q. is not moribund; let us say instead that he faces a life which is qualitatively atrocious, even torturous, by ordinary standards, and that it is quite unacceptable to him. Under such circumstances, would physicians then also have a professional obligation to provide him with some means of ending his existence?

The answer is, there well may be such obligation. Everyone has the right to freedom from torture. This follows from the principle of autonomy and respect for persons. A competent person may decide to terminate his or her life for qualitative reasons. Of course, so long as that person is physically able to end his or her life in a way that does not offend his or her dignity, there will be no reason for a physician to intervene or to provide assistance.

However, when that is not the case, because the means for bringing about what the patient considers a dignified death may not lie in the hands of the patient, then the matter is different. Not all patients consider starvation, the leap from a building or the use of firearms and nooses dignified means of exit. They may see drugs as a dignified and appropriate way to go. However, by prohibiting access to appropriate drugs except by order of a physician, our society has placed most of such means firmly under the control of medicine.

Logically, therefore, as Dr. Sidney Wanzer stated in a recent article in *The New England Journal of Medicine*,[78] this entails that the physician may well have the duty to assist the competent patient who wishes to die but who lacks appropriate and acceptable means, by "prescribing sleeping pills with knowledge of their intended use, or by discussing the required dosage with the patient." And this holds true even when the patient is not moribund. Because to deny patients the means for a dignified exit is, to use the words of Tristam Engelhardt, Jr., to force on the patient the "injury of continued existence."

Before we conclude this section, one final question: How does all this affect those who are cerebrally dead—or, for that matter, those who are wholly brain-dead. What is the situation here? In brief, the situation is radically different. The key presumption underlying what we have discussed so far is that the individuals in question are persons. Certainly Arthur Q. was a person. In these cases, then, the physician has to be conscious of moral principles and imperatives, and has to try to balance his or her own ethical position as a professional with the rights of the patient-person.

However, when the patient is decerebrate or even whole brain dead, the presumption of personhood no longer holds. The patient, if that is then still the right term, is then what one famous theologian has described as a living human body.[79] This radically changes the ethics of the situation. While the physician should accord respect to the *humanum*—to the human body (which means that he or she may not deal with it in any way whatever)—there is here no question of duty or right—certainly not a question of right-to-life. Therefore treatment may be discontinued as being medically inappropriate and useless.

But it may also be discontinued for another reason that centres in the ethics of resource allocation. Patients who are persons have a right to health care. If that right is impaired because the necessary resources are being used for someone who is not a person, then a perversion of rights has taken place. It is estimated that there are approximately 800 patients in permanent vegetative state (pvs) in Canada at the present time.[80] The aggregate cost of keeping them alive is approximately $20,000,000 per year.[81] If such expenditure seriously erodes the accessibility of ordinary patients to the health care they need, then the right of these patients takes precedence over the commitment to keep individuals in a pvs alive. That may be hard on the next-of-kin and relevant others. However, when it comes to a question of allocation of resources, the merely living body may be, indeed must be, allowed or made to die in order that persons may live.

Living Wills

There is one topic which we have only touched on but which lately has attracted a great deal of attention: living wills. Living wills or advance directives are documents prepared by people while they are still competent, in anticipation that at some future time they will no longer be competent and therefore will be unable to make health care decisions for themselves. To guard against the possibility that they might be treated or kept alive against their will or in violation of the qualitative standards that are the valuational focus of their lives, such people formally direct that under the circumstances they set out in the document, they should be allowed to die.

There are various versions of living wills or advance directives.[82] However, whatever the version, the important ethical question really is this: Is such an advance directive ethically binding on the physician?

The literature is full of arguments both pro and con. Not unexpectedly, the arguments against tend to stress the claim that it is impossible for a patient to specify with sufficient precision beforehand the exact circumstances under which the living will or advance directive should come into effect. They also tend to suggest that by laying down a specific course of action ahead of time, a document such as a living will would ignore the possibility that the patient has changed his or her mind.

Arguments for, on the other hand, tend to insist that the principle of autonomy gives every competent person the right to decide the course of their lives while they are still able to do so. Such arguments tend to point out that the difficulties raised by opponents of living wills really are more theoretical than practical in nature.

Both sides have valid points to make. Over 39 States in the U.S. still have such legislation on the books,[83] as do several countries.[84] Furthermore, in 1987 the Ethics Committee of the Canadian Medical Association passed a resolution that a certain form of living wills should find legal recognition;[85] and in 1988 the General Council of the CMA resolved that the CMA/CBA Liaison Committee should take appropriate steps to convince the relevant legislative authorities to enact such legislation.[86] Therefore, the medical community itself does not think that it is impossible to define the enabling conditions for (passive) euthanasia sufficiently clearly.

Still, the difficulty of specifying precisely the circumstances is a legitimate concern. While the fact of this difficulty does not detract from the ethical legitimacy of living wills, it would be unrealistic not to recognize its force. However, one could meet it by combining the notion of a living will with that of a surrogate decision-makers. A patient would designate someone to act as surrogate decision-maker in the eventuality that the patient should no longer be competent to make his or her own health care decisions. The patient could provide the surrogate decision-maker with a living will which would outline the values that the latter should follow in case the patient became incompetent and a decision had to be made. It would then be up to the surrogate decision-maker to follow these guidelines. The whole arrangement could also be formalized by giving the surrogate decision-maker durable power of attorney, to come into effect when the patient becomes incompetent. Nova Scotia has recently taken a step in that direction when it passed, and proclaimed, its Patient Consent Act. This Act allows a patient to give someone durable power of attorney for just such an eventuality.[87] In Canada, therefore, the first step in this direction has already been taken.

The combination of living will and durable power of attorney would have two advantages. It would meet the concern that living wills may not be applicable to the actual situations that arise. The surrogate decision-maker would be able to adjust the guidelines contained in the will to the situation at hand. It would also avoid the sort of situation where next-of-kin disagree over what should be done and where the physician is caught in the middle.

To this one could add that when no surrogate decision-maker has been designated, a living will should still be treated as an expression of the patient's will, and therefore should be considered binding. However, in order to facilitate decision-making one could establish the convention that in these cases the physician will take over the role of the surrogate decision-maker. This convention should of course be publicly known. It would then be up to the physician to interpret this will in light of the values expressed in it and in light of the medical facts. One could add that any apparent departure from the values or guidelines contained in the will would have to be legally justified when challenged. In this way, the living will would become an instrument that would allow the leeway necessary to accommodate changing circumstances while at the same time giving a reasonable guarantee that the values which shape the life of the individual would not be compromised merely because the individual is no longer able to insist on them him- or herself.

The possibility that the patient had a change of mind at the last moment does, of course, exist. However, there are other situations in which it holds as well, for example, when a patient is about to undergo an operation. It is always possible that just before the patient loses consciousness from the anaesthetic, he or she has had a change of heart and wishes to withdraw consent. No-one would suggest that because this is a possibility, therefore patients should not be operated on. Instead, the appropriate thing to do is try and make sure that such a change has not in fact taken place. So here too, the possibility always exists. The best the physician can do is try and make sure that it isn't the case, and then go on. Anything else would impose requirements of certainty that are accepted nowhere else, and its effect would be to rule out altogether the very possibility of ever following any directive.

Voluntary versus Non-Voluntary

Finally, there is a distinction which so far we have ignored in our discussion: the distinction between voluntary and non-voluntary euthanasia. Voluntary euthanasia is usually understood as the euthanatizing of a patient at his or her own request, where of course it is assumed that the patient who makes this request is competent at the time of making it. Non-voluntary euthanasia, on the other hand, is understood as the euthanatising of a person without that person having expressed such a wish.

The reason we have ignored this distinction is not that it is not valid, but that in a sense, our whole discussion has really dealt with some aspect or other of it. On the basis of our discussion we can now say that all other things being equal, voluntary euthanasia is ethically defensible. The only real question is whether anyone has a duty to act on a voluntary request for euthanasia if the patient is no longer capable of acting on it him- or herself by committing suicide. And here we have also suggested an answer.

As to non-voluntary euthanasia, our discussion implies that under certain circumstances it, too, is ethically defensible. For instance, it is ethically defensible in the case of congenitally incompetent persons who have never been in a position to formulate any values, let alone express wishes, and who find themselves in a situation where the continuation of their lives would amount to unmitigated and unrelenting torture. People who are in such a position should not be treated worse than people who have the good fortune to be able to make their own decisions. The rights of the incompetent should not be less than the rights of the competent solely because of their incompetence!

However, Yale Kamisar's impassioned argument against euthanasia here comes back to haunt us. Kamisar is right: There is the danger that once accepted in principle, non-voluntary euthanasia will become the justification for killing unwanted population, for emptying hospital beds or for ridding ourselves of people whom we consider undesirable. That must not be allowed to occur. Therefore any move to give legal recognition to euthanasia must provide some mechanism that would rule this out. This could be done by placing the power to make such a decision solely into the hands of the courts. The courts, exercising their *parens patriae* powers, could then reach a decision on the basis of argumentation on both sides of the issue and after examination of all appropriate evidence. Under such circumstances, non-voluntary euthanasia would be acceptable, not because the legal decision would make it ethically acceptable, but because the legal process would provide the safeguard that what is ethically acceptable *per se* would not be misused.

Conclusion

If what we have argued is valid, then under certain circumstances—circumstances that we have outlined—euthanasia is ethically acceptable.

However, the question whether something is ethically acceptable has to be carefully distinguished from the question whether what is ethically acceptable should be allowed by law. It is here that the slippery slope argument and the argument from analogy come into their own. Whatever their ethical and logical cogency may be, these arguments focus on the fact that there is another dimension to human beings: a dimension that allows them to depart from what is ethical. And the arguments are surely justified in making this claim. The historical facts are incontrovertible in that regard.

The question we have to ask is whether, given these facts, and given this potential for unethical behaviour, euthanasia should be legalized under carefully controlled conditions. Our answer is a qualified yes. Yes, for the reasons that we have already indicated in the course of our discussion. Qualified, because it all depends on the nature of the legislation that allows it. If it were legislation that allowed it to occur without judicial review, we would object. If it was legislation that had a built-in automatic judicial review mechanisms that included input from the public, the law, the health care-professions, handicapped persons and so on, we would be in favour. To this we would add that such a law should contain a clear indication that if the review process found that the act was not ethically justified, then the person who performed the euthanasia should be prosecuted under the relevant homicide sections of the *Criminal Code*.

ENDNOTES

[1] "Neither will I administer a poison to anybody when asked to do so, nor will I suggest such a course." Oath of Hippocrates, 460–370 B.C.

[2] CMA *Code*, Principle I.

[3] See H.E. Emson, *The Doctor and the Law* (Butterworths: Toronto and Vancouver, 1989) 2.5.2 and 10.2.2; Ellen Picard, *Legal Liability of Doctors and Hospitals in Canada*, (Toronto: Carswell, 1984); Janet Storch, *Patients rights: Ethical and Legal Issues in Health Care and Nursing*, (Toronto: McGraw-Hill Ryerson, 1982), 88; to mention but a few authors. For a more complete discussion, see the Law Reform Commission of Canada, Working Paper 28, *Euthanasia, Aiding Suicide and Cessation of Treatment* (Minister of Supply and Services: Ottawa, 1982).

[4] American Medial Association, Report A (A–77).

[5] For example, the report of the Council on Ethical and Judicial Affairs of the American Medical Association, June 1988.

[6] R.S.C. 1985 c. C–34, s.14.

[7] Based on a series of Toronto cases.

[8] *Mulloy vs. HopSang*, [1935] 1 W.W.R. 741 (Alta. C. A.).

[9] *Malette vs. Shulman*, (Ontario C. A.) 72 O.R. (2d) 417 [1990] O.3. No. 450 Section No. 29/88.

[10] See James Rachels, *The End of Life: Euthanasia and Morality* (Oxford: Oxford Univ. Press, 1986); Tristam Engelhardt, Jr., *The Foundations of Bioethics*, (Oxford: Oxford Univ. Press, 1986), 301-317; E.-H.W. Kluge *The Ethics of Deliberate Death*, (Port Washington, N.Y.: Kennikat Press, 1981) Chap. 1.

[11] *The Ottawa Citizen*, October 6, 1989 B7.

[12] Gallup poll released July 24, 1989. The poll involved a sample, of 1,029 persons and is considered accurate within 4% 19 times out of 20.

[13] S.H. Wanzer, D.D. Federman, S.J. Adelstein et al., NEJM (1989), 320: 844–849. For an opposing view, see J.R. Stanton and R.L. Maker, "The Suicide Sell," *Senior Patient*, Nov./December, 1989, 51–54.

[14] G.C. Garbesi, "The Law of Assisted Suicide," *Issues in Law and Medicine* (1987), 3(2): 93–111. This position was not upheld on appeal.

[15] Gallop released July 24, 1989.

[16] See the U.S. cases of *Superintendent of Belchertown State School vs. Saikewizc*, 373 Mass. 728, 370 N.E.2d 417 (1977); *In Re Storar*, 52 N.Y.2d 363, 420 N.E.2d 64, 438 N.Y.Sed, 266 *cert. denied*, 454 U.S.858 (1981); the Canadian case of *Bryanten*, etc.

[17] Position Paper on Abortion, Ottawa: Canadian Medical Association, 1987.

[18] *R. vs. Morgentaler*, [1988]1 S.C.R., 63 O.R.(2d)281, 26 O.A.1, 44 D.L.R.(4th)385, 82 N.R.1, 3 C.C.C.(3d)1, 31 C.R.R.1 (*sub nom. Morgentaler, Smolling and Scott vs. R.*)

[19] As note 18.

[20] Compare Medical Post reporting Gallup polls on public stance.

[21] See J.E. Magnet and E.H.W. Kluge, *Withholding Treatment, from Defective Newborn Children*, (Cowansville: Brown Legal Publications, 1985) chapters 3 and 4.

[22] The sanction against suicide was removed from the *Criminal Code* in 1972.

[23] Compare Bernard Haering, *Medical Ethics* (Fides: Notre Dame, Ind., 1973), 144.

[24] Oxford English Dictionary.

[25] Compare B.A. Ashley and K.D. O'Rourke, *Health Care Ethics: A Theological Analysis* (The Catholic Health Association of the United States: St. Louis, 1982), 375.

[26] As note 25.

[27] This is based on *Black's Law Dictionary*, 4th edition, rev.

[28] See American Medical Association, Report of the Council on Ethical and Judicial Affairs, No.19, "Persistent Vegetative State and the Decision to Withdraw or Withhold Life Support."

[29] "Prolongation of Life: Allocution to an International Congress of Anesthesiologists," Nov. 24, 1957; Pope Pius XII, *Osservatore Romano* 4 (1957).

[30] *Sacred Congregation for the Doctrine of the Faith*, Declaration on Euthanasia, Vatican City, 1980.

[31] See R. Veatch, *Death, Dying, and the Biological Revolution: Our Last Quest for Responsibility* (New Haven and London: Yale Univ. Press, 1970), 106; P. Ramsey "On (Only) Caring for the Dying," in The *Patient as Person* (New Haven and London: Yale Univ. Press, 1970), 120–123.

[32] *Mulloy vs. Hopsang*, [1935] W.W.R. 741 (Seter C.A.).

[33] I.e. one where neither experimenter nor experimental subject knows who is getting the placebo and who the active substance.

[34] These clauses, respectively read as follows: "12. An ethical physician shall, except in an emergency, have the right to refuse to accept a patient"; and 16. "when his morality or religious conscience alone prevents him from recommending some form of therapy will so acquaint the patient."

[35] Law Reform Commission of Canada, Working Paper 28, *Euthanasia, Aiding Suicide and Cessation of Treatment*. Ottawa: 1982.

[36] Report 20, *Euthanasia, Suicide and Cessation of Treatment* (Ottawa: Minister of Supply and Services, 1983).

[37] CMA, *Code of Ethics*, clause 18.

[38] R.M. Sade and A.B. Redfern, "Euthanasia," *New England Journal of Medicine* 292: 16 (April 17, 1975).

[39] J.R. Connery, "The Moral Dilemma of the Quinlan Case," *Hospital Progress* 56: 17 (Dec. 1975) 18–19.

40. D.N. Walton, *On Defining Death: An Analytic Study of the Concept of Death in Philosophy and Medical Ethics* (Montreal: McGill/Queen's University Press, 1979), 96f. See also T.L. Beauchamp, "A Reply to Rachels on Active and Passive Euthanasia," in Beauchamp and Perlin, *Ethical Issues in Death and Dying*, (Englewood Cliffs, N.Y.: Prentice Hall, 1978), 246–248.

41. Walton, ref. note 40, 170.

42. See also P. Foot, "Euthanasia," *Philosophy and Public Affairs* 6: 2 (Winter 1977).

43. James Rachels, "Active and Passive Euthanasia," *New England Journal of Medicine* 292: 2 (Jan 9, 1975) 78–80.

44. See above at p. 240.

45. Law Reform Commission of Canada, Working Paper 33, *Homicide*, 89 (italics added).

46. Law Reform Commission of Canada, Working Paper 46, *Omission, Negligence and Endangering* (Ottawa: Law Reform Commission, 1985) 41, no. 3.

47. As note 46, p.41 no.4(1)

48. As note 46, p.19–20.

49. For a comparable conclusion rejecting the difference between active and passive euthanasia, see James Rachels, "Active and Passive Euthanasia," *New England Journal of Medicine* 292: 2 (Jan. 9, 1975) pp. 78–80); and R. Macklin, *Mortal Choices* (N.Y.: Pantheon Books, 1987) 78ff.

50. *Revised Statutes of Quebec*, c. C–12.

51. Jonathan Bennett, "Whatever the Consequences," *Analysis* 26: 3 (1966) 83–97.

52. *R. vs. Fortier*, Nov. 17, 1980, File No.500–01–805, Superior Court, Longueil, Quebec.

53. See P.J. Fitzgerald, "Acting and Refraining," *Analysis* 27: 4 (1973) 133–139, for another analysis.

54. See also Otto Kirchheimer, "Criminal Omissions," Harvard Law Review, 55 (1942). See also *Omissions, Negligence and Endangering*, Working Paper 46, Law Reform Commission of Canada (Ottawa, 1985) Rec. 2–4, 6 for a discussion of some of these issues.

55. Walton, ref. note 40, 96 f.

56. Walton, ref. note 40, 96 f.

57. Walton, ref. note 40, 120.

58. On the notion of intrinsic value, see G.E. Moore, *Principia Ethica* (Oxford: Oxford Univ. Press, 1928).

59. Albert Schweitzer, *Kultur und Ethik*, 339 (author's translation).

60. I. Kant, *Foundations of the Metaphysics of Morals* (New York: Bobbs-Merrill, 1959), 47 (B422).

61. See Peter Singer, *Animal Liberation*, (New York: Random House, 1975). For a somewhat more mitigated view, see Tom Regan, *The Case for Animal Rights*, (Berkeley and Los Angeles: Univ. of California Press, 1983). See also, Thomas Regan and Peter Singer, eds., *Animal Rights and Human Obligation*, (Englewood Cliffs, N.J.: Prentice-Hall, 1976).

[62] Compare Anglican Church of Canada, *On Dying Well* (Anglican Church Information Office: Toronto, 1975); see Kluge *The Ethics of Deliberate Death* (Port Washington: National University Publications, 1980), 38f. for an analysis.

[63] This is the official position of organized Canadian medicine, although neither the Royal College nor the Canadian Medical Association have an official policy statement condemning euthanasia.

[64] Compare R.M. Veatch, *Death, Dying and the Biological Revolution* (New Haven: Yale Univ. Press, 1976); Paul Ramsey, *The Patient as a Person* (New Haven: Yale Univ. Press, 1970); Helmut Thielicke, *Theologische Ethik* (Tubingen, 1964); Richard Trubo, *An Act of Mercy* (Los Angeles: Nash, 1973).

[65] CMA Position, "Resuscitation of the Terminally Ill," CMAJ vol. 136 (Feb. 15, 1987).

[66] This is central to the so-called principle of double effect. For a classical discussion of the principle, see J.T. Mangan, "A Historical Analysis of the Principle of Double Effect," *Theological Studies*, 10 (1949), 40–61.

[67] The ethical implications of knowingly hastening death by using narcotic analgesics, etc. is ignored by the 1986 statement, "Treatment Decisions for Infants and Children" (1386–1) of the Canadian Paediatric Society.

[68] Reported in Daniel Maguire, *Death by Choice* (New York: Doubleday, 1974) 155; see also S. Lack and E. Lamerton, eds., *The Hour of Our Death*, (London: Chapman, 1975), 36f. and *On Dying Well*, 11 f.

[69] See also Veatch, ref. note 64, Chapter 5.

[70] J. Gould, "The Ethics of Euthanasia in J. Gould and L. Craigmyle, *Your Death Warrant: The Implications of Euthanasia*, (London: Chapman, 1971) v.88.

[71] Yale Kamisar, "Some Non-Religious Objections Against Proposed Mercy-Killing Legislation," *Minnesota Law Review* 42 (May 1958) 969–1042.

[72] See also the discussion of QUALY's, above at 228.

[73] David Hume, *Treatise on Human Nature*, L.A. Selby-Bigge, ed., (Oxford: Clarendon Press, 1967).

[74] Gerald Winslow, "Anencephalic Infants as Organ Sources: Should the Law be Changed? A Reply," *The Journal of Paediatrics* 115: 5 (part 1, November 1989) 829–832, 831.

[75] Francis Bacon, *The New Atlantis* (London, 1627).

[76] See "Dramatic Increase in Support for Euthanasia'" L. Bozinoff and P. MacIntosh, *Gallup*, Gallup Canada Inc. July 24, 1989. "In 1864, 66% of the public backed euthanasia." In 1989, "Seventy-seven percent of the public believes that when a person has an incurable disease that causes great suffering, then a doctor should be allowed by law to end the patient's life through mercy killing, if that person has made a formal request in writing." The regional distribution is as follows: 81% in Quebec, 77% in Ontario and B.C., 72% in Atlantic Canada, and 71% in the Prairie regions. The results are considered accurate within four percentage points 19 times out of 20.

[77] For tentative support, see L.E. and F.A. Rozovsky, "Suicide and the Law," *Canadian Critical Care Nursing Journal* 5: 3 (Sept/Oct., 1988) 24–25. "There may even be an argument that physicians, nurses and perhaps other health professionals have an ethical duty to relieve that suffering. Such relief would take the place of suicide."

[78] S. Wanzer et al. (ref. note 13), *New England Journal of Medicine* (March 29, 1989).

[79] H. Thielicke, "The Doctor as Judge of Who Shall Live and Who Shall Die," in K. Vaux, ed., *Who Shall Live? Medicine, Technology, Ethics* (Philadelphia: Fortress Press, 1970), 162 f.

[80] *Globe and Mail*, Aug. 23, 1989, quoting Dr. Leslie Ivan, professor of surgery, Univ. of Ottawa.

[81] Society for the Right to Die, *Handbook of Living Will Laws*, (New York: Society for the Right to Die, 1987).

[82] See *Handbook of Living Will Laws*.

[83] *Handbook of Living Will Laws*, at various points.

[84] Eg., Switzerland and Uruguay. The Netherlands have introduced enabling legislation for active euthanasia. That legislation has not been passed at this time; however, Dutch physicians by and large are acting as tough it had been, and they have been encouraged in this by the state itself. According to one estimate, at least 3–5000 deaths per annum are the result of active euthanasia in the Netherlands at the present time. See Doerflinger, listed in the bibliography.

[85] See Minutes of the CMA Committee on Ethics, 1989.

[86] See Proceedings of the 1988 General Council of the Canadian Medical Association, Resolution 88–39.

[87] Nova Scotia Patient Consent Act, 1990.

SUGGESTED READINGS

- The Canadian Medical Association. "Guide for the Treatment of Terminally Ill Patients." Ottawa: Canadian Medical Association, 1987.

    This is based on the "Joint Statement on Terminal Illness," subscribed to by the Canadian Nurses Association, the Canadian Bar Association and the Canadian Hospital Association. It contains guidelines that physicians should follow if they think it medically appropriate that death of the patient should be allowed to occur.

- Doerflinger, Richard. "Assisted Suicide: Pro-Choice or Anti-Life?" *Hastings Center Report* 19: 1(Jan/Feb 1989) suppl. 16–19.

    A look at assisted suicide in the Netherlands and an examination of the pros and cons of the issue by someone who knows the situation.

- Law Reform Commission of Canada, Report 20, *Euthanasia, Aiding Suicide and Cessation of Treatment*. Ottawa: Minister of Supply and Services, 1983.

    This report to the government of Canada examines the issue of deliberate death from the perspective of possible reform of the *Criminal Code*. While it recommends some alterations with respect to allowing death to occur, it retains the distinction between active and passive euthanasia and rejects the former.

- Rachels, James. "Euthanasia," from Tom Regan, ed., *Matters of Life and Death: New Introductory Essays in Moral Philosophy.* New York: Random House, 1980, 28–38.

    A classic discussion of both active and passive euthanasia by one of the premier authors in the field. Rachels rejects the active/passive euthanasia distinction as being ethically dubious.

- Schmeiser, Douglas A. "Living Wills and Medical Treatment of the Terminally Ill." *Health Management Forum* 2: 3 (Fall 1989) 32–37.

    A discussion of the use of living wills by someone who has experience as a hospital administrator and who can see some of the problems associated with the usual living will format.

11

Abortion and the Status of the Fetus

This chapter discusses abortion and sketches some of the major ethical issues that surround the status of the human fetus.

Some questions to focus on while reading are:

1. What does it mean to say that the fetus is or is not a person? Why is this question important? Is there any ethically relevant difference between saying that the fetus is a person and saying that it is a human being?
2. If a fetus is a person, does this mean that abortion is ethically unacceptable?
3. What about the rights of the mother in the abortion context? Of the father? Of society? How can we explain this in terms of one of the ethical systems sketched in Chapter 2?
4. Is there an ethical difference between types of abortions?

Introduction

Not all human pregnancies go to term. It is estimated that approximately 31% end in spontaneous abortions. Over half of these occur before the woman has even realized that she was pregnant.[1] Miscarriages or spontaneous abortions, therefore, are not at all uncommon. Furthermore, there is usually a good medical reasons why they occur. In about 54% of spontaneous abortions the fetus is found to be physiologically abnormal—usually to a degree incompatible with what is considered to be a reasonable and acceptable quality of life. Spontaneous abortions, therefore, might be called nature's way of correcting mistakes.

However, not all terminations of pregnancy are spontaneous. Here as in other areas, mankind has gone beyond nature. From early times, people have terminated pregnancies deliberately by inducing abortions. This is true in all cultures, all countries, and all religions,[2] and whether we are considering the historical past or the present setting.[3]

Of course, induced abortions have not always been judged in the same way. Not even in religious contexts. Christianity provides a good example. If we can take the writings of such people as St. Augustine (5th century A.D.) and St. Thomas Aquinas (13th century A.D.) as representative, early Christianity did not uniformly condemn abortion as murder. Instead, it maintained that one has to distinguish between the earlier and the later stages of fetal development. Their reasoning was simple and to the point. To kill a living being is not in and by itself murder. It becomes murder only when the living thing is a human being or person. However something is a person not because it has a certain type of body, or because it has a particular kind of parents. What makes it a person is that it has a human soul. A fetus does not have a soul from its very beginning. It acquires a soul only after it has developed sufficiently to be capable of sensation and mental activity. Until it has reached that point, therefore, to abort it is not to commit murder.[4] Needless to say, the position of the Catholic Church has since changed. The current position is that the human fetus is a human being in the moral sense, or a person, from the moment of conception; therefore to kill it deliberately is always murder.

The legal position of Western culture has also changed over the years. In Roman and Greek times, the law permitted abortion at the behest of the head of household.[5] In English speaking countries this situation persisted to the time of Blackstone (1765). According to Blackstone, it did not matter in who performed the abortion or at whose instigation it was done. Nor, according to Blackstone, did it matter whether the abortion was induced before or after "quickening." An induced abortion was simply a misdemeanour.[6] As time went on, inducing an abortion became an increasingly serious matter until in the 19th century it became characterized as murder.

Canadian law initially followed the English model. It considered induced abortions as murders until the proclamation of Section 251 of the *Criminal Code*. That Section allowed the induction of an abortion but only under certain conditions: It had to be approved by

> ... the therapeutic abortion committee for [an] accredited or approved hospital, by a majority of the members of the committee and at a meeting of that committee at which the case of such female person has been reviewed.[7]

and the committee had to certify in writing that in the opinion of the committee,

> ... continuation of the pregnancy of such female person would or would be likely to endanger (the woman's) life or health.[8]

From then on, the story becomes complicated. In 1988 the Supreme Court in *R. vs. Morgentaler*[9] struck down Section 251 as unconstitutional. In giving its reasons, the Court focused on the abortion committee requirement of Section 251. The Court rejected this requirement as imposing an unequal burden on woman in different parts of the country, and as advantaging urban women over rural ones. It also stated that

> Forcing a woman, by threat of criminal sanction, to carry a fetus to term unless she meets certain criteria unrelated to her own priorities and aspirations, is a profound interference with the woman's body and thus an infringement of the security of the person.[10]

It is of some interest to note that when the Supreme Court rendered its decision in *Morgentaler* it stated that while it considered Section 251 to be unconstitutional, it did not thereby intend to rule out the possibility of the federal government passing a statute specifically aimed at controlling abortion.[11] The only requirements the court suggested was that such a statute would have to be within the parameters indicated in *Morgentaler* itself. It would have to allow for the "priorities and aspirations" of women, and it could not impose undue and unequal burdens with respect to access.

This ruling of the Supreme Court effectively left Canada without any federal legislation targeted specifically at abortion. The only applicable laws left were statutes such as sections 45, 215 to 217, 222 to 226 and 229 of the *Criminal Code*. However, these deal with medical practice in general: the duties of the physician towards the patient, surgical procedures, duty of care and so on.[12] Therefore, the only restrictions on free and unhindered access to abortions that remained were provincial. These restrictions focused not on the criminality of abortion, which was a federal matter, but on funding and provisions of access. In most cases, they consisted in the refusal of the province in question to fund abortions as an insured service under the provincial insurance plans.

In the meantime, the situation had been complicated still further by a suit brought from a pro-life perspective by J. Borowski. That suit, initially decided in 1987 at the provincial appeals level in Saskatchewan, alleged that the fetus was a human being in the legal sense of the *Criminal Code* and the Charter of Rights and Freedoms from the very moment of its conception, and that therefore abortions *per se* should be considered murder in the eyes of the law.[13] That suit was decided in early 1989 against Mr. Borowski. The Supreme Court again was very careful in its ruling. It declined to decide the question whether the fetus was a human being or person in the eyes of the law. Instead, it said that this was a matter not strictly covered by existing legislation; and that rather than being a matter for the Court to decide, it was more properly the prerogative of Parliament to determine in a legislative fashion.

The government of the day had been trying to avoid having to come to grips with this thorny issue. The summer of 1989, however, saw two more court cases which catapulted the situation into the federal legislative arena. One came from Quebec, which, interestingly enough, had the most liberal abortion policy of any of the provinces. In both cases, men attempted to prevent their female partners from obtaining an abortion. In the first, *Murphy vs. Dodd*,[14] the courts refused to uphold what the plaintiffs claimed to be the rights of the father. The matter was settled at the lower levels and never reached the Supreme Court for determination.

The second case, *Tremblay vs. Daigle*,[15] did go all the way to the Supreme Court. In fact, the matter had become so contested and the Court saw the issue to be so important that it interrupted its summer recess and, sitting in full session, heard the appeal. It gave a decision on August 8, and handed its reasons down on November 11.[16] It was unanimous in the view that Ms. Daigle had a right to an abortion. Once again, however, the Court refused to rule on the status of the human fetus outside of the scope of existing legislation. As it put it:

> The respondent's argument is that a fetus is an "être humain," in the English "human being," and therefore has a right to life and a right to assistance when its life is in peril. In examining this argument it should be emphasized at the outset that the argument must be viewed in the context of the legislation in question. The Court is not required to enter the philosophical and theological debates about whether or not a fetus is a person, but, rather, to answer the legal question whether the Quebec legislature has accorded the fetus personhood ... . The Court's task is a legal one. Decisions based upon broad social, political, moral and economic choices are more appropriately left to the legislature.[17]

Finally on November 3, 1989, driven by public clamour from all sides and by the perceived political need to remove the issue from the federal scene, the government introduced Bill C–43, "An Act Respecting Abortion." The stated intent of that Bill was to fill the legislative void created at the federal level by the 1988 *Morgentaler* decision, to protect the fetus and to provide uniformity throughout the provinces. The Bill stated that:

> 287. (1) Every person who induces an abortion on a female person is guilty of an indictable offence and liable to imprisonment for a term not exceeding two years, unless the abortion is induced by or under the direction of a medical practitioner who is of the opinion that, if the abortion were not induced, the health or life of the female person would be likely to be threatened.
>
> (2) For the purpose of this section, "health" includes, for greater certainty, physical, mental and psychological health;
>
> medical practitioner, in respect of an abortion induced in a province, means a person who is entitled to practise medicine under the laws of that province;
>
> opinion means an opinion formed using generally accepted standards of the medical profession.
>
> (3) For the purpose of this section and section 288, inducing an abortion does not include using a drug, device or other means on a female person that is likely to prevent implantation of a fertilized ovum.[18]

The effect of Bill C–43 was to place the whole onus of decision-making on the medical profession in general, in terms of the standards it established and the professional guidelines that it promulgated, and on the observance of these standards and guidelines by individual physicians. By that very token, the status of induced abortions became a peculiarly and uniquely medical issue. The medical profession was given the role of gatekeeper. Whether an abortion was appropriate was to be decided in terms of medical judgements and standards. With this, the acceptability of induced abortions became a matter that could no longer be decided simply in terms of the standards of the individual physician. The ethics of the profession as a whole became involved. Is the indication of an abortion ethically defensible given the ethics of the profession?

Some Initial Considerations

The question cannot answered by pointing to the law. The fact that something is permitted or enjoined by a statute does not necessarily make it ethically acceptable. Neither does tradition, no matter how hallowed or well-entrenched, provide ethical guarantees. Nor, finally, is it possible to establish the ethical acceptability of abortion by citing the Policy on Induced Abortion put forward by the Canadian medical association and adopted by most of the provincial medical associations. The Policy Summary on Induced Abortion contains the following points:[19]

> There should be no delay in the provision of abortion services.

> No discrimination should be directed against doctors who provide abortion services.

These clauses contain no justification of abortion itself. They merely imply that so far as the CMA is concerned, abortion is ethically defensible. This does not address, let alone settle the issue. Without ethical justification, however, the position reduces to a mere announcement of policy. To the ethically minded physician, this would be insufficient.

Furthermore, this policy, like that of the Royal College, says nothing about the status of the human fetus. Consequently it ignores *the* question that lies at the heart of the abortion controversy. That is the question, "What is the ethical status of the human fetus?" (Where the term "fetus" is intended to cover the whole range of development from the time of fertilization to the moment of birth.) The question is crucial because how it is answered will determine the nature and limits of the actions and omissions that are permissible with respect to the fetus. The ethics of abortion will follow from this as a matter of course.

The Ethical Status of the Human Fetus

Three major ethical positions have been advanced in the debate over the status of the human fetus.[20] At the one extreme there is the view that a fetus is a person from the moment of fertilization, and that therefore it enjoys the same fundamental rights that belong to all persons.[21] The following statement illustrates this perspective rather well:

> We need to keep our eyes on the ball. I was once a zygote and so were you, and if we license experiments on pre–14-day humans we are licensing experiments on the likes of you and me. We are denying that it is our being that makes us human. But if not that, then what? ... if membership of Homo sapiens is not really what counts ... who is to decide what does?[22]

The implications of this position are severe. They involve prohibition against all actions that would prevent implantation from occurring; proscription of abortions except when they are done for the sake of the fetus itself,[23] or, in certain cases, when the life of the mother is threatened;[24] and a general opposition to actions that could not be defended in the case of other persons.

At the other extreme stands the position that a human fetus is not a person in any ethically relevant sense "until it has proceeded alive from the body of its mother."[25] This position finds its most radical expression in statements like the following, taken from an editorial in the *Newsletter* of the Federation of Medical Women of Canada:

> A woman is her fetus. Until the fetus is born, there is only one person, the mother ... say "no" to fetal personhood. Trust your instinct and assert your womanhood. Let us reestablish organic unity between the fetus and the mother through the recognition of only one person prior to childbirth, the mother.[26]

In fact, according to some who espouse this position, there is some doubt about the personhood of the child even after birth. According to them, not even the new-born child is a person. It will become a person only after it has acquired self-awareness and the ability to formulate life-plans.[27] According to this view abortion would be ethically permissible at any time. So would infanticide, until the child has attained self-awareness and has acquired the ability to formulate life-plans. In fact, this approach holds that any sort of action will be allowable so long as it does not interfere with the rights of someone who *is* a person, or with the rights of society.

We should add, however, that so radical a perspective is not a necessary consequence of denying fetal personhood. Even here, it is possible to adopt a middle ground and agree with the Law Reform Commission that:

> ... to decide whether to give the fetus criminal law protection we don't need to decide if it is a person.[There is nothing which limits criminal law protection to persons. Further, even those who deny that the fetus is a person might accept a measure of criminal law protection at some point in development.] Instead we can directly ask how far we should protect it. Indeed, the answer to this question—how to protect it, how to treat it, how to regard it from a moral standpoint—is itself part of the answer to the question whether morally it counts as a person.[28]

However, not only is the logic of this statement obscure, it also makes the personhood and ethical status of the fetus dependent on the criminal law—on what legislators decide. While some authors have explicitly embraced this consequence, (e.g. Engelhardt)[29] it is really out of place in ethical considerations. Its proper relevance is confined to argumentation touching the law.

A third view takes an intermediate position between the two. It holds that although the fetus is not a person from the moment of conception, it becomes a person at some time during its gestational development but prior to its actual completion. This position allows for some variations in the exact point when this stage has been reached. 12 and 20 weeks of gestation are the most common variants[30]. Its most important consequences, however, are these: Before the fetus becomes a person, the range of permissible actions is ethically constrained only by the competing interest and rights of members of society. These may include constraints based on the values that people hold, their interests in the continued existence of the fetus, and so on. The fetus itself, however, would have no rights. Of course, once the fetus has become a person, its rights and interests must be taken into account. More precisely, its rights will have to be balanced against the rights of all those who claim that a certain action (or omission), which conceivably would harm the fetus, should be allowed.[31]

Given this variety of views, we might usefully order our considerations around the following three sets of questions:

1. Is the fetus ever a person? And if so, at what point does it become a person?

2. If the fetus is ever a person, does it have rights? More specifically, does it have a right to life and the right to a certain kind of treatment?

3. If the fetus does have a right to life and the right to a certain kind of treatment, what is the relationship between these rights and the competing rights of the mother (and of relevant other persons)?

Let us consider these in turn.

Is the Fetus Ever a Person?

Ethical analysis must be internally consistent. Therefore, what we say in response to this question must not conflict with what we have already said in our discussion of death. The reason why considerations about death are germane here is that the question whether someone is already a person is really the other side of the question whether that individual is still a person. The two cannot be considered independently of each other. They are opposite sides of the same coin.

We discussed the conditions under which someone is still a person when we were dealing with the issue of death.[32] We said then that there are two distinct positions, depending on whether we define death in cognitive or in purely biological terms. If we define death in purely biological terms, then someone is a person as long as her or his body is still capable of integrated organic functioning. From that perspective, the individual will count as a person just as long as there is a functioning brain-stem; because as long as there is a functioning brain-stem, the organism as a whole is capable of integrated and independent survival. The case of Elaine Esposito and of others in a permanent vegetative coma illustrated the thrust of this approach quite well.

On the other hand, if death is defined in cognitive terms—not as death of a biological organism but as death of a human being in a psycho-social sense—then the purely biological capacity for continued organic survival will be insufficient to identify anyone as a person. It is the cognitive capabilities of the individual that are then important.

From this standpoint, someone is a person in an ethical sense just so long as he or she either is sapiently and cognitively self-aware or has the present capacity for such awareness without having to undergo a fundamental change in functional constitution. We also noted that neither sapient cognitive awareness nor the capacity for it are directly observable. From this we concluded that to be able to tell whether someone meets these conditions, we must have some criteria that allow us to say whether actual awareness or the present constitutional capacity for it are present in a particular case. We determined that overt behaviour inclusive of symbolic communication constitute such criteria, but went on to say that ultimately these are not always present—and sometimes cannot be identified as such. In any case, so we reasoned, the material basis for sapient cognitive awareness as well as for its constitutive capacity lie in the presence of a neurological system that is functionally sufficiently integrated and complex to be able to support the relevant sorts of cognitive functions. We therefore concluded that from this standpoint, the ultimate material criterion for ascribing personhood is the presence of just such a nervous system.

If we apply these considerations to the human fetus, we arrive at two distinct answers to the question, Is the fetus ever a person? If we adopt the biological approach—the approach that is correlated with the "whole-brain" criterion for death—then the fetus will meet the criteria for personhood just as soon as it has a functioning brainstem. In other words, we shall then have to say that the fetus becomes a person some at time around the twelfth week of gestation.[33]

On the other hand, if we accept the cognitive approach to death—that is to say, if we adopt the cerebral criterion—then the answer is, "As soon as the fetus has developed a nervous system that can provide the basis for sapient cognitive awareness." And here, of course, we have to keep in mind that we are not looking for actual or even developed awareness. What we are looking for, what this criterion requires, is the same level that we would find sufficient for the ascription of personhood in all other cases.

The important point to note about all of this, however, is that on neither interpretation does the human fetus count as a person from the moment of conception. In each case the reason is the same: A fetus does not have neurons, let alone a nervous system until much later. The brain stem appears and begins operating as an integrated neural unit controlling bodily functions somewhere around the twelfth week; and while rudimentarily identifiable cellular structures of the cerebral cortex appear at about 7.5 to 8 weeks, it is only during the 16th to 20th week that there is evidence of the layering organization characteristic of a neocortex. As one commentator put it in a slightly different context,

> The situation [of fetal development at 18 to 20 weeks] is roughly comparable to that assumed to exist in the stable comatose state displayed by Karen Ann Quinlan, a state short of the current definition of brain death.[34]

At 25 weeks the cortex shows neuronal cell bodies with distinct elongating processes but limited branching and few synaptic connections. By 33 weeks, however, branching of processes is extensive and synaptic connections are many.

Between 24 to 28 weeks, the cerebral cortex acquires its typically multi-layered structure.[35]

In other words:

> Integrated behaviour such as we associate with persons in the usual context seem to appear first midway in the third trimester, along with maturation changes in the upper brain. Professional behavioural observers have described this behaviour as though it indicated a rudimentary and fluctuating subjective awareness, possibly the first appearance of a conscious self.[36]

The upshot of all this is that we are faced with a choice. We can either follow the path indicated by the whole-brain criterion for loss of personhood and apply it consistently, with due alteration of detail, to the case of the fetus; or we can follow the path mapped out in our discussion of the cerebral criterion. Each option yields a different answer to the question, "Is the fetus ever a person?" If we follow the first, then the fetus will not be a person until it has a functioning brain stem; if we follow the second, it will not be a person until it has a rudimentary functioning cerebral cortex capable of sustaining sapient cognitive awareness at some level.

We advocate the second position. As we pointed out in our discussion of death, what turns a living biological organism of the species homo sapiens into a person is the present capacity for sapient cognitive awareness. The material basis for that capacity, however, is not the brain as a whole. It is the cerebral cortex. In light of this we have to say that the threshold for personhood can be crossed from two sides: once, when the essential features of an integrated and functioning cerebral cortex come to be in place; and once, when these features and functional capacities cease to exist. A consistent development of our underlying premises allows no other option. Therefore, the logic of our initial position on death forces us to say that fetus cannot be a person until cerebral development and functional integration have taken place.

If the data that we have referred to are correct, then at twenty weeks gestation the fetus typically is at a stage analogous to that of cerebral death. By 24 weeks, however, it will usually have passed that threshold, or at least will be in the process of passing beyond it. Once it reaches the seventh or eighth month, it will definitely have crossed it and will have become a person in this cerebrally defined sense.[37]

The reason we put it like this is that there are variations in individual development. This is true whether we are dealing with a human fetus or anyone else. Some will develop more slowly, others more quickly, and some not at all. Anencephalics would be good examples of the latter kind. An ethically acceptable policy, however, must not only be consistent. It must also allow for variations and differences between individual cases. In other words, not only must it identify the areas where the choice is clear, it must also recognize that there are grey zones where the particulars of the given case do not quite fit the general rule.

It is with this in mind that we suggest that from the cerebral standpoint, about 20 weeks would be a reasonable point at which to place the beginning of fetal personhood. That would put the limit at the lower end of the grey zone marking the fetal transition from non-integrated to integrated cerebral functioning. Here as elsewhere, if it is possible to do so without becoming unreasonable, it is better to err on the side of safety. Of course, if future discoveries should reveal that the capacity for cerebral functioning is present earlier, then lower limits for allowing abortions would have to be adjusted accordingly.

Does the Fetus Have Rights?

Which brings us to the second set of questions: If the fetus is a person at some stage of its development and before it is born, does it have an ethical[38] right to life? And, Does it have the ethical right to a certain type of treatment?

The two questions are closely connected but logically independent of each other. We shall therefore take them in turn. Beginning with the right to life, the logic of rights that we have outlined in the earlier chapters[39] entails a direct and simple answer: A fetus acquires rights just as soon as it becomes a person, whenever that may be. Prior to becoming a person it cannot and does not have rights. At least, not rights in an ethical sense. The law may wish to accord it statutory rights of a legal sort. That, however, is an entirely different matter and as such has no implications for ethics. It is a function of what a society considers appropriate for a particular context or situation.

So, both approaches agree. A fetus acquires rights when it becomes a person. When is that? We have already given the answer: When its neurological development meets the material and functional criteria for personhood. As to when that occurs, the two approaches to personhood that were identified above once more yield distinct answers. The whole-brain or brain-stem approach entails that the fetus will acquires ethical rights at some time around the 12th week of gestation; the cerebral approach entails that it acquires them at some time around the 20th week of gestation.

As to the right to life, little more needs to be said. The principle of priority entails that the right to life is fundamental. It is the logical prerequisite for any other right. If the fetus has any rights at all, it must have this right.

We can therefore say that the fetus acquires the right to life either at about twelve or at about twenty weeks of gestation, depending on which definition of personhood is accepted.

However, we want to add several caveats to all this. First of all, it is important that this conclusion not be misunderstood. It says nothing about whether the fetus who has this right to life, or, for that matter any other right, is *in utero* or has actually been born. It leaves that issue unresolved because from an ethical perspective it is utterly irrelevant. Where someone is located—one's place of residence, so to speak—has nothing to do with whether or not one is a person. The following case will make that clear.

> A seven month-old fetus at L.L. hospital has been diagnosed by sonogramme as having a surgically correctable congenital malformation of the kidneys. The paediatric nephrology team of L.L. hospital is prepared to correct the malformation by

removing the fetus from the uterus, performing the necessary repair, and then returning the fetus to the uterus once again. The team performs the operation, returns the fetus to the uterus, and the fetus continues to develop normally until it is born two months later.

The point of the case is that if where a fetus is did determine its ethical status, that is to say, if where it is did determine whether or not it was a person, then this fetus would not be a person prior to the operation, but would be a person during the operation while it was outside the uterus, would once again not be a person when it was returned to it, and finally would be a person once again upon being born. Such an analysis would be bizarre.

Legally, of course, the analysis would be different. According to current Canadian law, a fetus does not become a person until[40]

> ... it has proceeded, in a living state, from the body of its mother whether or not
> (a) it has breathed,
> (b) it has an independent circulation, or
> (c) the navel string is severed.

Therefore, according to current Canadian law the fetus would have become a person once it had emerged from the uterus because of the operation. However, it would then stay a person *even after it had been replaced* when the operation was finished; because once it has become a person, it would have to meet the criteria for death in order to stop being a person. That would mean that those fetuses who had been fortunate enough to have been removed from the uterus and then replaced would be persons, whereas the fetuses who had not been removed, because they did not need surgery, or whatever, but who were at the very same (or even greater) stage of development, would not count as persons! In other words, legally speaking a fetus would count as a person simply because it had briefly changed its place of residence, while other fetuses who had remained where they were would not even though they would otherwise be identical in development and constitution. But as we said, these are purely legal considerations, and only serve to underline the incoherence of the law as it stands.

The second point is this: Nothing we have said so far entails that there are no constraints that apply to the treatment of the human fetus. There are constraints; and they derive from two quarters. One finds its roots in the fundamental value that our society places on life in general and on human life in particular. This value is so fundamental that any deviation from it violates the sensibilities of everyone in society. Therefore, it would have to be justified in terms of the affront that it gives to the psychological integrity of members of society. Not to provide it would amount to psychological assault, which would be a violation of the principle of autonomy and respect for persons. Such justification might appeal to a still more fundamental value, or it might point to some fundamental right on part of some person that otherwise would be infringed. We shall explore these constraints further when we consider fetal experimentation.

The third point we want to make is that we have said nothing so far about the interrelationship between the rights of the fetal person and the rights of others. We only said that at some stage of development the fetus (normally) becomes a person, and that at that point it acquires rights in general and the right to life in particular. We still have to consider what strength these rights have, and how a conflict between fetal rights and the rights of others is to be resolved. And that, of course, is our next set of questions.

What Is the Relationship between the Right to Life of the Fetal Person and the Competing Rights of Others?

It would be an understatement to say that the answer is far from simple. But it would also be disingenuous to overplay the difficulty of the issue. Many of the difficulties that arise in this context derive not from the ethics but from the socio-political and psychological contexts in which the question is normally asked. These contexts tend to colour, and predispose, whatever answer we are likely to give (or receive). However, if we abstract from these parameters, and if we focus solely on the ethics, then the following considerations seem relevant.

First, no right is absolute. The principle of relevant difference and the principle of priority play a role here as anywhere else. This means that neither the rights of the fetus nor those of the pregnant woman can automatically be assumed to take priority. The circumstances under which the rights arise, and the conditions in which the rights are claimed, are crucial to any evaluation.

Second, the fact that a something is not allowed or forbidden by an ethical principle does not mean that there are no other parameters that constrain the relevant action. We have already seen that the values a society holds may function in such a constraining capacity.

Third, on a more practical note, we must always be careful to distinguish between what we would like to see happen in terms that are emotionally acceptable or that fit a particular agenda, and what is defensible in ethical terms.

Fourth, the fact that something is allowed are even mandated in law does not necessarily make it ethically defensible. The point is trite, but bears frequent repeating.

With this in mind, let us return to the question: "What is the relationship between the right of the fetal person and the rights of the pregnant woman?" The answer is that no-one can tell *a priori*. It depends on the nature of the circumstances, the strength of the competing rights and the values that are involved. What we can say is that when there is a conflict, we must approach the situation as free of emotional predispositions as possible and try to resolve the situation in ethical, not emotional terms.

However, although we cannot give a general and universal answer *a priori*, there are some general considerations that strike us as relevant. For example, it seems safe to say that the balancing process that we spoke of a moment ago is different in different stages of fetal development. In the early stages, it is more appropriately described as a balancing of the value of respect for life of the fetus as against the claim of autonomy and the right to self-determination on part of the woman. However, as the pregnancy progresses the fetus increasingly becomes an object of serious ethical concern until, when it acquires the capacity for sapient awareness (which occurs roughly at twenty weeks) that ethical concern becomes full-blown.[41] At that point, the balancing no longer centres in a weighing of respect for life against the principle of autonomy. Instead, it becomes a balancing of the right to life and to a certain quality of life on part of the fetus, against the right to self-determination on part of the pregnant woman. The existence of right-claims will no longer be at issue. What will be at issue will be their relative strengths.

Still, we must take care to make sure not to understand this notion of a balancing process in too restrictive a fashion, either from the side of the fetus or from the side of the woman. As Edward W. Keyserlingk put it in 1984

> ... two extremes must be avoided. One is that only the pregnant woman's health and welfare should count, but not that of the unborn child, the latter classified as simply a biological extension of the woman with no rights of its own. The other extreme to be rejected is that only the unborn child's health and welfare should count, but not that of the pregnant woman, the latter considered as essentially and only the incubator or support system for the unborn child, her own rights and health taking second place ... Both are (or should be) patients, but neither of them in a absolute or unqualified sense.[42]

The rights of both the fetus and the pregnant woman must be given due weight. However, it is also important to remember that rights provide only a framework of possible acts that may be requested from others. What action is chosen, and indeed, whether the right itself is claimed at all, depends on the values of the individual whose right is at issue. Therefore, when we come to balance rights, the strengths of these values have to be taken into account. The more strongly a value is held, the more likely that the person who holds it will want to insist that it be observed. The more likely also that they will be observed in a particular direction.

This creates a twofold problem. First, a fetal person cannot claim a right. It lacks the cognitive and physiological ability to do so. Therefore it follows that if the rights of a fetal person are to be translated into practically meaningful terms, there has to be a surrogate or proxy who exercises its right for the fetal person.

Second, a fetus does not have values. Therefore a surrogate will have no basis on which to decide whether to exercise a particular right for a fetal person, let alone in what direction. This presents a dilemma.

The solution to this dilemma lies in the fact that a fetus has instinctive drives: drives that it shares with all other human beings. In an inchoate form, these drives correspond to the motivational gradients that we have identified as values. This means that in the context of decision-making, the drives can function as analogues of the values that determine the actions of ordinary persons. Therefore, they can take the place of values in the decision-making of the proxy. Their estimated strength will govern the rigidity with which the surrogate has to insist on the relevant rights of the fetal person, and their nature will determine the direction. Since these drives become stronger and more defined as the fetus develops, we should see a corresponding increase in insistence on fetal rights as the pregnancy progresses.

We can therefore make some practical sense of the notion of fetal rights. What is more, we can talk about them in essentially the same terms that we talk about the rights of all other persons. We can even talk about balancing right claims by taking into account the strengths of the values that are relevant to a particular rights-claim.

All of which brings us to the next question: How can the competing right-claims of the pregnant woman and the fetus be balanced in induced abortions? The 1989 General Council of the CMA directed the Committee on Ethics to consider the proposition that "in the decision concerning a abortion, both parties must consider the existence of the unborn child and respect its rights."[43] How can this be translated into an ethically acceptable perspective?

Abortion

The answer is that we must distinguish between induced abortions performed on fetuses before they become persons, and induced abortions performed on fetuses after they have become persons. In the first case, there will be no problem of rights, only one of values. In the second case, there will be a problem of values as well as of rights. However, before explaining this, we should first become clear about what precisely we mean by the term "induced abortion."

The standard definition given to the phrase in Canada comes from the Canadian Medical Association's 1988 Policy Summary referred to above. It goes like this:

> Induced abortion, as interpreted by the CMA, is the active termination of a pregnancy before fetal viability. In this context viability is the ability of the fetus to survive independently of the maternal environment.[44]

After twenty weeks gestation one no longer talks about an abortion but rather about a premature birth.[45]

Nevertheless, despite the fact that this definition of abortion is generally accepted, it is seriously incomplete. It does not mention let alone take into account that abortions are not usually performed solely for the purpose of emptying a uterus. While this is not usually stated explicitly or, for that matter, clearly considered by many people, one of their central purposes of having an abortion is to kill the developing fetus.[46] This is clearly reflected in clinical discussions of abortion; discussions like the following:

> After twenty weeks we reverted to using the intra-amniotic method of urea combined with PGE 2, accepting a higher incidence of cervical trauma and the real possibility of coagulation disorder, since the method results in fetal death thereby minimizing unnecessary stress to both parents, patients and nursing attendants.[47]

It also finds expression in the claim that "the use of hypertonic saline alone or in combination with S/PG significantly reduced the frequency of live abortions" and the admission that for that reason it is preferred by some obstetricians and gynaecologists, since it tended to minimize emotional reactions on part of the staff.[48] It is also recognized clearly in psychiatric discussions of abortions and their effects on medical personnel:

> It appears that physicians will choose a procedure more dangerous to patients because it is less psychologically traumatic to themselves not to face the struggling fetus they just aborted.[49]

Therefore, while theoretically speaking one could go along with the CMA and define an induced abortion simply as the deliberate termination of a pregnancy prior to gestation, realistically speaking we should add "with the intent of killing the fetus."

To this we should add parenthetically that while the evacuation of the uterus and the killing of the fetus need not occur simultaneously, they usually do. To be sure, there are case in which the aborted fetus dies after the abortion. For instance, when the abortion is performed with prostaglandins[50] or even saline induction.[51] However, these are unusual circumstances. As we said, by and large the intent is to use a method that ensures the death of the fetus. Therefore, while on occasion induced abortions do result in living fetuses, and while most institutions in which or under whose jurisdiction abortions are performed do have guidelines that require that these fetuses then be treated in an appropriate medical fashion, such an outcome is neither desired no hoped for. In fact, when it occurs, it results in a great deal of concern and consternation.

Arguments in Favour of Induced Abortion

To return, then, to the question: Are induced abortions ethically acceptable? As we have already seen, there are arguments on both sides of the question. On the affirmative side, there is a whole series of arguments that find their focus in the claim that a woman has a fundamental and inalienable right to self-determination.

The argument that is encountered most often in this connection is that a woman has a right to her own body. Pregnancy is a condition of her body. Consequently a woman has the right to terminate her pregnancy. Otherwise the right to her own body would be empty. This sort of reasoning is sometimes combined with the contention that since a woman exists prior to the fetus, her rights take precedence over those of the fetus.

Then there are arguments that focus on how the pregnancy came about. For example, there is the argument from contraceptive failure. Even though both the woman and her partner may have taken due care to prevent a pregnancy from occurring, the fact is that contraceptive methods sometimes do fail.[52] Not to allow an induced abortion in such cases would be to punish the woman for something that is not her fault. The argument from rape goes in a similar direction. A wrinkle is introduced by the argument from incest. It contends that traditionally, abortions have been allowed in such cases. Therefore, to forbid them now would be to fly in the face of what society has always accepted.[53]

Health reasons have also been considered grounds for permitting abortions. When the health or life of the woman is threatened by a continuation of the pregnancy, an abortion should be permissible. Conditions like Eisenmenger's syndrome come to mind in this context, as does progressive renal failure and similar conditions. The argument here is that unless the woman herself has clearly understood the danger of the risks associated with pregnancy and has given a voluntary, competent and informed consent to its continuation, the fact that her health and life are threatened is sufficient to guarantee her the right to an abortion. Both the old Section 251 and the new Section 287 of the *Criminal Code* explicitly recognize such factors, and confer a legal right. A variant of this kind of argument focuses on the threat to the pregnant woman's psychological wellbeing and maintains that if her "mental or psychological health" is threatened or if she is likely to commit suicide in desperation, an abortion would be legitimate no matter what the stage of fetal development.[54]

The fetus has also been described as an "unjust pursuer."[55] The thrust of this observation is that therefore abortions should be allowed at any stage of fetal development because they simply amount to self-defense. Then there is the claim that a fetus is simply a part of the woman's body.[56] This, too, would allow abortion on demand.

Finally, we sometimes encounter the argument that every woman has the right to shape her life according to her wishes and aspirations. An unwanted pregnancy, however, would make the attainment of her life-goals impossible. Women are not mere fetal containers.[57] Therefore autonomy and respect for persons entail that she should be able to have an abortion if she so wishes. This sort of reasoning finds clear support in the Supreme Court judgement of *Morgentaler vs. the Queen*, where Chief Justice Dickson and Mr. Justice Lamer stated that

> Forcing a woman, by threat of criminal sanction, to carry a foetus to term unless she meets certain criteria unrelated to her own priorities and aspirations, is a profound interference with a woman's body and thus an infringement of the security of the person.[58]

On the other hand, sometimes it is argued that abortions should be allowed not only when health and life of a woman are in danger, but also when the health or welfare of the as-yet-unborn child are at risk. For instance, sometimes a pregnant woman is or is perceived to be a bad risk as a mother. Severe maternal mental handicap has been of special concern in this connection.[59] In these cases the argument has been made that if the woman were allowed to continue her pregnancy, the child that would be borne might well suffer in its quality of life. It might even become a grim statistic.

Somewhat differently, it has also been said that the knowledge or even well founded suspicion that the child-to-be would suffer from a congenital defect like Tay-Sachs disease, haemophilia, cystic fibrosis, trisomy, justifies abortion for the sake of the child.[60] The list of medical indications that have been identified in this connection is large and growing steadily.

Lastly, although by no means finally, there is the argument that abortion is acceptable because the fetus is not a person. It therefore poses no ethical problem whatever.[61]

Arguments against Induced Abortions

The arguments against abortion are equally as varied. For instance, it has been said that abortion is ethically indefensible because the fetus is a person. For the logic of this argument it is irrelevant whether the fetus is a person from the moment of conception[62] or only after it has passed a certain stage of development. On either perspective, it is said to have a right to life. It is then argued that its right takes priority over any competing right on part of the mother because utter helplessness demands utter protection.[63]

Other arguments against abortion have tried a different tack. They have attempted to invalidate the arguments in favour of abortion themselves. For example, some of the arguments in favour of induced abortion that we saw above have been based on the contention that abortions may be necessary in order to protect the mental health of the pregnant woman. As a matter of fact, between 85 and 95% of all abortions in Canada are done for psychiatric reasons ostensibly to protect the mental health of the pregnant woman.[64] The line of argumentation against this that we have just mentioned maintains that not only are the majority of so-called psychiatric indications for abortions spurious or even manufactured,[65] ("It seems that psychiatry was exploited in an attempt to satisfy a social need within the context of the medical model.")[66] but that women who had abortions for psychiatric reasons either did no better than those who had been refused abortions[67] or actually did worse than those whose requests for abortions were refused.[68]

Still other arguments against abortion maintain that to allow abortions contravenes the principle of respect for life, that it results in the brutalization of our society;[69] and so on. However, when all is said and done, the central question that we have to answer is really this: Does the deontological framework that we have developed so far, and which has allowed us to say that it ethically acceptable deliberately to bring about the death of a human being under certain circumstances, also allow us to say that abortion is also acceptable under certain circumstances?

Conclusion

The answer cannot be found by saying that there is a practical need to allow abortions so as to avoid the death of women caused by having them illegally. First of all, this claim is statistically false.[70] Second, and from an ethical perspective much more importantly, the fact that people will do something, or that they are likely to do something, does not constitute an ethical reason for approving of what they do.

Nor does an appeal to women's rights settle the issue. Without denying the validity of these rights, we must always remember that no right exists in isolation. The competing rights of other persons must always be kept in mind. As we have just seen, the human fetus becomes a person after a certain point of development. The question of abortion therefore is one that has to be addressed in terms of competing rights of *all* relevant persons. It also must not ignore the role of individual and societal values.

With this in mind, what should we answer? Our discussion of the status of the fetus points the way. Abortion, induced abortion, is ethically defensible but only within certain limits. From the point of the fetus, these limits are reached when the fetus has become a person. Until that point has been reached, abortion will not violate any fetal rights because until the fetus has reached that stage, it has no rights. At least, not ethical ones. The only ethical protection the fetus has prior to becoming a person derives from our society's fundamental value of respect for human life and the rights of others not to be psychologically assaulted. However, these values and rights may be overruled by the right to self-determination of the pregnant woman. That right, in turn, is basic because it derives from the principle of autonomy and respect for persons.

But here we must be careful. As we said a while ago,[71] no right is absolute. Each right is constrained by the conditions under which it arose and by the conditions under which it is claimed. The principle of relevant difference and the principle of impossibility must always be satisfied for a right to be effective. The right to self-determination, therefore, is not the right to arbitrariness. Neither is it the right to offend the sensibilities and values of others if there are reasonable alternatives available: alternatives that allow the woman to retain her autonomy and satisfy her life-plans within the context of society's values. If there are such alternatives, then the weight of this right will have to be balanced against the alternatives that are thus open to the woman.

What this means is that if the pregnancy is the result of competent and voluntary behaviour on part of the woman; and if society has made it possible for the woman to avoid becoming pregnant by providing free and easy access to contraceptive or other appropriate methods of birth-control; if, furthermore, society makes it possible for the woman to pursue her life-plans without abortion by offering her a reasonable alternative that does not amount to punishing her in an unjust fashion, then society has the right to refuse the woman access to abortion.

However, the fact of the matter is that these conditions are seldom met at the present time. Therefore, it would be unjust to deny women who have taken due care to avoid pregnancy, but who nevertheless find themselves pregnant, the right to an abortion. For their parts the health care professions must make sure that each woman has free, unhindered and reasonable access to abortion services prior to twenty weeks of gestation as an upper limit. This duty falls particularly on medicine. The fact that abortion is a medical act and that medicine is a service monopoly entails that the profession must make sure that this is the case.

As for society, not only must it make abortions readily accessible in the early stages of pregnancy, it must also fund them within the twenty-week time-frame. In fact, not only must it fund the procedure itself, society must also defray the costs that are incurred by a woman who tries to avail herself of this right. Travel and accommodation costs to the nearest facility that provides abortion services are implicated here. Economic status must not be allowed to invalidate a right.

At the same time, such funding need not be without strings. Induced abortions should not be seen as a method of birth control. To view them in that light would be to contravene our society's fundamental value of respect for life. Therefore, society may insist that repeat abortions that are sought for psycho-social reasons be funded by the person seeking the abortion. Failing that, society may prohibit repeat abortions. Such a move, however, would require that society also make adoption or appropriate other placement services available, and assist the woman to whom it has refused abortions in her nutritional and other requirements.

As to the twenty week limit on induced abortions, the deontological ethical position we have sketched makes it almost absolute. The only exceptions are fetal indications. It is discriminatory to suggest that a fetal person must await the onset of an unbearable existence before a decision to end that life can be made. No competent person is required to do so. While the decision to end one's life may be viewed with awe, concern or even misgivings, a competent person has the right to commit suicide before an incurable cancer, Huntington's chorea or other extremely debilitating diseases overtake her. The repeal of the suicide clause from the *Criminal Code of Canada* was at least partly based on a recognition of this fact. An incompetent person should not be placed in worse straits. "The rights of the incompetent should not be less simply because of the fact of their incompetence."[72]

In other words, what traditionally have been called medical indications in favour of abortion—that is to say, medical indications from the side of the fetus—are entirely appropriate. They merely empower the woman or other appropriate proxy decision-maker to use the qualitative criteria that are appropriately applied by competent decision-makers in their own case. The argument is relatively straightforward. Once the fetus has become a person, it is still an incompetent one. That fact of incompetence, however, does not entail that it has no rights. It merely means that these must be administered by proxy.

Proxy decision-makers, however (unless they are faced with a previous competent indication by the now-incompetent person), must use an objective reasonable person standard when administering the individual's rights. Objective reasonable person standards are quality standards. Medical prognosis, social expectation, etc., clearly enter in. Therefore, if according to the best data available under the circumstances, the quality of life of that the fetal person can expect will be so irremediably low as to not be worth living—Tay-Sachs, severe neural tube defects, cystic fibrosis coupled with severe handicaps, congenital abnormalities inconsistent with cognitive sapient and pain-free existence, for example, here come to mind—then the proxy decision-maker need not insist on the right to life. In fact, the proxy decision-maker would have a strong obligation to prevent such a life from materializing. Abortion in as painless a manner as possible should therefore be considered.

Under certain circumstances a woman simply does not have access to an abortion until the stage of fetal personhood has been passed. This is particularly true in rural areas. However, this does not constitute a deontologically defensible reason for extending the period within which abortions are defensible. What it does show is that society has an obligation to make sure those circumstances do not arise.

Finally, there are cases in which continuing the pregnancy foreseeably will result in the death of the mother. It might be thought that in such cases abortion would be acceptable as a matter of the woman's right even after the fetus has become a person. But this is not necessarily true. Once the fetus has become a person, the only way in which a preference for the life of the mother can be argued is by reference to the principle of relevant difference. Some have attempted to do just that: for instance, by arguing that the fetal and the maternal life are not on a par. The woman is more fully conscious, she has more fully developed life-plans;[73] her life includes lines of obligations towards others which are not present for the fetal person; and so on.

However, in the end all this means is that the fetal person has not yet had opportunity to make such connections. Lack of opportunity does not change one's ethical status. Furthermore, it may be argued that by allowing the pregnancy to progress to the point where the fetus has become a person, the woman has subordinated her rights to the right of the fetus. Therefore, once the fetus meets the conditions that are otherwise accepted as definitive of personhood, the life of the mother does not automatically take priority. A genuine balancing process must occur.

Still, the balancing process must not proceed independently of the principle of best action. The duty of the physician towards the woman is to do what is medically appropriate and best under the circumstances, assuming that she wishes this to be done. The fact that this best may involve a treatment of the woman which may have fatal consequences for the fetus does not make the treatment itself ethically unacceptable. Rather, it means that the physician has an obligation to look around for some treatment of the fetus that is appropriate under the circumstances to save its life.

Just as the woman's right to life does not give her the right to kill the fetal person, so the fetal person's right to life does not give it the right to kill the woman. The principle of best action therefore entails that the best possible under the circumstances should be done for each as a person. This may result in the death of the fetus; but that death will not be the result of inaction or even of a fatal action directed towards the fetus to save the pregnant woman's life. Instead, it will be the result of the imperfection of the techniques expended on the fetal person. Society may have an obligation to encourage and facilitate an increase in the success-rates of such fetal techniques, but the fact that they have not yet attained that stage does not redound to the ethical deficit of the physician.

In all of this we have ignored the potentiality inherent in the fetus even before it attains personhood. However, potentiality is just that: potentiality. Someone who potentially is a physician does not yet have the duties that physicians incur in virtue of becoming physicians. These will come later. Likewise with any other potentiality. What is potential does not have the same ethical status as what is actual. To assume otherwise is to beg the question.

We have also ignored that fact that the fetus exists *in utero* and is dependent on the woman for its life. Some people have argued that this makes a fundamental ethical difference.[74]

We have already dealt with the claim that where a fetus should is make an ethical difference to its status. It would make where someone is (which is to say, physical location) an ethically relevant consideration with respect to whether that individual is a person. That seems hard to believe, as we said before, if this were true, then if a fetus was removed from a uterus in the course of fetal surgery it would be a person while out of the uterus, but would cease to be a person once again when returned to it.

The second part of this reasoning does not fare much better. It would make the fact that someone is dependent on an *organic* life-support system, in this case the mother, an ethically relevant factor that turned the fetus into a non-person. Again, that seems difficult to accept. We do not accept this sort of perspective in other contexts. For instance, the respirator-dependent person's right to life is not lower than that of other person simply because he or she is on a respirator. Furthermore, it would be ludicrous to suggest that quality-of-life consideration on the part of the technicians who tended the respirator would or should outrank the right to continued care of the persons who depend on it. The fetal person is in an analogous position to the person on a respirator. The fetus depends for its life on the mother the way the respirator-dependent person depends on the respirator technician.

However, the reply to this would have to be that the two sorts of cases are quite distinct. It is the woman herself who functions as a respirator—and of course as a nurturer and medium of gestation. However, women are not machines. They are persons. And because they are persons, they have rights. Therefore their rights still outweigh the rights of the fetus, because the fetus does not have any.

The logic of this reply would be unexceptionable and cogent were it not for one fatal mistake. It simply *asserts* that a fetus has no rights, and it simply *insists* that the rights of the fetus play no fundamental role, because it simply *assumes* that at no point is a fetus a person. We have given reasons for maintaining the opposite. Until these reasons are successfully met by counter-argument, their position stands. At some point in its development, the fetus becomes a person.

Once the fetus has become a person, considerations of maternal quality of life are outweighed by considerations of the fetus' right to life. Of course, maternal quality-of-life considerations would be relevant prior to the fetus becoming a person. Even the fact that a woman may not have had the opportunity of access to abortion services prior to this time does not make feticide acceptable, any more than it would make infanticide acceptable. Instead, what it argues for is a change in social conditions.

Finally, a word about the appropriate treatment of fetuses who are not yet persons. We shall return to the subject in the next chapter, when we deal with fetuses as future persons. For now, suffice it to say that history is replete with examples where individuals have been denied appropriate treatment because they have been denied the status of persons. The fate of women themselves, prior to their enfranchisement, as well as slaves, ethnic and religious minorities and so on are all-too familiar examples.

Our society accepts certain values. These values may not be ethical in nature. Still, they function as fundamental principles of acceptable conduct. One of these values is respect for human life.

No human life, whatever its stage of development, may be deprived of the protection that this value affords without good reason. Therefore, all other things being equal, the human fetus, whatever its stage of development, is also entitled to appropriate and respectful treatment.[75]

From this it follows that even though a fetus may not yet have reached the stage where it becomes the object of full-fledged ethical concern, it is still entitled to the protection embodied in humane legislation directed towards the treatment of animals. The fact that a fetus does not have the same status as an ordinary member of human society does not mean that it has even less rights than non-human living beings. Therefore, a fetus, even before it becomes a person, may become involved in protocols that are of no benefit to itself only on the condition that there is some overwhelming ethical reason, rooted in the rights of extant and full-fledged members of society, that outweighs the considerations that stem from the principle of respect for human life. The human fetus, therefore, should not be involved in non-therapeutic endeavours or undertakings that are not mandated by overwhelming societal or individual ethical considerations.

ENDNOTES

[1] A.J. Wilcox, C.R. Weinberg, I.F. O'Connor, D.D. Baird, et al., "Incidence of Early Loss of Pregnancy," *New England Journal of Medicine* 319:4 (July 28, 1988) 189–194; compare H. Pilpel, "Personhood, Abortion and the Right to Privacy" in M. Shaw and A. Doudera, eds. *Defining Human Life: Medical, Legal and Ethical Implications* (Ann Arbor: AUPHA Press, 1983) 154; and J.B. Henry, *Clinical Diagnosis & Management by Laboratory Methods,* 18th edition (Philadelphia: W.B. Saunders, 1991) 478, for somewhat different figures.

[2] Compare I. Makdur, "Sterilization and Abortion from the Point of View of Islam" in *Islam and Family Planning,* vol. 2 (271); see also A. R. Omran, "Abortion in the Natality Transition in Moslem Countries," in the same text, 70.

[3] See Bernard Dickens, "Comparative Legal Abortion Policies and Attitudes Towards Abortion," in Shaw and Doudera, ref. note 1.

[4] Compare E.H.W. Kluge, "St. Thomas, Abortion and Euthanasia," *Philosophical Research Archives*, 1981/82.

[5] See Dickens, reference in note 1.

[6] Dickens, reference in note 1, p. 242.

[7] *Criminal Code of Canada*, Section 251 (4).

[8] *Criminal Code of Canada*, Section 251(4)c.

[9] *R. vs. Morgentaler*, [1988] 1 S.C.R. 30, 63 O.R. (2d.) 281, 26 O.A.C. 1, 44 D.L.R. (4th)385, 82 N.R. 1, 3 C.C.C. (3rd)449, 62 C.R. (3rd) 1, 31 C.R.R.

[10] As note 9.

[11] That statutory interference, however, would have to follow the principle of the least intrusive alternative as underlying the *Canadian Human Rights Act* S.C. 1976–7, c. 33; appealed to in *Re Eve* (1987), 31 D.L.R. (4th) 1 (S.C.C.) 2 S.C.R. 388; *Re Infant K*, Supreme Court of B.C. Jan. 30, 1985, Vancouver Registry A 842 616. See also David Chambers, "The Right to the Least Restrictive Alternative" in *The Mentally Retarded Citizen and the Law*, M.I. Kindred et al. eds., (New York: Free Press, 1976) 93, which says when government does have a legitimate communal interest to serve by legislating human conduct, it should use methods that curtail individual freedom to no greater extent than is essential for securing that interest.

[12] This has sometimes been represented as leaving Canada without any laws governing abortion. As should be clear from the articles of the Criminal Code that we have just cited, this was not really the case.

[13] *Borowski vs. Canada* (Attorney General), [1989] 1 S.C.R. 342, affirming on other grounds (1987) 33 C.C.C. (3d) 402.

[14] *Murphy vs. Dodd et al.*, 70 O.R. (2d) 681.

[15] *Tremblay vs. Daigle*, 62 D.L.R. (4th) 634.

[16] The situation was complicated by the fact that during the course of the Supreme Court hearing, Ms. Daigle's lawyer announced that he had received word that Ms. Daigle had undergone an abortion in the U.S. in defiance of the injunction from the Quebec Court of Appeals, which was still in effect at that point in time.

[17] *Tremblay vs. Daigle*, S.C.R. 21533, 18–19.

[18] Bill C–43, "An Act Respecting Abortion," 2nd Session, 34th Parliament, 38 Elizabeth II, 1989.

[19] CMA Policy Summary on Induced Abortion, CMAJ 1176A (1988).

[20] See MRC Guidelines on Human Experimentation.

[21] See Pope Paul VI, Encyclical Letter "Humanae Vitae," *Acta Apostolicae Sedis* LX: 9 (1968).

[22] "Embryos Again," Editorial, *Ethics and Medicine* 5: 2 (1989) 17.

[23] We shall address this issue later, from the perspective of therapeutic abortions to prevent what Engelhardt has called "the injury of continued existence."

[24] The so-called Doctrine of Double Effect enters here.

[25] Section 206(1) of the *Criminal Code*. The recent case of *Daigle* does not change this.

[26] Federation of Medical Women of Canada *Newsletter*, Vol.1 (October, 1989) 1.

[27] Michael Tooley, *Analysis of Abortion and Infanticide* (Clarendon Press: Oxford, 1983); and S.I. Benn, "Abortion, Infanticide and Respect for Persons," in Joel Feinberg, ed., *The Problem of Abortion* (Belmont, Calif.: Wadsworth, 1973).

[28] Law Reform Commission of Canada, Working Paper 58, *Crimes Against the Fetus*. (Ottawa: Minister of Supply and Services, 1989).

[29] H.T. Engelhardt, Jr., *The Foundations of Bioethics*, (Oxford and New York: Oxford Univ. Press) 236–237.

[30] Canadian Medical Association, "The Ethical Status of the Human Fetus: A Discussion Paper," (Ottawa: CMA, 1989).

[31] See note 30, above.

[32] See also note 30, above.

[33] See R.R. Llinar, ed., *The Biology of the Brain from Neurons to Networks* (New York: H.W. Truman, 1989).

[34] C.L. Grobstein, "A Biological Perspective on the Origin of Human Life and Personhood," in Shaw and Doudera, *Defining Human Life*, ref. note 1, 9.

[35] *Defining Human Life*, ref. note 1, 10.

[36] *Defining Human Life*, ref. note 1.

[37] Compare E. Milner, *Human Neural and Behavioural Development* (Springfield, Mass.: Thomas 1967) 67.

[38] The reason why we added the word "ethical" is that the difference between ethical and legal rights tends to get confused in a lot of the debate surrounding the status of the human fetus. Unless indicated otherwise, we are only talking about ethical rights.

[39] See Chapters 2, 9, 10 at various points.

[40] *Criminal Code* Section 223 [206].

[41] See Law Reform Commission Working Paper 58, pp. 40ff. and at other points for considerations along similar lines.

[42] Edward W. Keyserlingk, "Fetal Surgery: Establishing the Boundaries of the Unborn Child's Right to Prenatal Care," in Carl Nimrod and Glenn Griener, eds., *Biomedical Ethics and Fetal Therapy* (Waterloo, Ont.: Wilfrid Laurier Press, 1988) 81–105, at 102.

[43] Resolutions of General Council, Quebec City, 1989.

[44] CMA Policy Summary: Induced Abortion.

[45] *Williams Obstetrics*, 2, 745. For a somewhat different definition, see *Dorland's Medical Dictionary* (Philadelphia: W.B. Saunders Co., 1988) 27th ed., 210, which focuses on the word "premature" and therefore defines a premature birth as the "birth of a premature infant."

[46] Mary B. Mahowald, "Is There Life After *Roe vs. Wade?*" *Hastings Center Report* 19: 4 (July/August, 1989) 22–29, at 23.

[47] O.H. Smith, H.A. Twig and I.L. Croft, "Prostaglandins in Gel: A Method to Minimize Nursing Involvement," *British Medical Journal* 282: 2012, 1981.

[48] I.R. Pahl and L.E. Lundy, "Experience with Mid Trimester Abortion," *Obstet. Gynecol* 53: 587–590, 1979.

[49] See Ney p. 512, reference at note 64, below.

[50] See also N.H. Lauersen and K.H. Wilson, "The Role of Long-Acting Vaginal Suppositories of 15-ME—PGF 2x in first and second trimester abortion," *Journal of Advanced Prostaglandin Thromboxane Research* 8: 141–143, 1980.

[51] See F.J. Kane, M. Feldman, J. Susheila, M.A. Lipton, "Emotional Reactions in Abortion Services Personnel," *Archives of General Psychiatry* 28: 409–414, (1973) with respect to hypotonic saline solution because nursing personnel frequently the only ones around when the patient aborted.

[52] See Mahowald, p. 24, reference in note 46 above.

[53] See Nathan M. Simon, "Psychological and Emotional Indications for Therapeutic Abortion," in R.B. Sloane, ed., *Abortion* (New York: Grune and Stratton, 1971) 86f., for a brief discussion of related issues.

[54] For an explicit recognition of this (with the exception of the possibility of suicide) see *Criminal Code*, Section 287.

[55] Jewish law does not give a fetus the status of a person and in fact requires a 30-day post partum viability to decide legal matters pertaining to the newborn. Compare F. Rosner, *Modern Medicine and Jewish Law* (N.Y.: Yeshiva Univ., 1972), 66–9 and following.

[56] See reference at note 26 above.

[57] See George J. Annas, reference at note 75 below.

[58] *R. vs. Morgentaler* [1988] 1 S.C.R. 30 at 3.

[59] See *Re Eve*, *Re M*, etc.

[60] Compare Shaw and Doudera, *Defining Human Life*, ref. note 1. Chapter 15.

[61] A primary Canadian proponent of this is Christine Overall. See Christine Overall, *Ethics and Human Reproduction: A Feminist Analysis* (Bristol: Allen and Unwin, 1987).

[62] This is known as the position of immediate animation. For a historical discussion, see J.F. and S.J. Donceel, "Abortion: Mediate and Immediate Animation," *Continuum*, 5 (1967): 167–71. See also Kluge, *The Practice of Death*, (New Haven: Yale University Press, 1975), Chapter 1.

[63] Paul Ramsey, *The Patient as Person* (New Haven: Yale, 1970), 11–58.

[64] P.G. Ney and A.R. Wickett, "Mental Health and Abortion: Review and Analysis," *Psychiatric Journal of the University of Ottawa* 14: 4 (Nov., 1989) 506–516, at 506. See also B.K. Doane and B.G. Quigley, "Psychiatric Aspects of Therapeutic Abortions," CMAJ 125 (1981) 427–432.

[65] Ney and Wickett, ref. note 64, 506. According to an older study, suicide is rare among pregnant women: M. Sim and R. Neisser, "Postabortive Psychosis: A Report from Two Centers," in D. Mall and F. Watts, eds., *The Psychological Aspects of Abortion* (Washington: University Publications of America, 1979) 1–13.

[66] See also H.N. Babikian, "Abortion," in H.I. Kaplan and A.M. Freedman, eds., *Comprehensive Handbook of Psychiatry*, 2nd edition (1975) at 1496–1500.

[67] See S. Drower and E. Nash, "Therapeutic Abortion on Psychiatric Grounds," *South African Medical Journal* (1980) 54: 604–608 and 55: 643–647.

[68] Babikian, reference in note 66, above: "Women suffering from psychiatric illness before abortion showed no significant improvement after abortion and had more difficulties coping with the stress of abortion than psychologically more healthy women."

[69] See "Humanae Vitae," reference at note 21, above.

[70] Statistics Canada, vol. IV, 1965–84 will provide a useful check here. No pregnancy with abortive outcome has been reported as fatal in Canada since 1979.

[71] See Chapter 2 for more detail.

[72] Bracktenbach, *In the Matter of Colyer*, 660 P. (2d.) 738 (Sup. Ct. Wad. 1983).

[73] This is one of the central implications of Tooley, reference at note 27, above.

[74] Judith Jarvis Thomson, "A Defense of Abortion," *Philosophy and Public Affairs*, 1:1 (1971) 47–66.

[75] For a recent discussion indicating agreement with according the fetus some status, see George J. Annas, "A French Homonculus in a Tennessee Court," *Hastings Center Report* 19: 6 (Nov. Dec. 1989) 20–22, at 20 "Every national commission worldwide that has examined the status of the human embryo to date has placed it in this third category: neither people nor products, but nonetheless entities of unique symbolic value that deserves society's respect and protection." (For a Canadian judicial reflection of a balancing approach from a gradualistic perspective, see Madame Justice Wilson in *Morgentaler*, p.8.)

SUGGESTED READINGS

- Dickens, Bernard. "Comparative Legal Abortion Policies and Attitudes Towards Abortion," in M. Shaw and A. Doudera, eds. *Defining Human Life: Medical, Legal and Ethical Implications*. Ann Arbor Mich.: AUPHA Press, 1983.

  One of the most comprehensive discussion of abortion legislation by one of the foremost legal authorities on abortion in Canada.

- Foot, Philippa. "The Problem of Abortion and the Principle of Double Effect." *Oxford Review* 5.

  A classic discussion of the doctrine of double effect by someone who is not committed to the religious perspective which gave rise to the doctrine itself.

- *R. vs. Morgentaler.* [1988] 1 S.C.R. 30, 63 O.R. (2D.)281, 26 O.A.C. 1, 44 D.L.R. (4TH)385, 82 N.R. 1, 3 C.C.C. (3RD)449, 62 C.R. (3RD)1, 31 C.R.R.

  This is the classic Canadian case that struck down Canada's abortion law that required that abortions be performed only after they had been approved by a duly constituted abortion committee which found that the woman's life or health was seriously endangered by continuation of the pregnancy.

- Sacred Congregation for the Doctrine of the Faith. *Declaration on Procured Abortion*. Rome: Vatican, 1985.

  This treatise constitutes a formal promulgation of the Roman Catholic Church's rejection of abortion.

- Sumner, L.W. "Toward a Credible View of Abortion." *Canadian Journal of Philosophy* 4 (Sept., 1974) 163–181.

  An early article by a prominent Canadian philosopher on the subject of abortion from an analytical philosophical perspective. It contains a moderate view of abortion.

- Tooley, Michael. "Abortion and Infanticide." *Philosophy and Public Affairs* 2 : 2 (1972) 137–165.

  This paper antedates Tooley's book on abortion and infanticide, and contains the foundations of the argumentation contained in the book. It is based on a philosophical distinction between being a person and being a human being, and contains an analysis of what it is to be a person.

12

The Right to Have Children

This chapter deals with the right to have children. While its practical focus is the Canadian context, it attempts to discuss the issues that arise in terms of the general ethical considerations that have been developed in the preceding chapters. It also touches on the ethics of population control independently of the question of abortion, and tries to lay the groundwork for the discussion of the ethics of assisted reproduction that will be the focus of the next chapter.

In reading this chapter it will be useful to keep the following questions in mind:

1. Canada is a signatory of the Universal Declaration of Human Rights and the Proclamation of Teheran. What does this mean so far as Canadian society is concerned?
2. What are some of the arguments in favour of the universal right to have children? Some arguments against? Is there any one that strikes you as more convincing than others? Why?
3. What are some of the ethically relevant considerations that are raised by sterilization as a method of population control. Do incompetents present a special problem? Explain.
4. Is it ethically acceptable to sterilize incompetent individuals? Is it ethically acceptable to sterilize anyone else?

Introduction

Men and women of full age, without any limitation to race, nationality or religion, have the right to marry and found a family.

So reads Resolution 217A(iii), Universal Declaration of Human Rights. It was drafted in the aftermath of the eugenics program of Nazi Germany and of the politics of population control that had become an integral part of its policies. It was adopted by the United Nations General Assembly on December 10, 1948. Twenty years later, on May 13, 1968, the United Nations reiterated its position in the Proclamation of Teheran:

> Parents have a basic right to determine freely and responsibly the number and spacing of their children.

The usual interpretation of these statements is that the signatories agreed to recognize a universal, fundamental and unconditioned right to have children, and that they wanted to signal their conviction that this right ought not to be interfered with by the state.[1]

However, a close reading of these statements shows that they do not actually say this. They rule out state interference based on race, nationality and religion. However, they are silent about interference on the basis of age, mental or physical health, genetic endowment, and the like. This may not be coincidental. Parental age, as well as mental, physical and genetic endowment play an important role in the ability to bear healthy children and to raise them.

Furthermore, while the Proclamation of Teheran insists on the freedom of parents to determine the number and spacing of their children, it does not say that this freedom is absolute. It says that the determination of the number and spacing of children should be "responsible." This raises the possibility that the drafters of the Proclamation and those who ratified it did not envision this as an absolute and unconditioned right. In fact, it suggests that they believed this right to be subject to limitations and controls that centre on the notion of responsible child-bearing.

These considerations are not merely speculative and historical. If the usual interpretation is correct and everyone has an inalienable and unconditioned right to have children, then both society and the health care professions (and in particular physicians) are placed in a unique position. For society it means that it has a negative obligation not to interfere with that right. It may not sterilize anyone, as it has done in the past with the mentally handicapped[2] and criminals;[3] nor may it enforce birth control, as the Chinese state and Bangladesh[4] appear to be doing at the present time, and as has been done in some Canadian mental institutions. It also means that society has a positive duty to assist persons whose normal attempts to become biological parents have failed. This in turn entails an obligation to provide such services as Artificial Insemination (AI), *in vitro* (IV) fertilization, and so on.

For physicians it would mean an unconditioned duty to assist patients in their attempts to achieve biological parenthood. Physicians therefore could not take into account such factors as the mental or physical condition of a patient who seeks reproductive assistance, the social and developmental prospects that an offspring of such a patient might face, or similar considerations.

On the other hand, if the more limited interpretation is correct, then society may not only have a right but a duty to interfere in the reproductive activities of its members: in circumstances, namely, that could not be described as involving "responsible" reproduction. It would also allow physicians to consider the psychosocial parameters surrounding a patient's request for medical assistance, as well as the medical capabilities of the patient for meeting the requirements of being a parent.

It is therefore important to know which of these interpretations (if indeed any) is correct. Is there an unconditioned and inalienable right to have children? Or does that right, if right there is, have limitations and conditions? If there are limits, how are they to be drawn? Where? and, By whom? We shall consider some of these questions in the present chapter.

Historical-Legal Considerations

Canada is a signatory to the Universal Declaration of Human Rights as well as to the Proclamation of Teheran. This binds Canada as a nation in a moral sense. Of course, it is questionable whether that means anything within the context of Canadian law. In the end, it may express more of an attitude than anything else. However, there are clear indications that Canadian society does indeed accept a legally recognized right to have children, at least for women who are capable of bearing children. There are also clear indications that so far as Canadian courts are concerned, this right may not be interfered with by anyone except the women themselves.

This is clearly illustrated by the cases that deal with involuntary sterilization. They portray the involuntary sterilization of women as a violation of the equal treatment provisions of the Canadian Bill of Rights[5] and of those sections of the Charter that deal with the inviolability of the person.[6] The recent case of *Eve vs. Mrs. E* provides a good example of this. The Supreme Court of Canada quoted with approval the British case of *re D (a minor)*.[7] In that case Mdme. Justice Heilbron had condemned the sterilization of a child of seven as an operation

> ... which involves the deprivation of a basic human right, namely the right of a woman to reproduce, and therefore it would, if performed on a woman for non-therapeutic reasons and without her consent, be a violation of such a right.

Mr. Justice LaForest, writing the unanimous decision of the Canadian Supreme Court, echoed this position in the following words: .

> I cannot agree that a court can deprive a woman of that privilege for purely social or other non-therapeutic purposes without her consent. The fact that others may suffer inconvenience or hardship from failure to do so cannot be taken into account.

Therefore, in the eyes of the Supreme Court of Canada, there is a general legal presumption that a female person has the right to have children. The Court agreed that there may be situations in which this right can be interfered with by the state. However, the Court emphatically insisted that such an interference may occur only under very special circumstances and only for very special reasons. It may take place only when (1) there is a valid public claim that would override the woman's right; and when (2) the woman is incompetent and the interference with her reproductive capabilities is protective of the woman herself as an person.[8]

Historical accuracy demands the observation that this has not always been the position either of Canadian society or of Canadian courts. In fact, until quite recently, sterilization for non-therapeutic reasons had been accepted by the public with little if any protest. Several Canadian provinces had statutes that allowed such sterilization,[9] and the courts did not raise judicial objection to their implementation. Of course, physicians played an important role in this matter: not only as the individuals who actually carried out the sterilizations, but also as the ones who recommended them. It is only in the last few decades that the situation has changed.

Some Ethical Issues

Historical changes are one thing; the question of their justification is another. The fact that something has happened—that society and the courts have changed their attitudes and perspectives—does not necessarily mean that they were justified in doing so. Societies and its legislators have been known to make mistakes, just like any other persons; and judges are also subject to human failings.

Therefore, if we take legal and legislative actions as indicative of a change in social attitude towards the right to have children, then we really cannot assume that the matter is settled by looking at historical trends. That would be ethics by consensus. What we really have to ask is, Is this change in social attitude and law ethically justified? Does everyone really have the right to have children?

Once we ask those questions, we are immediately brought face to face with another question—one which so far has received little if any attention either in the literature or in public debate: What does it mean to say that everyone has the right to have children? Does it mean that everyone has the right to biological offspring of their own? Or does it mean that everyone has the right to be a parent? Does it mean a combination of these? Is there something else entirely that is here at stake?

These are not questions of mere lexicography. Different consequences follow, depending how the notion of a right to have children is understood. If it is understood as the right to be a parent, then nothing in principle would bar society from interfering in the reproductive capabilities of its citizens. So long as people were provided with children to parent, their right would be fulfilled.

Involuntary sterilization for reasons unrelated to the health of the individual person would therefore not be ruled out. Furthermore, as long as society provided anyone who wanted it, the opportunity to parenthood, society would not have any obligation to investigate and correct the causes of infertility. For the health care professions, this would mean that investigations into infertility etc. would not have to rank high on their research priority list. While infertility might well be a health issue, it would not be an important one.

On the other hand, if the right to have children is understood as the right to have biological offspring of one's own, matters would be quite different. Society would have an obligation to try to prevent or cure infertility. However, by the same token it would not follow that biological parents necessarily had any right to keep the children they had thus produced. This fact becomes particularly important in the contemporary context, where surrogate motherhood has become a reality.

For the health care professions, it would entail an obligation to assist those who are unable to have biological offspring of their own. Investigations into the causes of infertility would be a priority item, as would research projects aimed at ways of curing the problem. It might even entail an obligation to develop new techniques of reproduction for those who are inherently incapable of having children. Research into such things as "artificial placentas," "male pregnancies" and so on, would become entirely appropriate.

Finally, if the right to have children included both the right to have biological offspring of one's own as well as the right to be a parent to them, the picture would shift once again. Not only would society have an obligation to fund research aimed at eradicating or curing infertility, it would also have an obligation to help people in their efforts to function as parents—even if the people have difficulties parenting. This would become important in the case of mentally or otherwise handicapped persons. Similarly, for the health care professions it would mean that not only would these professions have an obligation to assist patients in their efforts to have biological offspring of their own, but the professions would also have an obligation to delve into the psychology of parenting, so that everyone could in fact realize their right to parenthood, and to delve into the social implications of and requirements for parenting and so on.

All of these interpretations of the right to have children have their supporting arguments. Which interpretation (if indeed any) is correct? Short of examining all of them, there is no way of telling. However, we are not going to do that. It would be too lengthy a process. Still, sometimes what people mean becomes clear from the reasons they give for what they say. Therefore, what we are going to do is look at some of the reasons that are advanced in defense of the claim of the right to have children. In that way we may gain insight into the nature of the claim itself, while at the same time developing a way of evaluating it.

Some Arguments for the Right to Have Children

Argument from Biology

One of the more traditional arguments in favour of the right to have children is based on the biological nature of the human species. The argument is very simple. The human species is a species of animal. That means that unless human beings reproduce, the species will disappear. Consequently the right to reproduce—which is to say the right to have children—is grounded in the biological nature of humanity itself.[10]

Even though this sort of argument is fairly traditional, it would be unwise to base a universal right to have children on it. Of course the biological facts are beyond doubt. Without reproduction, and therefore without children, the human species would disappear. However, while the facts are beyond doubt, the inference that is based on them is invalid. First of all, the fact that a species will disappear unless it does something (whatever that might be) does not entail either a right or a duty to engage in that particular kind of action. For that inference to go through, we would need another premise. We would need the premise that the species should continue to exist in the first place. However, we cannot simply assume that this premise is true. It has to be shown.

Second, the logic of this argument is faulty in another way. Even if we agreed that there is a right (or duty) to preserve the species, this would not entail that every member of the species—which is to say, every person—has the right to reproduce. In fact, the very opposite would follow. What would follow would be that all and only those people who could reasonably be expected to contribute to the survival of the species would have that right. That would certainly not include everyone. It would exclude all those who carry identifiable dominant lethal genes; those who carry genes that would not be advantageous in a changing global environment, or those whose reproduction would in any way compromise the survival of the species as a whole. Therefore, instead of grounding a universal right to have children, this sort of argument would entail a severely conditioned right: a right governed by the most rigorous eugenic and evolutionary standards. Very few advocates of the right to have children would accept such a position.

Argument from Desire

Another argument for the right to have children is based on the fact that most of us want to have children:[11] We have a desire for children, so to speak. From this the argument concludes that we therefore have a *prima facie* right to have children. That right may be overruled on certain occasions. But when it is overruled, there must a reason for it. It cannot simply be a matter of social whim.

It takes little imagination to see that this argument does not prove anything. Logically, a desire by itself does not secure a right. Not even a *prima facie* right. That conclusion would follow only if we assumed as an ethical premise that the existence of a desire itself is sufficient to give a *prima facie* right. That assumption is questionable at best. If there were true, murderers would have a *prima facie* right to their victims, robbers to their spoils and criminals in general would have a *prima facie* justification in committing their crimes.

Realization of Personal Potential

Still another argument for the right to have children settles on the notion of self-fulfilment. Human beings have the potential to grow as persons in the context of their own family: as nurturers and as providers of security, comfort and education to children. They also derive a sense of self-fulfilment from this. Without children, this potential will never be fulfilled; and without them, this sense of self-fulfilment will be missing. Therefore people have that right.[12] This sort of argument is similar to the one that we have just considered. Instead of making the desire to have children its focus, it centres around the notion of a personal potential. From the existence of this potential it concludes that there is a right.

The short analysis of this argument is that it does not work, any more than does the argument from desire. The mere existence of a potential does not establish a right—whether that be a personal potential or a potential for anything else. If it did, the potential surgeon would have a right to an operating room, the potential millionaire to her fortune, and the potential orator to the adoration of a crowd. All of these involve personal potentials. All of them involve the development of a capacity inherent in the individual. Yet few people would agree that the mere presence of such potential confers a right.[13]

But this argument does allow us to see several things. One thing that it allows us to see is that we have to distinguish between two claims—the claim that there is a right to experience pregnancy and childbirth, which is sometimes expressed in phrases like "the right to fulfil one's function as a woman"; and the right to parent. The first involves the biological potential of the individual as a biological organism; the second involves the mental or psychological potentials of the individual as person. The two may overlap in a particular line of reasoning. For all that, however, they are distinct; and any argument for the right to have children must be careful not to trade the one for the other.

The second thing this line of reasoning allows us to see is that the whole issue of the right to have children cannot be discussed simply in terms of the perspective of the right-holder. The fact is that this claim is a claim to a right whose fulfilment inherently involves *children*. However, children are not objects. They are persons. Therefore, any argument for the right to have children must be careful not to deteriorate into an argument for the claim that it is ethically acceptable to use persons as a means for realizing one's own potential—or for anything else.

Of course, the argument from the realization of personal potential need not be interpreted in this way. We could say that what the argument really aims at is the conclusion that we all have the right to avail ourselves of the opportunities for self-realization that are normally present in society. We could then say that these opportunities for self-realization normally include the right to sexual expression: i.e., the right to engage in intercourse. This is recognized and accepted as entailed by the right to self-determination. Intercourse normally leads to pregnancy, which leads to children, which in turn leads to parenting. We could then say that the argument gets to the same conclusion after all, only by a different route.

This way of interpreting the argument would avoid having to treat children as objects. However, it would not ground a right to have children in any real sense. It is simply false that intercourse normally leads to pregnancy; just as it is false to say that pregnancy normally leads to the birth of a child and hence to parenting. Contraception is widely practised in our society; and abortion, both spontaneous and induced, severely reduces the number of pregnancies that go to term. So the logical linkage that is supposed to lead from the facts to the conclusion is at best on shaky grounds.

But that aside, the argument still would not establish the unlimited and unconditioned right that was claimed in the original position. The original position claimed that there is a right to have a child, not that there is a right to an opportunity for sexual intercourse in the hope that children might result from it. It may be that people have the right to an equal opportunity for self-expression. It may also be that this includes the opportunity for intercourse as a special case. Such a right to intercourse would then impact on society in terms of guaranteeing equality of opportunity. This would be important in terms of the development of and access to sexual counselling and reproductive technologies, since at least part of their raison d'être is to provide equality of opportunity in this matter.[14] However, the original claim is explicit in focusing on children as fulfilling the right itself. That is what is missing from the present interpretation.

A final word about logic of the argument from potential. Even if we did allow that the existence of a personal potential guaranteed the right to realize it, this would not establish an unconditioned right to have children. It would only establish that there was such a right when such a potential was present.

The recent Manitoba court case of —*vs. Child and Family Services*[15] is interesting in this regard. The case concerned mentally handicapped parents whose child was to be taken away from them because the parents allegedly lacked the capability of parenting—in our terms, because they allegedly lacked the relevant potential. The lawyer for the parents brought a Section 15 Charter argument—that is to say, an argument based on the equality section of the Charter of Rights and Freedoms. He argued that taking a child from parents with mental disability is "justified only if the parents are unable to provide appropriate care despite the provision of supportive services." The child was ultimately returned to the parents because the lawyer was able to persuade the court that the Manitoba provincial *Human Rights Code* requires reasonable accommodation provisions. "All of the relevant evidence points to the capability of the parents to care for their child, and the parents are willing to accept reasonable conditions as to monitoring and supervision."

The point of mentioning this case is threefold: *First*, it shows that even in the legal context the argument from personal potential is considered successful only if in fact there is the relevant potential. This means that the argument could not be used to establish a right to have children for people who are so severely handicapped that they cannot "provide appropriate care" to their children even with assistance. *Second*, and by that very token, it shows that even when it is based on this premise, the right to have children is not absolute. *Third*, it suggests that the notion of equal opportunity has to be considered within the overall social context. It cannot be considered merely in the context of the individuals themselves. We shall return to this point later.

Argument from Social Expectation

The argument from social expectation is one of the more powerful arguments for the right to have children. It contends that there is a universal and unconditioned right to have children because having children is something that we normally expect as members of society. We normally expect that we will have the opportunity to reproduce and parent, and we normally expect others to have children.[16] In that sense, the right is very much like the right to health care.

However, as it stands the conclusion the argument draws is too strong and the inference does not follow. We could easily admit that there is a general and socially sanctioned presumption that people in society normally will have children. We could even admit that this presumption is built into the very nature of social existence, so that the mere fact of being a member of society would license this expectation as a matter of right.

However, none of this would establish the existence of a right that was absolute and unconditioned. What it would establish is something much more limited: a right that was subject to parameters that derive from the nature society itself.[17] More precisely, it would show the existence of a right that was conditioned by (1) the nature of the circumstances that are presumed to be the normal conditions of its fulfilment, and (2) by the competing rights of others.

What (1) amounts to is this: Rights that arise in a social context do not arise in isolation. For instance, the right to health care arises in a context that includes the medical sophistication of the society, the availability of resources, its socio-economic capabilities, other needs of members of society, and so on. There is also an historical background that leads up to the recognition of these rights.

Furthermore, rights are recognized in a certain social climate that determines their direction. For instance, formal recognition of the right to health care takes into account the fact that there is a history of providing certain types of health services as a matter of course, that there are other competing rights that are equally as legitimate, such as the right to education, and so on. It also has an eye to the capabilities of the society insofar as the right can be translated into access to types of services, for example. We identified these factors previously as parameters of embedding.

Finally, the context of embedding also includes the valuational perspective of society itself. This perspective may not always be clearly formulated. Nevertheless, it is present as a conditioning moment. The parameters of embedding affect all socially grounded rights. These parameters include the expectations that society considers normal with respect to the exercise of a given right. For example, it is a normal expectation of society that people will not unnecessarily and irresponsibly expose others to harm. Therefore, the right to freedom of action is limited by this expectation. This means that we may not shout "Fire!" in a crowded theatre. Nor may we expose others to the risk of infectious diseases just because we feel that the guideline that would prevent such a spread of infection constitute a restriction of our lifestyle.

Therefore, if we understand the right to have children as a socially guaranteed right, then the limiting conditions that affect rights in general apply to it as well. If we then say that the right to have children flows from the expectations that are normally present in our society, this means that the conditions that normally surround that expectation must apply as well.

However, the normal conditions that surround this expectation include the assumption that in all likelihood the children will be normal. That is to say, even though people may be aware that there is a statistical chance that their children may be abnormal, the usual expectation is to the contrary. After all, the usual expectation is geared to the norm of experience.

Therefore, if the right to have children is understood in this way, then it comes with the built-in limiting conditions of the societal norm in terms of expectations about infant health. Consequently anyone whose expectations do not fall into that norm could not claim to have a right to have children.

We have to be careful not to misunderstand this. The norm is not a unique and precise set of characteristics that is fixed and that endures forever—something like a specific weight, a particular colour, size, neurological functioning or the like. Nor is it something that a particular society decides as matter of social whim. It refers to the range of characteristics that are usually encountered in children in the context of a particular society: the sorts of health conditions or functional characteristics that one could normally expect of or for them. This means that the norm-range, the range of normal expectations, may not be the same for all communities.

Furthermore, it follows that if the right to have children involves this expectation, then some communities may consider as normal a child who in another setting would be considered defective. But it would still follow, on this interpretation, that if people have reasonable grounds to believe that the children they might have would probably fall outside this norm-range—whatever it might be—then they could not claim a right to have children. In their case, the operant condition of this right would not be met.[18] Consideration (1) therefore entails that if the right to have children is going to be argued in this way, there will indeed be such a right, but this right will be heavily conditioned.

Consideration (2) also accepts the idea that there is a socially guaranteed right to have children. And like consideration (1), it entails that this right is heavily conditioned. It differs from consideration (1) in the way in which it arrives at this limitation. Instead of looking at norms and expectations, it looks at competing rights. It is based on the contention that no right is absolute. All rights are conditioned by the equal and competing rights of others. Therefore, even if there is a right to have children, it will be a *prima facie* right only. There is no guarantee that it will be effective in a particular setting.

For instance, suppose that a society was so impoverished as to food, water, medical resources, and so on, that the introduction of another member into the community and supplying for its needs (the birth of a child) would imperil the very existence of the people who are already on the scene. The people who are already on the scene have a right to life as well as a right to have children. All other things being equal, the right to life is more fundamental than the right to have children.[19] Any members of that society could therefore say that their right to life outweighs the right of anyone in that society to have children. Therefore on this assumption having a child would not only be pragmatically unwise but ethically objectionable. It almost goes without saying that if this train of reasoning is correct, the implications for individual societies as well as for the overall global context are tremendous.

The consequences of consideration (2) extend even further. They also touch the notion of quality of life. For example, suppose that the socio-economic resources of a society are so strapped that the society can barely support its present members. While the advent of more children would not necessarily mean the death of some of these members, it would seriously lower the quality of life that people could normally expect. Universal and chronic malnutrition would become rampant, health levels would drop seriously, life-expectancy would be radically lowered, and so on.

If the argument from social existence were to be taken seriously, it would follow that the competing rights of others might here come into play once again. A society that accepted the fact of social existence as the basis of the right to have children would have to come up with a ranking mechanism that compared the right to have children with the right to a certain quality of life. The fact that no society has as has done so is no reason to say that it couldn't—or shouldn't.

Interim Considerations

The considerations that we have just canvassed suggest the following conclusion: There is indeed a right to have children. That right is derivable from the fact of social existence and the expectations that normally are legitimated by such existence. However, such a right is neither absolute nor unconditioned. It is not absolute because it is a *prima facie* right. It is conditioned by and subject to the competing rights of others. If others have rights that are more basic or more fundamental, they will overrule the right to have children. In this they are like all other rights.

It is also conditioned in that it presuppose that certain requirements are met: once from the side of society, and once from the side individual who claims the right. From the side of society, it presupposes that the society is materially capable of providing the opportunity for sexual expression and for supporting the children that foreseeably will result from it. It also presupposes that the other members of society are willing to subordinate their other rights if and when the need arises. From the side of individuals, it presupposes that they are able to treat the children that might result from their sexual activities as persons.[20]

Furthermore, this right must not be understood like the right to have an object or an animal. Children are persons. Therefore they must be treated as persons. Therefore, the right to have children is better understood as the right to take advantage of those opportunities that are offered to everyone in society as a matter of course. One of those opportunities involves the expression of human sexuality, which under normal circumstances results in the production of children. The presence of these children then constitutes an opportunity for realizing those human and personal potentials that are involved by parenting.

Again, it is not at all clear that these conditions are always met. Consider the social condition centring around competing rights. It would be unjustified to assume as a matter of course that all members of society will automatically subordinate their legitimate rights to a certain quality of life, or even to life itself, to the right of sexual expression and what flows from it. After all, these other rights are also sanctioned by society.

What is more, the right to life is more basic. This becomes especially obvious when we consider the sort of limited-resources scenario that we have sketched. One cannot simply assume that individual members of society would want to subordinate their right to life—or even their legitimate expectations of a certain level of health care—because someone else wants a child. There has to be some concrete indication of such an implied consent.[21]

Furthermore, any assertion of the right to have children cannot confine its considerations to the effect that such an assertion would have on adult and competent members of society. It must also take its effect on children and congenitally incompetent persons int account. They are also members of society; and they also have rights—including the rights that we have just mentioned. The state in its *parens patriae* role (or, for that matter, any other appropriate proxy decision-maker) has a duty to protect them against unjustified infringements of their rights.

We cannot simply assume that when these proxy decision-makers exercise their responsibilities properly they will automatically subordinate the rights of these incompetents to the wish of someone else to have a child. To assume this would be ethically irresponsible and would contradict the very principles on which the whole notion of proxy consent is based. Of course it may happen, but we have to look and see.

Finally, if society does guarantee its members an equitable opportunity of sexual self-expression (where that predictably will lead to children), then society also has an obligation to make sure that the children who will be borne will be treated as persons. The principle of autonomy and respect for persons entails such a duty. Furthermore, the principle of equity and justice entails that society has an obligation to try to make sure that these children will also be treated equitably. This conclusion can also be derived from the logic of the Crown's argument in the celebrated case of *Eve*:[22]

> The Crown's *parens patriae* jurisdiction exists for the benefit of those who cannot help themselves, not to relieve those who may have the burden of caring for them.

The fact is that infants are also individuals "who cannot help themselves." Therefore, the Crown has a duty to exert its *parens patriae* powers on their behalf as well. This means that when society has overwhelming grounds to suppose that the infants who will be borne will not be treated as persons, and when society cannot intervene in an assisting capacity to change the situation, it cannot stand by idly. Under such circumstances society must place conditions on allowing such self-expression and realization: conditions whose function is to ensure that the children that foreseeably will be borne will be treated as persons, not as objects of personal satisfaction and gratification.

Of course, these conditions will have to be equitable and just. Furthermore, they may not be conditions of mere convenience.[23] Nevertheless, they will be justified. Furthermore, not everyone will be able to meet them. Therefore, biology notwithstanding, not everyone will have the right to have a child. There is no right to have a child under any and all conditions.

Argument from the Right of Personal Integrity

But what about the claim that the right to have children has nothing to do with the social context? That the social context is in fact absolutely irrelevant? That what is really important is each individual's right to the integrity of their person?

The Supreme Court's decision in *Eve*, to which we have referred before, provides a good example of this sort of reasoning:

> The importance of maintaining the physical integrity of a human being ranks high in our scale of values, particularly as it affects the privilege of giving life. I cannot agree that a court can deprive a woman of that privilege for purely social or other non-therapeutic purposes without her consent.[24]

(In the interest of equality and justice we shall assume that, with due alteration of detail, the Court also meant this to apply to male persons.)

However, when we consider this closely, we can see that if this is how the argument is understood, then the logic of the reasoning does not hang together. The principle that underlies this position is of course unassailable. It is the principle of autonomy and respect for persons. However, the fact that the principle is unassailable does not mean that it can be used to establish the right to have children. At best, what the argument shows is that it may be ethically unjustified to violate the personal integrity of anyone without appropriate consent.

But even this has to be seen in context. While the principle of autonomy and respect for person is fundamental to medical ethics, it is neither unconditioned or absolute. As we discussed in chapters 2–3, the fact that people have a fundamental right to self-determination does not mean that they may exercise their autonomy in a way that would harm others.

To put it by way of an example: A physician does not have the right to request isolation for a patient under normal circumstances. However, if that patient has an infectious disease, and if society cannot be protected from becoming infected unless the individual is isolated and treated, then the physician does have the right to request this. And society has the right to curtail the freedom of that patient. In fact, we can put the point more strongly: Under such circumstances society and medicine have not only the right to insist that the patient be isolated and treated but also the duty, so that others will not be put at risk.[25]

Likewise, a nurse does not have the right to physically restrain a patient. However, when the patient is a danger to others because of psychotic episodes and if there is no other way of handling the situation, then the nurse has the right to ask for appropriate restraints.

We must therefore agree with the courts that everyone has a fundamental right to the integrity of the person. However, we cannot agree that this right is inalienable and unconditioned. It is limited by the rights of others to the security of their person. We also cannot agree that this right entails the right to have children. That right has to be established on other grounds.

Control of Reproduction

This of course moves the issue of limits and conditions centre stage. How can this notion of limits and conditions be translated into actual practice? and, What are the implications of all this for physicians and other health care professionals?

However, before going any further we should correct an impression that we may have created. It may seem that we have argued that everyone in fact wants to have children and that society may step in to control the process as a matter of course.

Nothing could be further from the truth. First of all, not all people want to realize their biological potential for parenthood in the full-blown social sense that we have just discussed—even if they should have that potential. Some people only want to experience the satisfaction of the sexual act. On the other hand, while some people want to realize this potential, they may have personal reasons for not going ahead. These reasons may range from the feeling that they cannot adequately provide for children, to the fact that they carry a genetic load which they do not want to pass on to any offsprings.

Second, society neither is nor should it be in the business of controlling the reproductive acts of its members as a matter of course. It should contemplate such a move with extreme caution, and it should attempt control only when it is ethically mandated. Even then, its attempt should always be in keeping with the principle of the least intrusive alternative.[26]

That is to say, society should never interfere with the integrity and autonomy of its members beyond the minimal degree necessary to achieve the end that is ethically mandated. This means that even if control of reproduction should prove to be ethically appropriate on a given occasion, it should not involve sterilization if contraception or other means would serve the same purpose.[27] In the words of the Law Reform Commission:

> The application of this principle would require that coercive regulations could be applied only when non-coercive methods would not achieve the same goals ... In practice, this would mean that it would have to be demonstrated that an individual either could not be taught to use ... other forms of birth control, or was not responsible enough to use them even if capable.[28]

However, it is important to note that with this the Law Reform Commission accepts that there may be circumstances under which society has both a right and an obligation of control. It may be impossible to delineate this area absolutely and with complete precision. Circumstances change. What may be appropriate on one occasion may not be appropriate on another, precisely because the circumstances are different. The best one can do is outline the ethical parameters that mandate interference, and the reasons for them. This we have done. What we now have to do is look at the means that society may use to discharge its obligation.

To reiterate: Social interference will be indefensible if it violates the principle of the least intrusive alternative. That is to say, it may not impose stricter limits on the actions of its members than are mandated by the conditions that require the interference in the first place. If it does, it exceeds the warrant given to it by the principles that mandate the interference.

Birth Control

What options are open to society if and when it is legitimate for society to contemplate control? Probably the best way to answer this question is to consider the methods of birth control that are available to the ordinary person under ordinary circumstances. We can then ask which one, if any, society may employ (if and) when it has a right/duty to interfere. We shall therefore begin by taking a brief look at birth control in general. We shall then return to our initial question.

When we say, "which methods are available to ordinary persons in society" we of course mean which options are *ethically* available. If some method was unethical in itself, then the mere fact that it was available would not allow society to use it even if some of its members did. So we shall look at the methods of birth control only from this ethical perspective.

There are two ways in which birth control may become ethically problematic: when there is something unethical about the fact of such control itself, or when there is something unethical about the way in which that control is practised in a given situation.

Birth Control as Such

The control of birth becomes ethically problematic *per se* only when there is an obligation to procreate or when the fact of control itself infringes on someone's right. It is difficult to see on what ethical principle the claim that there is an obligation to procreate could be based. The mere fact that without procreation the human species would disappear does not impose an obligation on anyone. In order to transform this fact into an obligation requires a premise that says that the human species ought to remain in existence, and that its members therefore have a duty to make sure that it does. Since this is the very thing that requires proof, this way of arguing merely begs the question. We discussed this reasoning before, so we shall leave it at that.

It could of course be argued that reproduction is a natural function of human beings, and that therefore the control of reproduction in any fashion would violate human nature. However, the trouble with this sort of reasoning is that if it were successful it would prove too much. For instance, it would also prove that human beings do not have the right to control their own reproductive urges. After all, these urges may well be seen as expressions of the reproductive drive that is part of human nature. That in turn would mean that therefore the rapist and the pederast would be ethically excused, and that, at least *prima facie* speaking, incest, and so forth, would be acceptable.

Such consequences are difficult to accept. Fortunately we are not driven to this extreme. As we pointed out a little while ago, the fact that something is natural does not mean that it is ethically mandated.

It seems, then, that there is no *a priori* reason why the control of reproduction in and by itself is unethical. Of course, it is true that such control might violate some religious precepts. For instance it might violate the Judaeo-Christian-Islamic injunction to be fruitful and multiply. However, such considerations would take us out of the realm of ethics and into the realm of religion. We shall therefore not pursue them.

Methods of Birth Control

If the control of reproduction is not unethical in itself, what about the possibility that such control may be unethical because there is something unethical about the *way* in which that control is practised in a given situation?

Here we have to distinguish two things: (1) the type of control that is practised, and (2) the relationship of that control to someone's rights. We should also add that we are here not concerned with birth control in the full sense with which the terms is usually used. We are only concerned with the type of control that prevents conception. All other methods are variations of abortion. They include chemical means such as RU–486[29] or the various estrogen-based pills, mechanical means like IUD's, and so on. We have already dealt with these in the preceding chapter, if not directly, then by implication. What we want to consider here are contraceptive methods.

Type of Control

Abstention

Technically the easiest and at the same time the most effective method of birth control is abstention from intercourse. Ethically, there is nothing to be said against it. Voluntary abstention harms no-one and violates no-one's rights. Even most religions agree that abstention is unexceptionable. Therefore, as a method of controlling reproduction it presents no ethical issues.

Contraception

Contraceptive methods are those that prevent fertilization. In their usual forms they involve either mechanical devices (condoms, diaphragms, etc.), chemical agents (foam, jellies), a combination of both (eg., sponges impregnated with spermicidal solutions) or hormonal means (various sorts of contraceptive pills). Ethically, there is nothing to distinguish between them. They prevent fertilization from occurring either by killing sperm outright or by preventing sperm and ova from coming into contact with each other.

The reason they strike us as ethically unproblematic is simple: neither the death of a sperm nor the death of an ovum is an ethical event. Neither an ovum nor a sperm is a person.[30] They are not even potential persons. Both lack the necessary genetic requirements. Therefore killing them, as happens by the use of spermicidal techniques, is not in itself unethical. It may involve a violation of a religious injunction—but as we said, that is another matter.

As to not allowing conception to occur, again there are no ethical objections. The only real opposition once more comes from the religious quarter. Some religions maintain that the sexual act must always remain open to the transmission of life.[31] Since we are not here concerned with religious ethics, we shall not pursue this any further.

Sterilization

Sterilization is an extremely effective method of birth control. Next to total abstention, it is the surest. It is also the most popular method of contraception in Canada at the present time.[32] With sterilization, conception is prevented either because the union of ovum and sperm is made biologically impossible by surgical means (e.g., by tubal ligation, hysterotomy or vasectomy) or because the organs which produce them are removed (e.g., by castration, removal of the ovaries or radical hysterectomy).

Sterilization is usually considered more drastic than the other methods of birth control we have mentioned. It involves a surgical invasion of a person's body: what the law calls a "trespass to the person." It also has less of a chance of being reversed than the other methods. To this we can add that traditionally sterilization in any of its forms has been considered mutilation.

Does this mean that therefore sterilization in itself is ethically objectionable? We would like to suggest that the answer is "No." Let us consider the notion of trespass to the person. Normally, the law does not condone such a trespass. However, the law contains a rider: It normally does not condone such a trespass *without the consent of the individual toward whom the trespass occurs*. When the person has given consent, the law is generally silent. There is a legal maxim dating from Roman times: *Volenti non fit iniuria*. "No harm is done to him who agrees to it."[33] Therefore, someone who (competently and freely) agrees to being injured cannot claim to have been harmed by that injury being committed.[34] But this is not merely a matter of legal tradition. The principle of autonomy entails the same thing. If someone voluntarily agrees to being harmed, and if the act in question does not violate any fundamental principles or violate anyone's rights, then the act of being harmed does not constitute an unethical act.

But therein lies the rub: "if the act in question does not violate any fundamental ethical principles or violate anyone's rights." It has been suggested that the act of sterilization does violate a fundamental ethical principle, and that it does violate someone's rights: It violates the principle of respect for persons. It also violates the right of the individual to integrity of the person even if that person had agreed to it.[35] For there are certain things to which one cannot agree, and this is one of them.[36] To allow oneself to be sterilized voluntarily is to allow oneself deliberately to be rendered dysfunctional in one of the most fundamental human characteristics. Therefore, to agree to sterilization bespeaks either an absence of competence or a deliberate ignoring of the fundamental inviolability of the human body. On the other hand, to sterilize someone non-consensually is to treat (read: mutilate) that person as an object. Neither is acceptable. Even the law, so it is argued, recognizes this fact. It insists that we cannot agree to all acts. For example, it is illegal to murder someone even though that person agrees to it.

> No person is entitled to consent to have death inflicted upon him, and such consent does not affect the criminal responsibility of any person by whom death may be inflicted upon the person by whom consent is given.[37]

With due alteration of detail, the same thing applies to sterilization.

However, closer consideration of this reasoning reveals that both the ethical and the legal position are somewhat different from the way it is portrayed. As the Law Reform Commission put it in its Working Paper 24, *Sterilization*:

> Although English case law has suggested that contraceptive sterilization may be contrary to public policy, Canadian courts have indicated otherwise ... Indeed, most legal opinion holds that the legality of such a procedure will be unquestioned provided it is performed on a fully informed consenting adult ... However, ambiguities and uncertainty as to the legal position may again result from the nature of the informed consent and the representation and warranties made to the patients by physicians before performing the procedure.[38]

Sterilization on the basis of informed consent would therefore seem to be juridically defensible. As to the ethics of autonomy and respect for persons, it deals with persons and not with bodies. From this perspective, therefore, there is nothing inherently wrong with controlling the functioning of our bodies. The fact of control of the body does not in itself amount to disrespect to the person.

Relationship to People's Rights

We began by saying that we have to distinguish between two issues: Is the method of birth control itself unethical? and, Is the way in which such control practised or imposed unethical? We have just dealt with the first of these. What we suggested was that it is not. We now have to address the second issue. In retrospect, it is really the central issue.

To begin with sterilization. Here we have to distinguish between voluntary sterilization and sterilization that is non-voluntarily imposed. It could reasonably be argued that if the decision for sterilization is made voluntarily and on an informed basis by competent persons then it is ethically unobjectionable. It then is simply an exercise of the right to self-determination. Therefore, when a competent young adult woman asks to have her tubes tied, or a competent young man asks for a vasectomy, in and of themselves such requests cannot be considered in any way unethical demands.

Of course it may be unreasonable for these people to ask to be sterilized when there are less intrusive and less drastic methods of birth control are available. However, that would not make the sterilization itself unethical. It would make it imprudent. Furthermore, there may be a contractual agreement not to be sterilized; for instance if these people are married and had entered a marriage-agreement not to be sterilized. But that is a different matter. It does not affect the ethics of voluntary sterilization per se.

There is a reply to this line of reasoning. We mentioned it before when we talked about birth control in general terms. It focuses on the fact that sterilization for non-medical reasons is a voluntary biological insult to the body. Therefore, it is ethically objectionable in itself.

However, this line of reasoning demands that we accept a certain premise: the premise, namely, that it is ethically objectionable to harm a functioning human body for purposes other than health. This premise may well be acceptable. We shall not debate it here. However, the way it has to be used here is too restrictive in its scope. It construes the notion of health too narrowly. It is important to understand that health includes more than simply physical health. Psychological parameters are also implicated. Therefore if we take a holistic approach to health, then we could reply that under certain circumstances, for the sake of the psychological health and wellbeing of an individual, an insult to the biological functioning of the human body may be justified. Which means that voluntary sterilization would not unethical after all.

As to non-voluntary sterilization, that is a different matter. It is different because the principle of autonomy and respect for persons forbids any unconsented-to violation of the integrity of someone's person. Of course there are cases where the strength of this principle must give way before the rights of others. We have already mentioned control of infectious diseases by vaccination. Years ago, the right of others not to be infected with smallpox overruled the right of a minority to refuse, and we could think of similar cases.

However, non-voluntary sterilization is quite different. Vaccination does not remove a natural capability that is definitive of the individual as biological organism. Sterilization is a much more drastic and extreme interference with personal integrity than vaccination. Therefore, unless there are weightier rights that overrule the *prima facie* right of the inviolability of the person, non-voluntary sterilization cannot be defended.

The same reasoning applies to birth control in general. Non-voluntary birth control is ethically acceptable as long as it does not violate the principle of autonomy. The issue here is simply not *what* is done, but *how*.

Sterilization of the Mentally Handicapped

A brief word about sterilization of the mentally handicapped. The thing to keep in mind in this context is that the material act of sterilization is the same, whether it is done on someone who is competent or on someone who is not. The important ethical question is one of process: "The rights of the incompetent must not be less than those of the competent." In other words, the ethical issue here is whether a proxy decision-maker is ever ethically justified (or, for that matter, obligated) to opt for the sterilization of an incompetent ward.[39]

In the last few years, Canadian law has tended to give a negative answer. By and large, the decisions have been that when control of fertility is mandated, there are other less invasive and less mutilative procedures and/or modalities that could be employed to the same effect.[40]

Furthermore, the law has usually sided with the pleas of the various associations for the mentally handicapped who have suggested that to sterilize the mentally incompetent, either in a particular instance or as a matter of course, is to deprive them of their right to have children. The associations have usually argued, and the courts have agreed, that it is to deprive the mentally handicapped of that right for no reason other than the fact that they are incompetent. This is unjustifiable discrimination. The only acceptable circumstance would be where the life (welfare) of the incompetent was seriously threatened and no less drastic a course of action would work. In other words, only "therapeutic" sterilization is acceptable.

But is this the reasoning really valid? Consider the following two cases:

(a.) A profoundly mentally retarded 14 year old is admitted to a small community hospital scheduled for a hysterectomy. This is being done at the request of the mother who provides 24 hours a day care for this child, who tends to "smear" stool and will presumably do the same with her menstrual flow. A nurse on the ward notifies the local pro-life group who picket the hospital. The physician quickly calls the surgery and discharges the girl. The mother is frustrated and angry. She says she would like to see one of those "do-gooders" cope with her child 24 hours![41]

(b.) J.K. was a severely retarded female of 12 years of age about to start her menstrual periods. According to her mother and two psychiatrists, she had an abnormal fear of blood which, to the best understanding of the psychiatrists, would not yield either to the various retraining and reconditioning therapies that existed nor was it likely that she would be able to overcome her fear and aversion in any fashion. The mother, therefore, wished the daughter to be sterilized by hysterectomy. She cited not only the daughter's psychological aversion problem, but also the fact that the daughter was incapable of looking after her own hygiene and therefore could hardly be expected to look after a child should she ever get pregnant.[42]

When we consider these cases, there are several things that we should keep in mind. First, the position that sterilization should never be authorized for non-therapeutic purposes, as was stated in *re Eve,* is difficult to pin down. The notion of therapy requires more precise definition. Does it focus only on the here-and-now?

on the present medical condition of the person? Lord Oliver, in *Re B (A Minor)*, expressed this very well:[43]

> ... I do not, for my part, find the distinction between "therapeutic" and "non-therapeutic" measures helpful ... for it seems to me entirely immaterial whether measures undertaken for the protection against future foreseeable injury are properly described as "therapeutic."[44]

Second, sterilization is a procedure that is available to the competent as a matter of choice. Justice therefore demands that in principle it must be available to the incompetent as well.[45] As the Alberta Institute for Law Research and Reform put it:

> In our view the law should not add to the social disadvantages experienced by mentally incompetent persons by denying them the use, in a proper case, of the method of birth control most popularly chosen by persons in the general population. The denial would not be consonant with either the goal of normalization or the principle of equality.

We cannot automatically assume that the sterilization of an incompetent is unethical simply because it would be performed on incompetent persons. That would be to discriminate against the mentally incompetent solely in virtue of their incompetence. And that would be unethical.

As to the concept of "normalization" mentioned by the Institute for Law Research and Reform, social policy at the present time promotes the "normalization" of mentally disabled persons. The goal is to move them out of institutions and into the community so that they may experience as normal a life as possible.[46] However, unless there are effective methods of preventing conception, this goal cannot be achieved. Sometimes sterilization is the only appropriate and effective method.

As Lord Oliver put it in the British case of *Re B (A Minor)*, the issue

> ... is not ... sterilization for social purposes; it is not about eugenics; it is not about the convenience of those whose task it is to care for [the incompetent person] or the anxieties of [the] family ... It is about what is in the best interests of this unfortunate [person] and how best she can be given the protection which is essential to her future well-being so that she may lead as full a life as her intellectual capacity allows.[47]

Furthermore, a blanket rejection of sterilization for the mentally handicapped for contraceptive purposes would ignore the fact that health involves more than physical parameters. It also involves psychological factors. It may well be that sterilization is the preferable option from a psychological perspective precisely because of its permanent nature, even for the handicapped persons themselves. We cannot decide that a priori. We have to look and see. If we decided the matter out of hand, we should indeed be discriminating in an unacceptable fashion.

Finally, chemical methods of birth control carry quantifiable risks in terms of increased morbidity and mortality;[48] especially if the incompetent person is on medication. It may well be that there are circumstances where on balance these risks outweigh the intrusiveness and irreversible nature of sterilization. The British case of *re B (A Minor)*[49] is particularly noteworthy in this regard. In this case the House of Lords upheld a lower court's ruling that it would be appropriate to sterilize a mentally handicapped and epileptic girl of 17. The reason was that contraceptive medications would react with the medicines necessary to control her epilepsy and mental instability. Under those circumstances, sterilization would in effect be mandated by the principle of best action and the principle of the least intrusive alternative.[50]

The Incompetent's Right to Have Children

We will now return briefly to the right to have children. How do the considerations that we have just raised affect the position of the mentally severely handicapped? The Law Reform Commission of Canada has stated that "There is nothing inherent in mental handicap that determines whether or not a person is competent to raise children."[51] It has also argued that

> Without some proof (beyond simple mental handicap) that a person is unable to care for children, the justification for state intervention in the procreative ability, that is the state's interest in protecting those unable to protect themselves, does not appear adequately established.[52]

In principle, these considerations strike us as appropriate. However, in some situations there may be proof that a specific mentally handicapped person is unable to care for children—and we would add, "for children as persons." Therefore in these cases we would expect the Law Reform Commission to agree with the stance that we have suggested.

However, we do differ with the Law Reform Commission on one very important point. We cannot agree that the right to have children is the right to an "opportunity to develop one's full potential."[53] To connect the two together in this way is to suggest that children may be treated as objects. We have already rejected this position earlier. The unethical nature of this stance would not be improved by the fact that those who would be treating the children as object are handicapped.

The fact is that very young children are incompetent *persons*, and they are unable able to protect or take care of themselves. If the state's mandate is to protect "those unable to protect themselves," then it must protect not only the adult handicapped but the children as well. This cannot be done by allowing one group of incompetents to violate the rights of the other group so that the first group's wishes may be satisfied.

Another way of putting this point is like this: Just as the right of the incompetent must not be less than those of the competent simply in virtue of their incompetence, so they must not be more. Especially if there is no ethically relevant difference that would mandate the greater right. That would amount to reverse discrimination. Mental incompetence is a handicap. Therefore, it is an acceptable reason for using greater care and consideration when evaluating the lengths to which we should go in implementing the rights held by such persons. However, this is different from saying that the handicap entails rights that others who do not have that handicap do not have. That would require separate justification.

We are here back to the sort of consideration we raised a moment ago when we talked about self-determination. On occasion, not to overrule a right to self-determination may threaten the very life of other members of society or may violate their fundamental rights in an egregious fashion, whereas no corresponding degree of harm would befall the other person if the right to self-determination were to be limited in its expression. The example that we gave was of a society that experiences such a scarcity of resources that any increase in its population would mean starvation[54] for the members of that society. We supposed that there was no way in which that starvation could be prevented if the population did increase; and we supposed further that some persons were either unable or unwilling to control their reproductive drives in such as way as to prevent an increase in population. We suggested that under these circumstances the society would be justified in interfering with the autonomy and freedom of these persons in order to prevent such an increase. If it should turn out that the only way in which the reason for that interference could be achieved was by compromising their physical integrity of these people, then society has that duty and that right. The right to personal integrity would be outweighed by the right to life of the other members.

With due alteration in detail, this analysis would apply in the present context. The right to self-determination and even self-fulfilment is not absolute. There are circumstances where society may have an obligation not only to impose limits but also to ensure that these limits are observed. However, this does not mean that the society may interfere with the integrity of its members because it finds it the more convenient course of action. In particular, it does not mean that society may interfere because it does not want to provide assistance that would allow these persons to function appropriately as parents. We can only echo the Supreme Court's reasoning in this regard:

> The argument relating to fitness as a parent involves many value-loaded questions. Studies conclude that mentally incompetent parents show as much fondness and concern for their children as other people; ... Many, it is true, may have difficulty in coping, particularly with the financial burdens involved. But this issue does not relate to the benefit of the incompetent; it is a social problem, and one, moreover, that is not limited to incompetents. Above all it is not an issue that comes within the limited powers of the courts, under the *parens patriae* jurisdiction, to do what is necessary for the benefit of persons who are unable to care for themselves. Indeed, there are human rights considerations that should make a court extremely hesitant about attempting to solve a social problem like this by this means.[55]

The state may interfere with the integrity of their person only if the right that is violated by not interfering is weightier or more effective than the right that is violated by the interference itself. Furthermore, even then it may do so only if there is no other way that society can prevent such a state of affairs from materializing. There must be a balancing of competing rights. Therefore society must always evaluate very carefully whether there are other medical ways in which such an outcome can be avoided. Usually, there are. For instance, the physician could instruct his patients in proper and effective methods of birth control. Sterilization is rarely if ever called for. The principle of the least intrusive alternative always applies.[56] To quote the Institute of Law Research and Reform once more:

> ... sterilization should be permitted only as a last resort, other alternatives having first been shown to be inadequate for the intended purpose.[57]

Conclusion

All persons of full age, without regard to race, religion or nationality, have the right to have children. In suitably amended form and with the conditions that we have indicated, this is surely correct. However, in the pursuit of this right, we should never lose sight of the fact that children are persons.

It would also be well if we remembered something that was said by the early proponents of female equality: biology is not destiny. The fact that someone cannot or does not want to take advantage of this right to have children should not be seen as a negative reflection on that person. There are ways of fulfilling our potential as persons without necessarily having biological offspring. And while society should not unfairly deprive anyone of taking advantage of the opportunities for having biological offspring that would normally be available to people as a matter of course, by the same token it should also not create a climate where the failure to take advantage of that opportunity, or the inability to do so, becomes the basis of value judgments. It is important that we do not forget that limits to our abilities to function in certain ways do not detract from our value as individuals; and that the exercise of our autonomy is a matter of fundamental right.

ENDNOTES

[1] Compare Great Britain, Dept. of Health and Social Services, *Report of the Committee of Enquiry into Human Sterilization and Embryology*, edited by M. Warnock (London, Her Majesty's Stationer's Office, 1984): "The Warnock Report."

[2] See Angus McLaren, "The Creation of a Haven for 'Human Thoroughbreds': the Sterilization of the Feebleminded and the Mentally Ill in British Columbia," *Canadian Historical Review*. 1986 67(2): 127–50. Similar sterilization laws existed in Alberta. See Alberta Institute for Law Research and Reform, ref note 32.

[3] This usually included dangerous sex-offenders. The statutes of Alberta and British Columbia in particular were implicated in this regard.

[4] Gail Vines, "Bangladeshis Coerced into Sterilization," *New Scientist* 1985 Sept. 19; 107(1474) 21–22.

[5] Canadian Bill of Rights, S.C. 1960, c.44, s.1.(b)

[6] Canadian Bill of Rights., S.C. 1970, c.44, s.1(a).

[7] *Re D*, [1976] 1 All E.R. 326 (Fam. D.). However, see *In re B (A Minor)*, [1987] All E. R. 206–219 (H.L.). The House of Lords affirmed a lower court's decision to allow sterilization

of a mentally retarded and epileptic 17-year old girl because it was in her best interests, because she had no understanding of the relationship between the sex act and pregnancy, and because she was considered incapable of coping with birth and raising a child. Evidence was led that she lacked the mental capacity to cooperate with contraceptive drugs—which incidentally could also interact with the medication necessary to control her epilepsy. For a commentary, see Andrew Grubb and David Pearl, "Sterilisation and the Courts," *Cambridge Law Journal* 1987 46(3): 439–464.

[8] See *Re Eve* (1987), 31 D.L.R. (4th) S.C.C., [1987] 2 S.C.R. 388 (S.C.C.)

[9] See Alberta Sexual Sterilization Act, S.A. 1928 c.37 (revised 1937 and 1942 to include as reasons neurosyphilis, certain epilepsies and Huntington's chorea.) repealed 1972 (S.A. 1972 c. 87); Sexual Sterilization Act, S.B.C. 1933, c.59.

[10] This is one of the strands of the so-called "natural law" arguments.

[11] This seems to underlie the U.N. Resolution and the Declaration of Teheran. See also *Report of the Commission of Inquiry into Human Fertilisation and Embryology*, M. Warnock, chairman (London: Her Majesty's Stationery Office, 1984) at 8–9.

[12] See *Re Eve*, reference in note 8.

[13] See the discussion of the right to have children, ref. in note 8, *Re Eve*.

[14] See Chapter 13.

[15] *- vs. Child and Family Services* Manitoba Court of Queen's Bench, 1989, unreported; *Canadian Human Rights Advocate* V: 10 (December, 1989) 10.

[16] See "The Warnock Report," reference in note 1.

[17] The principle of relevant difference is implicated here.

[18] For a critical analysis of some aspects of this reasoning, see R.H. Kenen and R.M. Schmidt, "Stigmatization of Carrier Status: Social Implications of Heterozygote Genetic Screening Programs," *American Journal of Public Health* 68 (1978) 116–120.

[19] See the discussion of ranking of rights, chapters 2 and 9.

[20] For a discussion of some aspects of this, notably the notion of "suitability" to be a parent, see M. Somerville, "Birth Technology, Parenting and 'Deviance'," *International Journal of Law and Psychiatry* 5 (1982) at 123. For a discussion of the issue in relation to techniques of assisted reproduction, see British Columbia, Royal Commission on Family and Children's Law, *Ninth Report of the Royal Commission on Family and Children's Law* (Victoria: 1975) 10, and elsewhere; and Ontario Law Reform Commission, *Report on Human Artificial Reproduction and Related Matters* (Toronto: 1985) 153ff.

[21] See the discussion of consent in Chapter 5.

[22] *Re Eve*, ref. note 8.

[23] See *Re Eve*, ref. note 8; see also Law Reform Commission of Canada, Working Paper 24, *Sterilization: Implications for Mentally Retarded and Mentally Ill Persons* (Ottawa: Minister of Supply and Services, 1978).

[24] *Re Eve*, ref. note 8.

[25] See the discussion of third-party obligations, chapters 3 and 4.

[26] See D. Chambers, "The Right to the Least Restrictive Alternative," in M. Kindred et al., eds., *The Mentally Retarded Citizen and the Law* (New York: Free Press, 1976).

[27] See Institute of Law Research and Reform, *Report for Discussion No.6* "Sterilization Decisions: Minors and Mentally Incompetent Adults," (Edmonton, Alta: 1988)at 87 and elsewhere.

[28] See *Sterilization*, at 71, ref. note 38.

[29] RU–486 interrupts pregnancies by opposing the action of progesterone at several sites in the uterus, leading to an eroding of the endometrium. The embryo is consequently detached and expelled along with the endometrial tissue. See L. Silvestre, C. Dubois, M. Renault, Y. Rezvani, E. Baulieu and A. Ulmann, "Voluntary Interruption of Pregnancy with Miferistone (RU–486) and a Prostaglandin Analogue: A Large-scale French Experience," *New England Journal of Medicine* 322: 10 (March 8, 1990) 645–648.

[30] I.e. they are not even potential persons, since they will never develop into persons, no matter how long they are allowed to live.

[31] Compare *Casti Connubii*, 1930; *Humanae Vitae*, 1968.

[32] See Institute of Law Research and Reform, *Report for Discussion No. 6*, "Sterilization Decisions: Minors and Mentally Incompetent Adults," (Edmonton, Alta: 1988) 33–4. According to a 1984 survey, of the 68.4% of Canadian women aged 18 to 49 who were using contraceptives, 35.3% had resorted to sterilization, 28% used the pill, 9.1% condoms, 8.3% I.U.D's. 13.2% of women had a male partner who was sterilized.

[33] See W.L. Prosser, *Handbook of the Law of Torts*, 4th edition (Minnesota: West Publishing Co., 1971) 101.

[34] For discussion of some of the issues associated with this, see M. Somerville, *Consent To Medical Care*, 43 and elsewhere. Currently, murder is not covered by this: The issue of the legalization of euthanasia is implicated here (ref. note 36).

[35] See the opinion of Lord Denning in *Bravery vs. Bravery* [1954] All E.R. 59.

[36] Compare Margaret Somerville, *Consent to Medical Care*, Study Paper for the Law Reform Commission of Canada (Ottawa, Ministry of Supply and Services 1980).

[37] *Criminal Code*, R.S.C. 1985, c.C–34, 14.

[38] Law Reform Commission of Canada, Working Paper 24, *Sterilization: Implications for Mentally Retarded and Mentally Ill Persons* (Ottawa: Minister of Supply and Services, 1978), 59.

[39] See also Somerville, *Consent* at 92f. (ref. note 36).

[40] For instance, by the use of subcutaneous implants, etc.

[41] Thanks to the Paediatric Nursing Group of the RNABC, Burnaby, B.C. 1990.

[42] This is based on a case that was before the B.C. Court of Appeals.

[43] *In re B (A Minor)* at 219; see also Lord Hailsham, *In re B* at 213 (ref. note 7).

[44] See also Lord Bridge, *In re B* at 214 (ref. note 7).

[45] See Institute of Law Research and Reform at 35 (ref. note 32).

[46] B. Nirje, "The Normalization Principle and its Human Management Implications," in R. Kugel and W. Wolfensberger, eds., *Changing Patterns in Residential Services for the*

Mentally Retarded (Washington: President's Committee on Mental Retardation, 1969); R.A. McCormick, Health and Medicine in the Catholic Tradition (New York: Crossroads, 1984) 149: "The principle of normalization involves an effort to ensure the complete rehabilitation of the disabled person by providing an environment as close as possible to the normal."

[47] Re B (A Minor), 219 (ref. note 7).

[48] See statistics associated with contraceptive medication and heart attacks in older women.

[49] In re B (A Minor), 206 (ref. note 7).

[50] Compare Canadian Human Rights Act S.C. 1976–7, c. 33; In the matter of Eve, Re Infant K, Supreme Court of B.C. Jan. 30, 1985, Vancouver Registry A 842 616. See also Chambers, (ref. note 26) 93, who says when government does have a legitimate communal interest to serve by legislating human conduct, it should use methods that curtail individual freedom to no greater extent than is essential for securing that interest.

[51] *Sterilization*, at 68 (ref. note 38).

[52] *Sterilization*, at 62 (ref. note 38).

[53] *Sterilization*, at 63 (ref. note 38).

[54] It does not have to be starvation. It may involve a severe reduction in life expectancy, quality-of-life, and so on.

[55] See *Re Eve*, ref. note 8.

[56] Chambers, at 93 (ref. note 26).

[57] See Institute for Law Research and Reform, at 87 (ref. note 32).

SUGGESTED READINGS

- Alberta Institute of Law Research and Reform. Report No.52, "Competence and Human Reproduction." Edmonton, 1989.

    This is one in a series of publications by the Alberta Institute of Law Research and Reform—the Alberta version of the Law Reform Commission. It takes a serious look at the hypothesis that the right to have children is predicated on certain presumptions. It also contains some draft proposal for new sterilization laws.

- Grubb, Andrew and David Pearl. "Sterilization and the Courts," *Cambridge Law Journal* 1987, 46(3): 439–464.

    This papers contains a general discussion of sterilization orders in Canada, the UK and the USA. It makes interesting comparison reading in the light of *Eve*.

- Ontario Law Reform Commission. "Is There a Right to Procreate?" *Report on Human Artificial Reproduction and Related Matters* 2 vols. Toronto: Ministry of the Attorney General, 1985, 41–45.

    The report of the Ontario Law Reform Commission is one of the most extensive treatments of techniques of new reproductive technologies available. Although somewhat dated, the reasoning it contains is still fundamentally sound. The section mentioned here considers the right to have children from a legal perspective.

- *Re Eve* (1987), 31 D.L.R. (4th) S.C.C., [1987] 2 S.C.R. 388 (S.C.C.).

  This sterilization case provided the Supreme Court with the opportunity to address the question of non-consensual sterilization of incompetent persons, and the question of the right to have children. In the course of its reasoning, the Court also rejected the concept of substitute judgement for Canadian jurisdictions.

- Wilson, R.W. "Voluntary Sterilization: Legal and Ethical Aspects," *Legal Medical Quarterly* 3 (1979) 13–23.

  This paper examines the ethical and legal aspects of voluntary sterilization by competent adults as a method of birth control. It constitutes a good complement to the discussion in *Eve* and of the discussion in Grubb and Pearl.

13

Genetic and Pre-Natal Screening

This chapter deals with the ethics of genetic and pre-natal screening. Its main purpose is to sensitize the reader to various issues involved in this rapidly developing area of reproductive technology. It touches on such subjects as screening for carrier status, pre-natal screening for various diseases as well as to determine the sex of the offspring, and the concept of wrongful life.

Questions to consider while reading this section include:

1. What is the ethical status of genetic screening for carrier status? What role (if any) should such screening play in the delivery of health care?
2. What is the ethical status of prenatal screening? What role (if any) should such screening play in the delivery of health care?
3. What is meant by "wrongful life?" Should the law admit actions brought on the basis of a wrongful life claim on behalf of a child?
4. Is eugenics ethically defensible?
5. Is it ever ethically appropriate to try to predetermine the sex of a fetus?
6. How could one balance the economic costs of screening against the value that Canadian society attaches to the human person?

Introduction

From the earliest times, people have known that what living organisms are like depends at least partly on the characteristics of their parents. They put this knowledge to use by breeding selectively for desirable traits in cereals, vegetables, fruits and livestock. They knew *how* to do it, but they did not know *why* it worked. The primary nature of the mechanism that was responsible began to be unravelled only in the 19th century with the work of Gregor Mendel[1]. Mendel traced the physical characteristics of peas through controlled cross-pollination for several generations. His work marked the beginning of the study of genetics.

Statistical tools for understanding inheritance became ever-more sophisticated, and genetics as a scientific discipline assumed an increasingly important role in animal husbandry, plant breeding and so on. In 1959 Krick and Watson discovered the double-helix nature of deoxyribonucleic acid (DNA). With this discovery, our understanding of the mechanisms of inheritance took a quantum leap forward. Subsequent decades saw the discovery of recombinant DNA techniques—of ways of ways of manipulating DNA by excising a bit of DNA here and splicing in a bit there in order to change the genetic code. With this, human kind acquired the ability to manipulate directly the blueprint for life.

The initial involvement in genetics and in the application of the knowledge it provided was confined to animal models. However, pressure soon mounted to extend it to the human sphere. The reasoning went something like this: Human beings are biological organisms. Therefore, if it is possible to identify and detect genes that code for specific characteristics in plants and animals, this should be possible for human beings as well.

Genetic screening—the identification and detection of debilitating and/or fatal human congenital conditions—soon became a legitimate area of medical research. In recent years, it has become one of the most successful and promising areas of scientific development. Already the list of human conditions and diseases that can be identified and detected numbers well over a hundred and it is growing steadily.[2] It includes Tay-Sachs, haemophilia, cystic fibrosis, sickle cell anemia and the like. In 1988 the U.S. Government funded research to construct a map of the whole human genome in order to provide geneticists with a base line of knowledge. The project potentially will allow for the identification of most genetically determined human defects.

Such knowledge may not come easily. Many human characteristics are poly-genetically determined. That is to say, they are encoded on more than one gene. Others are polymorphic, which means that they exist in more than one variation. Furthermore, the process faces severe technical problems with respect to detecting and identifying the relevant genes.[3] Nevertheless, the potential is there.

The question therefore arises whether we should engage in such research at all. If the point of the project is it simply to amass information about where the markers for genetically determined diseases are located, then from a purely pragmatic perspective the prudence of the undertaking has to be questioned. The study is expensive. Information is nice—but given the price-tag that attaches to this kind of research, it would merely drain badly needed funds away from other areas of endeavour. The start-up costs for the human genome project are in the neighbourhood of $1 billion U.S. How could such an expenditure be justified in the face of the need of those already living their lives: people who suffer from poverty, malnutrition and correctable bad health? Public health measures are the most successful means for raising the level of health in any society. Furthermore, 13% of the people in the U.S. have no health insurance and no appropriate access to health care.[4] In many other countries, Canada included, the level of health care could be substantially improved without this costly research.

On the other hand, if this sort of study is going to have practical implications then we have to ask ourselves how this knowledge is going to be applied. Using it to detect genetic flaws on an individual and voluntary basis may be one thing; using it in a mass genetic screening program would be quite another. That has something ominous about it. Furthermore, what would count as a genetic flaw? What would count as a medical indication for initiating screening in the first place? Can these notions even be defined in a value-free way?

Further, once these so-called genetic flaws have been identified, what should we do with this information? The genetic technology that is being developed in other areas does not offer any means of "curing" genetic "flaws" in human beings. What good does it do to know these things if there is nothing we can do about them? Should we practise eugenics? That is to say, should we enact laws that would prevent people who carry defective genes from having children? Or should we simply tell people about their genetic inheritance? If so, what precisely is it that we should tell them? Should we tell them that if they reproduce there is the possibility that they may have defective offspring? What effect would this have on their psychological perception of themselves? On the way in which they are perceived by others? On their right to have children?

Or should we continue to develop recombinant DNA technology and apply it to human beings to the point where we can repair (or improve on) nature? As we shall see later, there are distinct moves in that direction, and in some areas we are on the verge of success. However, this immediately raises a whole series of other questions about the nature and extent to which we should interfere with the very nature of future generations. Recent developments in medicine have given us almost god-like powers over life and death. In many cases we can determine who will live and who will die, who will be healthy, who will be functional—and to what degree. Should we now expand this role by playing Creator and controlling the very image of humanity itself?

Some Historical Considerations

It is not easy to find answers to these questions. We can look to history for a start. Humanity has always sought to shape its own image, even before the advent of modern genetics. Such attempts may not have occurred on purpose or with full consciousness of the fact. (Nevertheless, mate-selection has functioned in this way.) All cultures and races have held to standards of beauty and of what was considered the norm. Genetically, this has channelled mate-selection into certain lines. Steatopygia among the Bushmen-Hottentot is a well-known and perhaps extreme example. Great height among the Watussi and rounded body-shape among the Inuit are two more examples. There are numerous others. However, social planners have considered the notion for a long time. Utopian social planners toyed with the idea of incorporating these ideas into deliberate breeding programs. For instance, Plato argued that we should use our knowledge of breeding better and healthier animals and apply it to the human race.[5]

For over two millennia, this sort of perspective remained idle theory. Then, around the turn of the century, the ideas that had been proposed first by Plato and then by people like Galton began to surface in the arena of politics. At first in Great Britain[6] and then in the U.S.,[7] prominent public figures came out in favour of the notion. Eminent jurists such as Oliver Wendell Holmes, and politically influential figures such as F.D.Roosevelt publicly supported it and welcomed the knowledge and techniques involved as useful instruments of social policy.

The eugenic movement was born. It maintained that the removal of deleterious genes from the gene pool was essential to the survival of the human race. On a positive note, it encouraged the perpetuation of "beneficial" genes as necessary to its salvation. The movement acquired such popular support that in 1911 sterilization laws began to be enacted in the U.S. and continued for decades.[8] Canada followed in the 1920s and 1930s.[9] When in the late 1920s Germany became interested in the issue as a matter of social policy, it turned to the U.S. for information and advice.[10]

The eugenics movement had two sides to it: positive and negative. Positive eugenics was the active encouragement of those with "good" or "desirable" genes to have children. The population policies of Nazi Germany provide a good example of positive eugenics. Women—"Aryan" women—who had more than 10 children were honoured with special decorations by the state. Negative eugenics was the active attempt to delete what were identified as undesirable genes either by sterilizing those who carried them or by being discouraging them from having children.[11] The sterilization policies of Nazi Germany again provide the standard example, but the sterilization programs and statutes in the U.S.[12] and Canada[13] also illustrate this approach rather well.

However, eugenics was not just a political program with a popular base. It also enjoyed support from the scientific community. Scientists who were motivated solely by concern for human society advocated both negative and positive eugenics. However, they did not think that statutes were the appropriate way to achieve the aims of the program, or that force or coercion should be used. They envisioned a voluntary program based on the responsible exercise of human freedom.

J. Mueller, one of the foremost geneticists of his time and one of the most outspoken scientific proponents of eugenics, emphasized this clearly when he rejected any attempt to impose forcible control by the state.[14] However, his pessimism about the success of such a voluntary program is reflected in the following passage:

> However, it seems asking almost too much to expect those individuals who are really less well equipped than the average in mentality or disposition to acknowledge to themselves that they are genetically inferior to their neighbours in these respects and then publicly to admit this low appraisal of themselves by raising no

family at all or a smaller one than normal, especially since at the same time they would often be thwarting a natural urge to achieve the deep fulfilment, accorded to their superiors, that go with having little ones to care for and bring up. Moreover, those with physical impairments would likewise tend to rationalize the situation, by thinking that they possessed some superior psychological qualities that more than compensated for their physical defects.[15]

In other words, Mueller foresaw the ironic possibility that the very nature of the program envisioned would lead to its failure. People with the very traits to be enhanced—depth and scope of intelligence, curiosity, genuineness and warmth of feeling, joy in life and in achievements, humanness of appreciation, facility in expression, and creativity[16]—would be motivated by a sense of social responsibility; and since they would be aware that social resources are limited, they would practise restraint in their reproductive habits so as not to stretch those resources beyond the limit.[17] On the other hand, those who lacked such feeling and such appreciation would propagate like lemmings.

Scientists were not the only professionals who became involved in this area. Lawyers also entered the lists. As recently as 1973 the Chicago Bar Association proposed a screening law for all marriage-licence applicants to test their eugenic suitability for producing future members of society. One proponent of this bill characterized the perspective that underlay the proposal like this: " ... [W]e are going to have to try to reduce the number of non-productive members of our society."[18] Presumably, this was to be done by preventing those who were genetically so deviant and defective as to be congenitally incapable of being anything more than a drain on the public purse from having children!

Of course, not all proponents of eugenics focused on considerations of the public good. In recent times, some have approached it from the perspective of the offspring. Purdy,[19] for example, has argued that it is immoral for us to reproduce if we know that there is a high risk that we will have children with severe genetic damage and whose quality of life will be very low. Joseph Fletcher[20] has argued that we have a duty to the unborn to engage in genetic screening. Parents who carry a lethal, deleterious or debilitating gene have a moral duty to not to procreate. Not surprisingly, he has also maintained that people who run a greater-than-average risk of chromosomal damage because of their age (and therefore of having defective offsprings)—women over 35 and men over 65—have a moral duty not to have children. To have children under such circumstances would be to take the deliberate risk of condemning them to a low or subhuman type of existence.

We should also mention that not all arguments in favour of using our increased knowledge of genetics are eugenic in the original sense of the term. That is to say, not all of them advocate a eugenically oriented breeding program. Nor do they focus on screening for carrier status. Some advocate what is called pre-natal screening: the screening of fetuses in utero for genetic and other defects. Their main thesis is that since we can detect these defects in utero by the use of amniocentesis,[21] chorionic villi sampling,[22] etc., we should abort all fetuses who are found to be genetically defective before they become persons and begin to suffer. We owe it both to the children as well as to society itself.[23]

Some Arguments Against

However, right from the very beginning, the development and use of genetic screening techniques and related technologies met with stiff opposition. This opposition began in earnest in the 1930s and gained momentum as time went on. It opposes all eugenically motivated interference in reproduction, whether it be through genetic screening of the parents or through prenatal screening of the offspring. In its most extreme form, it even opposes the development of screening techniques themselves. This opposition can be sketched in terms of two sorts of arguments: arguments that focus on carrier status, and arguments that focus on prenatal screening.

Arguments Against Screening for Carrier Status

One of the major objections to identifying someone as a carrier of deleterious genes is that the exercise is essentially pointless. People cannot change their genetic heritage. Therefore, if they find out that they carry a lethal or deleterious gene, there are only three things they can do: (1) they can ignore the information; (2) they can accept it and decide not to have any biological offspring; or (3) they can accept it, procreate anyway but screen the still developing offspring in utero for inherited genetic defects.

Alternative (1) would make the whole exercise rather pointless[24]—especially given the cost involved in screening. Alternative (2) would penalize the persons who are identified as genetically deviant for an accident of fate. Alternative (3) would make sense only if the developing fetus was in fact aborted if the test showed genetic abnormalities. However, so it was argued, that would inculcate a rather callous attitude towards human life in general and towards handicapped persons in particular. It would amount to saying that the life of such a handicapped person was not worth living.

Furthermore, some identifiable genetic defects are associated with ethnic minorities. For instance, Tay-Sachs is 100 times more frequent among Ashkenazi Jews than in the non-Jewish population;[25] sickle cell anemia is associated particularly with Italians, Blacks, and certain other ethnic minorities. Consequently it has been argued that if genetic screening was to be used to identify carriers of certain genes, it might result in racial discrimination. These groups might be singled out for restrictive breeding laws. And even if they were not singled out explicitly, the effect of any laws in that direction would be the same. These groups would be discriminated against. And even if no such laws were enacted and even if this information were not acted on, the groups would be stigmatized by the identification of the carrier state itself.[26]

It has also been argued that the cost of genetic screening programs for carrier status is out of all proportion to the return. The Canadian experience in the case of Tay-Sachs illustrates this only too well. In one study, 21,071 individuals were screened.[27] This resulted in the detection of 24 couples who were both carriers, three pregnancies were monitored and one fetus was aborted at the cost of over $100,000. While the cost for other programs such as sickle cell anemia may not be quite as high, it may be argued that in view of the scarcity of medical resources such programs are extravagant.

Another argument has pointed out that the data that could be derived from genetic screening for carrier defects are useless from a preventive standpoint. Mutations occur at a low but constant rate in the human population. Therefore, new instances of genetic defects will be produced all the time. The rate may be small, but it is not insignificant.

Still another consideration has centred on the complexity of the mechanisms of inheritance. Most genetic characteristics are cross-linked with other characteristics. That is to say, they are genetically interconnected in such a way that the elimination of one entails the elimination of the other. Therefore, to eliminate these cross-linked deleterious genes would mean that we would lose desirable characteristics as well. But then the whole point of the of eliminating deleterious characteristics would be gone. We would be "improving" the genotype by making it worse.

There is also the fact that the notion of what counts as a deleterious gene is not at all clear. Like the notion of health, it might be functional in nature. This would mean that under certain circumstances what are seen as deleterious genes would in fact be advantageous. The gene for sickle cell anemia is a case in point. When the person who inherits it is not heterozygous[28] for it, it makes that person more resistant to malaria. It therefore confers an advantage on that person in malaria-infested areas.

Furthermore, there is quite a bit of uncertainty about the connection between a particular gene and what is identified as an undesirable characteristic. The XYY controversy is a good example. Earlier studies had suggested that people who carried an XYY chromosome were more likely to be criminal.[29] Subsequent investigations showed that this was not the case: that the connection that had initially been detected between the two was wholly fortuitous.

In other words, we may be mistaken in what we identify as a deleterious gene or in what we take to be its impact. Therefore we might irreparably damage the human gene-pool. We do not really know what is good and what is bad, what is useful and what deleterious. By deleting the one, we may in fact be deleting something that is necessary for survival of the species.

Arguments Against Pre-Natal Screening

As to the screening of fetuses for genetic defects, that also has not gone unopposed. Leon Kass is one of the more prominent figures in this counter-movement. He has argued that prenatal genetic screening has only one purpose: to kill those who are detected as genetically deviant. That, however, so he argues, strikes at the very core concept of our society: the concept of the ultimate worth of the human person. As he put it:

> What may be at stake here is the belief in the radical moral equality of all human beings, the belief that all human beings possess equally and independent of merit ... the right to life.[30]

Others go even further. They see a danger in the possession of the knowledge itself. They maintain that such knowledge may be misused to discriminate against those offspring who are identified as being at risk but who are not in fact aborted.[31]

Furthermore, they go on to say that while pre-natal genetic screening by amniocentesis will identify certain circumstances and conditions (e.g., Down's syndrome, haemophilia, etc.) there is no way to treat these other than by abortion. This is objectionable to many prospective parents. Therefore the knowledge gained would not only be useless to them, it would also throw them into the depths of despair. On the one hand they would know that they will have a radically defective offspring; on the other hand, there is nothing their private morality will allow them to do about it.

Those who argue against prenatal genetic screening also point to the following: Even when the parents think that abortion is morally acceptable, the fact is that the severity of the debility cannot always be determined by the genetic screening alone. The screening may give an indication that something is wrong. However, it cannot always give any firm guide as to how wrong this wrong actually is. The various trisomies[32] are here excellent examples. The fact that a trisomy—for instance Down's syndrome—is present does not give any indication about how severely it will be expressed by that particular person. Often the degree of severity can be determined only at birth. Therefore parents who base their decision on information they receive from genetic screening may find that although the aborted fetus was genetically flawed, it was functionally essentially normal because the defect did not express itself to any large extent.

Finally, as an ultimate warning, we are told that we should always keep in mind that some of the greatest persons who have ever lived would not have existed had genetic screening been in place and had the relevant action been implemented. Beethoven is merely one of many significant examples.

Some Considerations About Genetic Screening

The debate is far from over. However, we would like to suggest that the following considerations are relevant for the ethics of genetic screening, whether that screening be prenatal or for carrier status.

The overriding logical fact is that our lives and the life of society constantly require decision-making. Decision-making, in turn, if it is done rationally, involves considering and weighing competing options. However, options are not really options if they are not known. We cannot choose what we do not know. Furthermore, in order to make a truly informed choice, we also have to able to evaluate the relative strengths and weaknesses of the options from which we are to choose. Therefore knowledge and understanding are the key to rational decision-making and informed consent.

Knowledge and understanding are also key elements in the exercise of autonomy. If we are unaware that certain choices exist, we cannot figure them into our life plans. That means that our range of choices will be limited. If that limitation is the result of not having information that we could have, then our autonomy has been curtailed.

Carrier Status

These considerations obviously apply to screening for carrier status. To illustrate, let us take screening for a particular disease: Huntington's disease, for example. Let us suppose that we can screen potential victims of Huntington's disease prior to the actual onset of the disease process itself.[33] The disease is irreversible and ultimately fatal. It is also incurable at present. However, it would be premature to say that knowing that someone actually has the relevant genetic defect would be inappropriate, demeaning or useless. The people who are at known risk of having the disease may themselves want to know whether they actually have it. They might want to prepare for its onset. To set their house in order, so to speak. To deprive them of that opportunity would be to limit their options. By that very token, it would be to violate the principle of autonomy.[34]

Furthermore, the potential carriers may not as yet have had any children. Therefore they might want to know whether they would be at risk of passing on the disease to their offsprings. The knowledge that they do not have the disease might alter their future life-plans. The absence of the genetic determinant would mean that they could not pass the disease on to their offspring. Therefore they might decide to have children after all, whereas previously they would not have had any. On the other hand, the knowledge that they do carry the diseases might also affect their reproductive behaviour. They might decide not to run the risk of burdening future offspring with the condition. Autonomy and responsibility are at stake.

In general terms, the more we know about our own condition, the more informed our life-decisions will be. Of course there is the danger that the availability of genetic screening will make people feel that they have to use the technology: that they have no choice. By and large that is something that society should strive to avoid.

But autonomy always has limits; even here. Knowledge about carrier status should be voluntary as long as ignorance in that department does not detract from the legitimate rights of others and as long as it does not put others unnecessarily and disproportionately at risk.[35] When it does interfere with their rights, or when it does put them at risk, autonomy in that regard ceases. For example, while we might prefer to remain ignorant of our status as typhoid carriers, that preference does not amount to a right. When there is a justified suspicion that we are typhoid carriers we have to test that suspicion. We do not have the right to remain ignorant, because our preference would be putting other people's lives at risk, even if only the lives of future generations. This is what may underlie a recent statistic that shows 33% of Canadian physicians thought that patients should be informed about the test results for Huntington's disease even if they did not want to know it.[36]

Pre-Natal Genetic Screening

With due alteration of detail similar considerations apply to prenatal genetic screening. Prenatal genetic screening is a tool for providing us with data about the child-to-be. If we do not use such screening when it is appropriate, we will be embarking on a policy of deliberate ignorance. We will be placing ourselves and others knowingly and deliberately into a position where our decisions have to be made without relevant data: data that could have been available and that would have been material to the case. The result may well be decisions that we would not have made if we had known the data.

It is true that at the present time, the knowledge that is gained through genetic screening usually cannot be translated into curative efforts. Gene therapy is still very much an experimental technique that as yet has little application to human beings.[37] But again, this does not mean that the knowledge we can gain through screening would be entirely useless. There are many human diseases or health conditions that we cannot cure in a causal sense, but whose symptoms we can treat if the disease is detected early enough. This applies to pre-natal genetic screening as well. PKU screening is a case in point.[38] Infants who are identified as being at risk can be put on a special diet so that the severity of the disease process is minimized. Lives that otherwise would be severely reduced in quality are thereby given a chance for normalcy.

Of course, not all diseases that are detectable by prenatal genetic screening can be dealt with in this way. Tay-Sachs,[39] Friedreich's ataxia[40] and Lesch-Nyhan disease[41] are examples of diseases that cannot. There is no effective treatment for them. However, this still does not mean that the information would be useless. To say so would be like saying that because there is no effective treatment for people who have diseases like poliomyelitis or AIDS, we should not test for them; and even if we did test, we should not use the results of these tests. Knowing that a disease is present allows people to prepare for its onset and to ameliorate its effects: not only on the affected individuals themselves but also on others.

Knowing that their offspring will have a genetically determined disease that is incurable allows parents[42] (and the medical and nursing staff) to prepare for the fact that their child will be severely affected. It will also allow them (and the medical and nursing staff) to prepare for palliation if they so choose. To withhold this information is to deprive them of the opportunity to prepare. It also limits their domain of choice. The parents might want to abort the affected fetus. Therefore, the impact that the information can have on their life-plans may be tremendous.[43]

This last argument invites two replies. One is that if this sort of policy had been followed in the past, human society would have been the loser. People like Woody Guthrie would have been aborted because he suffered from Huntington's disease. The other reply is that abortion as a response to the pre-natal detection of genetic deviance is a sad commentary about our view of handicaps. It effectively marks those who suffer from genetically determined handicaps as second-class citizens whose lives are not worth living.

However, the first response is itself ethically objectionable. Certainly from a deontological perspective. Let us not quibble about whether Woody Guthrie is a good example, or whether it should be someone else. Let us focus on the logic of the argument itself. The argument rests on the contributions that Woody Guthrie (or some other cultural hero) has made: the important place that he occupies in the history of human culture. The argument would be less persuasive if we replaced the name of Woody Guthrie with that of Hitler, Al Capone or Attila the Hun. But that only shows that the argument's persuasiveness rests on equating Woody Guthrie with his usefulness to humanity. It is this perceived usefulness that drives it. However, this means that the argument really is utilitarian in nature. It covertly asks us to balance the good that could be derived from not aborting someone because of a genetic defect, against the price that we would have to pay by aborting that entity. That is to treat people as objects.

Furthermore, the argument asks us to do this balancing without having quantifiable parameters. We do not know what the likelihood would be of aborting an Al Capone or a Hitler or a Woody Guthrie if the parents aborted on the basis of genetic screening; just as we do not know what the likelihood would be of preserving one if the parents did not abort. In other words, the argument really reduces to an appeal to emotions, not facts.

The same thing is true about the second argument: that aborting fetuses that have a serious genetically determined condition is to reject handicapped people who suffer from such diseases, and to brand them as second-class citizens. This situation would also be true if the same policy were to be extended to handicapped people already on the scene. That is to say, it would be true if the same sort of treatment were suggested as appropriate for handicapped persons. However, no-one is suggesting that; and the logic of this reasoning does not entail it. The fact is that the fetuses aborted would not yet be persons and this makes a fundamental difference.

Furthermore, the reason for abortion is not that it is seen as a cure for the disease, but as a preventive measure. It is seen as preventing an injury from becoming complete when the fetus is born as a person. This puts the whole thing onto a different footing. It is not possible to prevent the injury of those who are already born and who are handicapped because of their genetic condition. In their case, what is called for is treatment and palliation. However, to suggest that something which is appropriate as a preventive measure thereby automatically will be used as a curative or palliative effort is to stretch logic beyond its limits. It would be like saying that because fluoridation of teeth is appropriate as a preventive measure, it should also be used for dealing with cavities.

Which brings us to the crux of the whole issue. Saying that something is a handicap or saying that it would be better if we could prevent people from suffering from a particular handicap instead of trying to find ways to deal with after it has occurred, is not to say that those who suffer from the handicap are worthless as persons. Nor is it to brand them as second-class citizens. To say that something is a handicap is to say just that: that it is a handicap. This is not a comment about the person who suffers from the handicap but about the condition of that person. Society has to find ways to deal with that handicap and so does the person who suffers from it. Otherwise we could simply ignore it. Therefore the fact that we want to do something about a handicap does not mean that we consider the person who suffers from it any less of a person. On the contrary, precisely because we consider that individual worthy as a person we want to do something about it.

There are three ways of dealing with a condition that involves suffering. We can ignore it, we can address its roots, or we can play catch-up. Ignoring suffering is clearly unethical. We have to try and deal with it. This leaves the other two options. The principle of best action entails that we should prevent suffering if it is at all possible, because prevention is usually more effective, less harmful and more dignified for the person who suffers from a particular condition. Aborting a fetus who has a severe disease before it becomes a person is preventive. It also does not harm a person. The fetus is not yet a person. On the other hand, to allow the fetus to develop until it becomes a person and then to try and ameliorate its condition is to allow that new person to come to harm first, and then to try and correct the harm that has been done. This does strike us as unethical.[44]

Fetal Diagnosis: Non-Genetic Prenatal Screening

So far, we have concentrated on prenatal screening that is genetic in nature. There are also methods of screening fetuses for defects that do not focus on its genetic condition. They include testing the maternal blood for alpha-fetoproteins. An elevated presence of these proteins is a good indication that the fetus suffers from a neural tube defect like anencephaly or spina bifida. Another technique is ultrasound sonography. It can be used to develop a visual image of the fetus. It allows us to determine whether the fetus has internal organic or external physiological malformations. Fetoscopy, which involves inserting a light-conducting tube through the woman's abdominal wall and into the womb, is sometimes used to visualize the fetus directly. It allows a visual inspection of the fetus for malformations.

However, whatever the method of prenatal diagnosis and whatever the reason for using it, the points that we raised a moment ago about prenatal genetic screening apply to prenatal screening in general. One of the central stake-holder in all of this is really the child—or more correctly, perhaps, the child-to-be. It is the child-to-be that carries the defect, and it is the child-to-be that will be aborted—or born—if the parents so decide. What we are doing when we do prenatal screening is testing the as-yet unborn individual for seriously debilitating conditions. We have identified some reasons why parents might want to do that, and why society should not prevent them. But there are also reasons why it is appropriate to do this from the perspective of the unborn individual.

The reason lies in the duty to prevent harm to persons. We talked about that before, when we dealt with the notion of causality. In the case of pre-natal screening and diagnosis, harm will be prevented if that new person is not born defective. What we are saying is that if the only way that this harm can be prevented is by aborting the child-to-be, then the child-to-be should be aborted before it becomes a person.

This line of reasoning underlies what in the last few years has come to be known as the notion of wrongful life. The concept is a legal one. Wrongful life actions are actions brought on behalf of a congenitally severely deficient children for having been born defective when it was known that they would be at high risk for being born that way and where this outcome was preventable by abortion.

Wrongful life actions have generally failed.[45] The judicial position is well summed up by George Annas:[46]

> 1. " ... to be damaged one needs to be worse off after the negligent act complained of than before it" and there is here no comparable situation *ante rem*; and
> 2. there is no right to be born healthy *simpliciter*.[47]

According to Annas, one can argue that the parents were unfairly saddled with a severe burden of support. The diagnostic procedures on which they relied when making their decision about whether or not to go ahead with the pregnancy were negligently carried out. Therefore, they have a right to recover for damages. And in some cases they have succeeded.[48] What can not be argued is that the child was worse off for having been born defective than for not having been born at all.

However, that is only one side of the argument.[49] A somewhat different position is taken by Marjorie Shaw.[50] She expands the notion of wrongful life beyond merely negligence in prenatal diagnostic procedures and the effect that this has on the parents. She disagrees with Annas in his fundamental premise. She maintains that to be born radically defective is to be worse off than not to be born at all.[51] She therefore claims that a woman who abandons her right to an abortion when she is informed of the risk of having a severely defective neonate is irresponsible and should be held liable by the child.

Shaw's reasoning focuses on the ethical question that is central to the whole issue of prenatal screening from the perspective of the offspring. Can one defend the claim that there is an obligation to prevent a low quality of life for individuals who have not yet been born? More strongly still, can one defend the claim that to be born radically defective is worse than not to be born at all? Annas says no; Shaw says yes. Who is right?

Let us agree that negligence and disregard of appropriate professional standards is always a matter of justified complaint. To that extent, wrongful life actions are always appropriate against a company or against a professional who engages in prenatal screening in a sloppy way. Therefore if someone suffers or incurs a burden as a result of professional carelessness, etc., the negligent party should be liable.

Having said that, it leaves unresolved the central issue between Annas and Shaw. Marjorie Shaw maintains that to gamble deliberately with the life of a child in terms of quality-of-life is unethical; and she does not care whether that gamble is taken by the company engaged to do prenatal screening or by the mother who decides to ignore the risks. Nor does she care whether the child is born or not. The fact is that an injury would occur if the child were to be born under these circumstances. For Shaw, that is sufficient. George Annas maintains that there cannot reasonably be any talk about an injury to the child. After all, the child had no prior undamaged mode of existence. Furthermore, there is no right to health but only to health care. Therefore how could a child—and an unborn child at that—possibly claim the right to be born with a certain level of health?

A possible way to resolve this disagreement is again to look at the legal notion of an injury becoming complete: this time from the perspective of the child-to-be. An injury may be potential until a certain set of circumstances arises. When it does, the injury becomes actual or complete. The very same injury merely has a protracted causal antecedent chain of events. The length of the antecedent causal chain does not change the fact that there is a real injury.

This reasoning can be illustrated by the infamous thalidomide case. Several years ago, thalidomide was prescribed to pregnant women to combat morning sickness. It transpired that although the drug was not injurious to the pregnant women, it had serious side-effects on the developing fetus. Specifically, it interfered with limb-development to such a degree that many of the children of women who were treated with the drug were born with only vestigial arms or legs.

The manufacturers and distributors of thalidomide were sued for damages by the children who were born thus defective. Their claim was effectively upheld, and damages were paid. The reasoning was this: those who were affected by the drug were not persons at the time that their mothers took the medication. Consequently they could not argue that they were injured at that time. Nevertheless, the taking of the drug initiated a chain of events. The outcome of that chain of events was a state of affairs that would not have existed if the drug had not been taken. That state of affairs, in turn, would have been described as a state of injury. In other words, the children were injured at the very time at which they became persons because at that point the injury initiated by the taking of the drug became complete. Becoming a person and being injured, although logically distinct, occurred temporally simultaneously.

If we now return to prenatal screening, we can see that Annas is correct when he argues that a fetus who is not a person does not have a right to be born with normal health, uninjured, and so on. But Annas is wrong when he suggests that the matter rest there.[52] A person has the right not to be injured. It does not matter whether the injury occurs at the very time that the individual becomes a person or at some later date. All that matters is the fact of injury itself. Therefore, as soon as a fetus becomes a person, it has the right not to be injured.

The chain of events that leads up to the infant's being born defective is simply a protracted causal sequence that culminates in an injury at the moment the fetus becomes a person. Therefore, if someone is aware that an injury will occur if the pregnancy continues, and if that person deliberately continues with the pregnancy, then that person becomes morally responsible for the outcome.[53]

This leaves the issue of abortion as a way of preventing this outcome. There are two claims here. One is that life itself is such a good that no matter what the circumstances, life itself is better than no life at all. The other is that the suggested cure for the problem is worse than the disease itself. To kill is also to injure. In fact, it is the greatest injury of all. Therefore, if being born defective is an injury, how much more so being killed in order to avoid that injury.

The reply to the first is that it follows only if the principle of vitalism is true. That is to say, it follows if and only if it is true that any kind of life is better than no life at all. We have already seen that this principle is not acceptable for adult persons. Parity of reasoning entails that it should not be accepted in the case of children either. To insist that it should hold in their case is to insist on discrimination.

The claim that killing is the greatest injury of all also misses the point. It involves the confusion of an action with an act. An action is the material activity involved in doing something. An act is the action together with its ethical significance in the context in which the action takes place. The two are not the same. Consider, for instance, cutting someone's face. It is assault and battery when done out of spite; it is an appropriate act of medicine when done in the course of cosmetic surgery while repairing a burn.

Bringing about someone's death also has to be considered from this perspective. To insist that bringing about someone's death is always to commit the ultimate injury is to say that the ethical nature of the activity is independent of the context in which it occurs: that it is always the same, no matter what the circumstances. But that is to confuse the action with the act. The context may make all the difference—and we are here not thinking simply of things like self-defense. If we are going to evaluate an action ethically, then we have to look at it in context. That means that we cannot always say that killing someone is committing the ultimate injury. Sometimes the very opposite is true. If the only thing a person can look forward to is a slow and agonizing slide into death or an undignified mode of existence that no reasonable person would want, then to insist that this person experience the full range of that agony is to insist on torturing this person. Diseases like Tay-Sachs are very much like other excruciating terminal diseases. Those who suffer from them will inevitably die a slow and agonizing death. In these contexts, the appropriate course of action is to shorten that suffering, since death is certain anyway. The point is that under such circumstances termination of life is ethically acceptable. Abortion is therefore not ethically inappropriate in such cases.

Sex-Determination

So far we have discussed prenatal screening from the standpoint of injury detection. However, it is not always used in that way. Sometimes it is used to determine the sex of the fetus.

There are situations in which knowing the sex of a fetus may be important from a medical perspective. For example, in the case of haemophilia. The gene for haemophilia is on the X chromosome. Therefore, it is important to know whether the fetus has a Y chromosome. If it does—which is to say, if it is a male child—and if there is a history of haemophilia in the family, then there is a good chance that the male child will also have haemophilia. Knowing whether the fetus is male will therefore be important to the parents. They may decide to abort the fetus in order to spare the child-to-be this severe handicap.

But there is also another use of prenatal sex-determination. For some people, and in some cultures, the sex of their children is very important;[54] particularly with respect to the order in which the children are born. For some, male children are preferred;[55] for others, female.[56] Prenatal sex-determination can be used to find out the sex of the fetus. When the fetus is not of the desired sex, the fetus is aborted. Sex, however, is not a disease or disease process. We therefore have to ask whether this use of prenatal screening is ethical.[57]

Actually, we are here faced with three questions. One is whether it is ever ethically acceptable to try to find out the sex of an offspring. Prenatal screening is here implicated. The other is whether it ethically acceptable to make sure that offspring will have a certain sex. The third is whether is it ethically acceptable to use abortion to this end.

We have already answered the first question in the affirmative. Sometimes it is very important to find out the sex of an offspring. Haemophilia is an obvious example.[58] But our desire to know the sex of an offspring need not be motivated by the suspicion that the offspring may have a sex-linked disease. It may merely be motivated by curiosity. That may not make knowing its sex beforehand a matter of overwhelming importance. However, just because knowing something is not important does not mean that knowing it, or trying to find it out, is unethical. Knowledge *per se* is ethically neutral. What is not ethically neutral is what is done with that knowledge.

Here we have to turn to the second question: Is it unethical to try to make sure that offspring will have a certain sex? The long and the short of it is that it all depends. The example of haemophilia again illustrates the point rather well. If the screening indicates that there is a good chance that the offspring will suffer from a sex-linked and debilitating disease, then there is nothing wrong with acting on the basis of that knowledge. It is simply a matter of preventing harm.

On the other hand, if there is no medical reason for preferring one sex over another, the matter is not quite so clear. It is tempting to agree with those who have argued that what we are dealing with in these cases is sexism, pure and simple:[59] that it is the height of discrimination on the basis of sex alone; and that it is unethical.

But the matter is not that simple. Sexism really is unethical only when it is directed towards persons. When persons are not involved, the situation is different. It is not unethical to prefer female cats over male cats, male dogs over female dogs, or whatever. Nor is it unethical to kill kittens or puppies that are not of the desired sex. It may be callous, and it may violate the principle of respect for life. It may even be injudicious, because it might run the danger of introducing a sex-imbalance into the population. However, none of these make sex-selection unethical.

A possible reason for viewing non-medical sex-selection with suspicion is the fact that it costs money. If the money has to come from health care plans, then there really are more appropriate uses for these funds. Health care funds should be used only for the delivery of health care. Sex is not a health condition. Therefore sex-selection should not be funded by the public health care system.

However, this still leaves the nagging feeling that there is more to the matter. And the interesting thing is that this feeling remains even when the sex-selection is paid for out of private funds, and even when it is not achieved through abortion. We experience the same unease when we consider techniques of sex-selection that deal only with gametes. These are techniques that either filter sperm that carry a Y-chromosome, or that concentrate sperm with Y-chromosomes, and so on.[60]

The fact is that there is something very disturbing to most Canadians in the idea of selecting the sex of children. Perhaps it is because we feel that the sex of a child should not be a matter of choice; that it should be left to chance. We cannot choose other characteristics of our children; so why should we be able to choose their sex?

What is unsettling about this is that sometimes we *do* choose the sex of our children; and society does not and has not objected. We choose the sex of our children when we go to an adoption agency and ask to adopt a girl or a boy. If choosing the sex of a child were unacceptable *per se*, and if having a preference for a child of one sex over a child of another points to a fundamentally sexist attitude which ought to be discouraged, then it we should also find it unacceptable in the case of adoption. We cannot have it both ways. Of course this does not entail that therefore sex-selection is alright after all. It may merely mean that current practice in this regard has to be reviewed. It may be that our social practice has not yet caught up with our ethical convictions.

Perhaps our rejection of sex-selection is itself a culture-bound and value-based phenomenon. Other cultures certainly find nothing wrong with sex-selection.[61] But even if is true, the fact that sex-selection is generally accepted as unproblematic would not necessarily make it ethically right. There is the strong suspicion that if there is such a marked preference for one sex over another in the case of children-to-be, then that preference must have a deeper root. It probably bespeaks a much deeper and fundamental sexist perspective in general. It is this sexist perspective that we have trouble with. We would like to think that all persons are equal and that they should be treated equally; that the sex of a person really does not matter; and that what matters is the person him- or herself.

Conclusion

According to Greek mythology, when Pandora opened the box given to her by Zeus, she inadvertently released upon humanity all sorts of evils. We might well ask whether developing and employing techniques of genetic and prenatal screening is not like opening a Pandora's box. Does the knowledge that we can obtain in this way carry a similar price-tag?

Once we have acquired information through the use of these techniques, can we ethically afford not to use it? Does the mere possession of such knowledge not impose on us an obligation to act, lest by not acting we become co-responsible for the negative outcomes that might have been avoided had we acted on that knowledge?

On the other hand, if we did act on that knowledge or did develop techniques that would allow us to act in some appropriate fashion, in what direction should we act? The answer, so it could be argued, is far from clear. Therefore, given uncertainty in this area, and given the unforeseeable consequences of any of our actions, would it not be better if we did not use techniques of genetic and pre-natal screening at all but simply let nature take its course?

These are considerations that ask us to err on the side of safety; and the concerns they express are certainly valid. However, as we have tried to show, both using the technologies and not using them carries its own ethical price-tags. In our estimation, the price-tag for not using the technologies is greater than that of using them. It seems to us that accidentally bringing about harm in the attempt to prevent harm to others is defensible, but that deliberately and knowingly allowing preventable harm to occur is not. We have an obligation to try to prevent harm to others. This obligation grows out of the principle of autonomy and of respect for persons. It goes almost without saying that when we try to prevent such harm, we should take every possible care not to produce new harm through our actions. This follows from what we called the principle of best action. Therefore, it seems to us that the use of genetic and pre-natal screening is entirely appropriate, and that the relevant technologies should be developed further but only with a strong overriding condition: their development should proceed only in the most circumspect and responsible way possible. The guidelines about biological experimentation in general, and about human experimentation in particular, should be most strictly adhered to. Furthermore, we should attempt the use of these techniques only if this can be defended as a species of health care. Anything else should be interdicted.

ENDNOTES

[1] Gregor Mendel, 1822–1882, an Austrian monk who, through experimentation on peas, laid the foundation of modern genetics. His work had a posthumous impact.

[2] Compare Leon Rosenberg, "Towards Newer Genetics," in M. Shaw, and A. Doudera, eds., *Defining Human Life: Medical, Legal and Ethical Implications* (Ann Arbor, Mich.: AUPHA Press, 1983).

[3] For a discussion, see any good contemporary text on genetics.

[4] See President's Commission for the study of Ethical Problems in Medicine and Biomedical and Behavioural Research, *Securing Access to Health Care* (Washington, D.C.: U.S. Government Printing Office, 1983) 3 vols; vol. 1.

[5] Compare Plato, *Republic* B 458f.

[6] By persons like Galton, Huxley, etc.

[7] See Jon Beckwith, "Social and Political Uses of Genetics in the United States: Past and Present," in R. Munson, ed., *Intervention and Reflection*, (Belmont, Calif.: Wadsworth, 1979) 384-392.

[8] As above at 385.

[9] See the sterilization statutes of Alberta and British Columbia, p. 305.

[10] Beckwith, full ref. note 7, 386ff.

[11] Beckwith, full ref. note 7, 385-387. For discussion of contemporary views along similar lines, see T.M. Powledge, "Genetic Screening and Personal Freedom," in R. Munson, ed., *Intervention and Reflection*. (Belmont, Calif.: Wadsworth, 1979), 371-375.

[12] Barry Mehler, "Eliminating the Inferior: American and Nazi Sterilization Programs," *Science for the People* 19: 6 (1987) 14–18. For a classic discussion with limited bibliography by someone who advocated such a program in the U.S. see H.E. Barnes, *The Repression of Crime: Studies in Historical Penology* (Montclair, N.J.: Patterson Smith, 1969; reprint of the 1918 edition.) especially at 180ff. Barnes also followed McKim in suggestion euthanasia for the "feebleminded" etc.: "Most states have begun to make some pretence at custodial segregation of the worst types of the idiotic and the feeble-minded, and sixteen, following the Indiana precedent of 1907, have legalized the sterilization of the hopelessly defective and the habitually criminal, but the laws have not been applied with any thoroughness except in California. The plan suggested by McKim of painlessly exterminating the idiotic, hopelessly insane and habitually criminal classes is probably as remote from practical adoption *as it is wise and desirable*." (ital. added).

[13] See ref. note 9, p. 305.

[14] H.J. Mueller, "Genetic Progress by Voluntary Conducted Germinal Choice," quoted in Paul Ramsey, *Fabricated Man: The Ethics of Genetic Control* (New Haven and London: Yale University Press, 1970) 162 n.24.

[15] H.J. Mueller, "Human Evolution by Voluntary Choice of Germ Plasm," in R. Munson, ed., *Intervention and Reflections*, (Belmont, Calif.: Woodsworth), 352.

[16] Mueller, ref. in note 15, 354.

[17] Mueller, ref. note 14.

[18] Quoted in Beckwith, full ref. note 7, at 389

[19] L.M. Purdy, "Genetic Diseases: Can Having Children Be Immoral?" in J.J. Buckley Jr., ed., *Genetics Now: Ethical Issues in Genetic Research* (Washington D.C., University Press of America, 1978).

[20] Joseph Fletcher, *The Ethics of Genetic Control* (New York: Doubleday, 1974).

[21] Amniocentesis involves the withdrawal of amniotic fluid surrounding the fetus by means of a hollow needle that is inserted through the abdomen and the uterine wall. The fetal cells that are shed by the fetus into the fluid are examined to detect certain fetal abnormalities. Amniocentesis usually won't be done before approximately 12 weeks gestation, and the results of the test are usually not immediately available.

[22] A technique by which chorionic cells (which originate from the fertilized ovum) are aspirated through the vaginal opening and tested. This can be done as soon as the chorion forms, and requires only days for analysis.

[23] Kass, ref. note 30, 465. A different perspective is offered by the Sacred Congregation for the Doctrine of the Faith, Instruction on Respect for Human Life in its Origin and Dignity of Procreation, (Rome: Vatican, 1987) pp. 14ff.

[24] Compare Karp, ref. note 56, 458–64; and Leon Rosenberg, "Toward an Even Newer Genetics," in Shaw and Doudera, ref. note 2, esp. p. 311.

[25] E. Goodman and D. Goodman, "The Overselling of Genetic Anxiety," *Hastings Center Report*, 12: 5 (Oct. 1982), 21.

[26] Compare R.H. Kenen and R.M. Schmidt, "Stigmatization of Carrier Status: Social Implications of Heterozygote Genetic Screening Programs," *American Journal of Public Health*, 68 (1978), 116–120.

[27] See also J.H. Swint, V.L. Carson, L.W. Reynolds, G.H. Thomas and H.H. Kazazian, "The Economic Returns to a Community and Hospital Screening Program for a Genetic Screening," *Preventive Medicine*, 8 (1979), 465–470. See also J.T.R. Clark, "Screening for Carriers of Tay-Sachs Disease: Two Approaches," *Canadian Medical Association Journal*, 119 (1978), 450.

[28] I.e., when the person has not received the same gene from both parents.

[29] "The XYY Man: Do Criminals Really Have Abnormal Genes?" *Science Digest* 79 (Jan. 1976), 33–38. But see A.A. Witkin, et al., "Criminality in XYY and XXY Men," *Science* 1983 (Aug. 13, 1976), 547–55. For a good discussion of the various aspects of genetic determination of criminality, etc., see A. Milunsky and G.J. Annas, eds., *Genetics and the Law* (New York: Plenum Press, 1976); D. Bergsma, ed., *Ethical, Social and Legal Dimensions of Screening for Human Genetic Disease*. Birth Defect Series, vol. 10 (New York: Stratton-Intercontinental).

[30] Leon Kass, "Implications of Prenatal Diagnosis for the Human Right to Life, in T.A. Mappes, and J.S. Zembaty, eds., *Biomedical Ethics* (New York and London: McGraw-Hill, 1978), 465. A different perspective is offered by the Sacred Congregation for the Doctrine of the Faith, *Instruction on Respect for Human Life in its Origin and Dignity of Procreation* (Rome: Vatican, 1987), 14H. For a similar solution but ultimately to the same effect, see also *Declaration on Procured Abortion* (Rome: Vatican, 1985) 14ff.

[31] See Kass, ref. note 30, 464-468; and R.F. Murray, "Problems Behind the Promise: Ethical Issues in Mass Genetic Screening," *Hastings Center Report* 2 (April 1979), 46–7.

[32] A trisomy is a genetic condition where there is an extra version of a chromosome. It is usually associated with a diagnosable health condition.

[33] The disease involves a gradual progressive and incurable neurological deterioration that ultimately leads to death. Although some markers have been identified, their identification is line-contingent and cannot as yet be used as a general tool for diagnosis.

[34] See D.C. Wertz and J.C. Fletcher, "Moral Reasoning Among Medical Geneticists in Eighteen Nations," *Theoretical Medicine* 10: 2 (June 1989), 123–138, at 126f., for the prevalence of autonomy as the central guiding principle in genetic counselling.

[35] See Michael D. Bayles, *Reproductive Ethics* (Englewood Cliffs, N.J.: Prentice-Hall, 1984); see also M.D. Bayles, "Harm to the Unconceived," *Philosophy and Public Affairs* 5:3 (1976).

[36] See Wertz and Fletcher, ref. note 34, 123–138, at 133.

[37] See Medical Research Council of Canada, 1989. See also Gregory Fowler, Eric T. Juengst and Burke K. Zimmerman, "Germ-Line Gene Therapy and the Clinical Ethos of Medical Genetics," *Theoretical Medicine* 10: 2 (June 1989) 151–165, at 151ff.

[38] Rosenberg, ref. note 2, 307 and elsewhere.

[39] Tay-Sachs affects 1 in 3,600 infants born to Ashkenazi Jewish parents. It is a progressive and irreversible degenerative disease of the central nervous system causing blindness, severe mental retardation, seizures, paralysis and death usually occurs by age 5.

[40] A progressive and incurable degenerative neurological disease in which certain groups of nerve fibres gradually deteriorate. It manifests itself in loss of co-ordination of movements and lass of balance, and affects the ability to stand still, speak, walk and use the arms.

[41] Lesch-Nyhan disease involves severe neurological disorders including spasticity, aggressive behaviour, retardation, self-mutilation, kidney failure, etc. It ultimately leads to death.

[42] And society, by preparing appropriate support measures.

[43] Rosenberg, ref. note 2, 311.

[44] Compare M.D. Bayles, "Harm to the Unconceived", *Philosophy and Public Affairs* 5:3 (1976).

[45] Compare *Curlender vs. Bio-Services Laboratories*, 165 Cal. Reporter 477 (Ct. App. 2d, Dist. Div. 1, 1980).

[46] George Annas, "Righting the Wrong of 'Wrongful Life,'" *Hastings Center Report* 11: 1 (Feb. 1981). See also *Gildiner vs. Thomas Jefferson University Hospital*, 451 f. Supp. 692 (E.D. Pa. May 25, 1978).

[47] Annas, ref. note 46, 9.

[48] Annas, ref. note 46.

[49] See Clifton Perry, "Wrongful Life and Comparison of Harms," *Westminster Institute Review* 1: 4 (1982), 7–9.

[50] Margery Shaw, "Preconception and Prenatal Tests," in A. Milunsky and G. Annas, eds., *Genetics and the Law II*, (New York, Plenum Press, 1980).

[51] See M.D. Bayles, "Harm to the Unconceived," *Philosophy and Public Affairs* 5: 3 (1976), 295.

[52] For a somewhat different analysis but to the same effect, see Bayles, *Reproductive Ethics*, ref. note 35, Chapter 2.

[53] See American Fertility Society, "Ethical Considerations of the New Reproductive Technologies," *Fertility and Sterility* 46: 3 (Sept., 1986) Supplement, Chapter 9. See also Ramsey, ref. note 14, and Haering, *Medical Ethics* (Notre Dame, Ind.: Fides Pub.1973).

[54] N.E. Williamson, "Boys or Girls? Parents' Preferences and Sex Control," *Population Bulletin* 33: 1 (January 1978) 3–35.

[55] Roberta Steinbacher, "Futuristic Implications of Sex Preselection," in H.B. Holmes, B.B. Hoskins and M. Gross, eds., *The Custom-Made Child? Women-Centered Perspectives*, (Clifton, N.J.: Human Press, 1981) 188 and elsewhere.

[56] See L.E. Karp, "Prevental Diagnosis of Genetic Disease" in T.A. Mappes, and J.S. Zembaty, eds., *Biomedical Ethics* (New York and London: McGraw-Hill, 1978) 458-64.

[57] For an interesting analysis of the prevalence of disclosure by physicians of the sex of fetuses to the parents, see Wertz and Fletcher, ref. note 34.

[58] See Michael Bayles, *Reproductive Ethics* (Englewood Cliffs, N.J.: Prentice-Hall, 1984) 37.

[59] See Bayles, ref. note 58 above, 38.

[60] See M.R. Netwig, "Technical Aspects of Sex Preselection," in *The Custom-Made Child*, at 181–186, (full ref. in note 55 above).

[61] Asiatic cultures tend to favour boys, as do most European cultures. African cultures present a mixed picture of preference and non-preference.

SUGGESTED READINGS

- Bayles, Michael. *Reproductive Ethics*. Englewood Cliffs, N.J.: Prentice-Hall, 1984.

    This is a good introductory discussion of some of the philosophical issues that arise in the context of human reproduction and the use of new techniques of reproductive technology. It is written by a former director of the Westminster Institute, in Ontario.

- Ethics Committee of the American Fertility Society. "Ethical Considerations of the New Reproductive Technologies." Suppl. to *Fertility and Sterility* 46: 3 (Sept. 1986).

    This paper represents the official position of an influential group of U.S. physicians specializing in the use of new reproductive technologies.

- Lappe, Marc. "The Limits of Genetic Inquiry." *Hastings Center Report* 17: 4 (1987) 5–10.

    A fairly recent and thoughtful discussion of genetic technology that has become available in recent years an its application to the human context. The practical details tend to be American in nature, but the ethical reasoning is relevant to any context irrespective of nationality.

- Law Reform Commission of Ontario. *Report on Artificial Human Reproduction and Related Matter.* Toronto: Ministry of the Attorney General, 1985.

   The classic standard Canadian discussion of the status of techniques of reproductive technology. The perspective is juridical, but the discussion also deals with ethical considerations.

- Overall, C. *Ethics and Human Reproduction: A Feminist Analysis.* Boston: Allen and Unwin, 1987.

   An extended treatment of the ethics of human reproduction by a feminist Canadian philosopher.

- Powledge, Tabitha and Joseph Fletcher. "Guidelines for the Ethical, Social, and Legal Issues in Prenatal Diagnosis." *New England Journal of Medicine* 300: 4 (1979) 168–172.

   As the title suggests, an discussion of guidelines for the use of pre-natal diagnosis. One of the more important issues that is addressed is the issue of responsibility in the face of negative diagnostic results.

- Tormey, J.F. "Ethical Considerations for Prenatal Genetic Diagnosis." *Clinical Obstetrics and Gynecology* 19 (December, 1976) 957–963.

   A discussion of prenatal genetic diagnosis from the perspective of a physician. An interesting companion piece to the article by Powledge and Fletcher.

14
New Techniques of Reproductive Technology

Recent advances in the biological sciences are reshaping the process of human reproduction. We considered some of the factors involved when we dealt with genetic and prenatal screening. The aim of this chapters is to give a brief overview of the ethical considerations relevant to such techniques as artificial insemination, *in vitro* fertilization, genetic engineering and cloning. We shall also take a brief look at the ethics of surrogate motherhood.

Questions that might usefully guide the reader include the following:
1. Do the ethical considerations that apply to artificial insemination differ from those that apply to natural insemination?
2. What is the ethical status of *in vitro* fertilization?
3. What is genetic engineering? What are some of the arguments for and against genetic engineering? Would the job of a health care professional be easier if we practised genetic engineering?
4. What is eugenics? Is it ethical?
5. What is the ethical status of surrogate motherhood?
6. "Man should not play God!" How would one defend—or attack—this claim in the context of genetic engineering, abortion, contraception, surrogate motherhood and the practice of medicine in general?

Introduction

The last few years have seen an explosion of interest in new reproductive technology. Implicated here are such things as *in vitro* fertilization, artificial insemination, cryo-preservation of ova and sperm, gene therapy (both somatic and germ line), cloning, artificial placentas, surrogate motherhood and the like. Internationally, commissions have been set up by various countries and by their professional organizations, and reports and recommendations have proliferated. In Canada, provincial governments have struck commissions to investigate the legal and social aspects of this technology,[1] various professional associations have formed committees to consider it,[2] and most recently the federal government of Canada established a Royal Commission to look into its social, legal, ethical and other implications.[3]

The reason for this explosion of interest lies in the realization that while the advancement of knowledge is a desirable thing and while its application serves to advance the state of humanity, such advancement is desirable only if it is not bought at the price of unethical behaviour, and that its application is to be welcomed only if it does not imperil the fundamental ethical position of society itself.

People are beginning to realize that scientific and technological developments do not occur in isolation but in a social context. The fact is that any scientific or technological development has societal implications. The context makes them possible, but is influenced by them in turn. This is particularly true in the realm of bio-technology, because the very nature and survival of humanity may be implicated. People are also beginning to understand the importance of a balance between what society can do in terms of scientific and technological capabilities, and what it should do in terms of ethics—between what society should encourage, allow and forbid.

There is also the realization that achieving such a balance is not a matter of serendipity. It is the product of a deliberate process that strives to understand conflicting concerns and attempts to harmonize them. It requires the identification of relevant issues, the reconciliation of distinct perspectives, and the determination of their importance and weight. Without this, the pace of development may outstrip the appreciation of its significance and surpass the understanding of its implications. When that occurs, the process assumes control and the subject matter begins to determine the direction of society itself.

In Vitro Fertilization and Associated Techniques[4]

General Comments

Many of the new reproductive technologies involve in vitro fertilization. The technique consists of gathering human gametes, ova and sperm, and of combining them under controlled conditions outside of the body of the woman to effect fertilization. This process usually occurs place in a petri dish, which is made of glass. Hence the name: "in glass" fertilization. The fertilized ova are often incubated for a while to ensure that fertilization has indeed taken place. The developing embryos, or "pre-embryos" as they are sometimes called, are then inserted into the cervix of the woman who is going to bear the children.[5]

The ova that are used are usually produced by using various drugs to induce[6] super-ovulation in a woman. These drugs stimulate the ovaries to produce more than one ripe ovum at a time. The ova are then harvested, usually by a technique called laparoscopy. Neither the stimulation nor the laparoscopy are without risk to the woman.

We should add that the ova that are used in vitro fertilization need not be those of the woman who will ultimately bear the child. They may come from a donor. Likewise, the sperm that are used need not be those of the legally recognized spouse of the woman who will bear the child. They may come from someone other than the legally recognized spouse of the woman who is to have the child. That person is also referred to as a donor. When it is the sperm from the legally recognized spouse, it has usually been treated to render it more fertile.

It should be clear that these are merely variants of techniques known as AID and AIH respectively.[7] In AID (Artificial Insemination by Donor), the sperm of a donor is inserted into the cervix of the woman; in AIH (Artificial Insemination by Husband), it is sperm from the legally recognized spouse (husband).[8]

We should also mention that the uterus in which the fertilized ovum will develop need not be that of the woman who will ultimately raise the child; nor need the ovum be biologically hers. When the uterus is not that of the legally recognized female partner, but the child, when born, is taken by a legally recognized couple, then the arrangement is often called surrogate motherhood.[9] In rare cases, both ovum and sperm come from the couple who will take the child, and the uterus-of-implantation is merely a womb for rent.

Finally—there is the possibility of allowing a fertilized ovum to develop in an artificial womb. This is sometimes referred to by the misnomer of artificial placenta.[10] However, so far this has been tried only on animal models, and is still very much in the experimental stages.[11]

All of these methods of assisted reproduction have been criticized. AID and AIH have been criticized for introducing an unnatural element into what should really be a natural function.[12] They have been portrayed as leading to psychological damage to children when they discover their origin.[13] They have also been criticized for encouraging the attitude that any problem that people encounter in their lives must be fixed. This, so it is argued, destroys the value of humility and does away with the opportunity for others to develop compassion.[14] Surrogate motherhood has also been criticized as the modern version of commerce in human beings,[15] and as destructive of the nuclear family which is the backbone of Western culture.[16] Furthermore, it has been criticized as demeaning to women by turning them into walking incubators.[17] It has even been suggested that the legal recognition of surrogate motherhood would allow the upper socio-economic classes to prey on socio-economically underprivileged women and lead to the development of two female classes: those who bear children, and those who can afford to raise them.[18]

These are serious charges, and they merit careful consideration. However, the considerations that are involved here are so complex that we cannot deal adequately with all of them. We shall therefore focus our discussion on in vitro fertilization and the technologies it enables. Aside from surrogate motherhood, it is these that are seen as the most serious.

One of the more traditional critiques of in vitro fertilization is reflected in the following passage from a text-book on bioethics by Ashley and O'Rourke:[19]

> ... in vitro fertilization and other procedures (like it) are ethically objectionable because they separate reproduction from its parental context and involve the production of human beings, some of whom will probably be defective because of experimental failure and who will probably be destroyed. This contravenes the basic principles of ethical experimentation with human subjects.[20]

Other objections come from the social sciences. For instance, it has been argued that in vitro fertilization procedures dull human sensibilities for one of the most important human functions—that of reproduction. Another suggests that it may lead to fundamental disruption of the ties of motherhood: to its "dismemberment."[21] Still another focuses on the fact that the availability of such techniques would allow single women or women who are lesbian in their sexual orientation to have children. This would jeopardize one of the most important institutions of our society: the nuclear family.[22] And in the same vein, some objections consider the technology as the beginning of slippery slope to a totally impersonal, inhumane reproductive policy where women are seen as biological incubators: as reproductive animals without any dignity and value.[23]

Other objections focus on the status of the fertilized ovum outside of the body;[24] on the use of spare fertilized ova that result,[25] the ownership of these ova, and so on. Pragmatic difficulties have also been raised. For instance, concerning the so-called quality of the sperm:[26] What guarantee is there that the sperm will not be genetically defective, or that it will not carry some disease like AIDS? Questions of record-keeping have been raised: What if the donor of the sperm (or the ovum) later turns out to have a congenital disease.[27] What provisions are or should be made for tracing? Or, for that matter, for allowing the children who have been produced by these techniques to seek out their genetic ancestors if they so wish?[28]

From the legal perspective there are issues of parental responsibility that require settlement. For instance, there are questions that deal with obligations of care and support of the children that result from such practices. The whole structure of current family law in this area is far from clear.[29] There is also the fear that legal complications of legitimacy and associated problem of inheritance may result. Again, the issues are not yet fully settled.

Finally there is a whole array of issues that centre around the ethics of the experimental protocols necessary to develop the techniques.[30] They also involve the material dangers inherent in such proceedings. In particular, in the aspiration of ova, fertilization in vitro and subsequent cryo-storage for future implantation[31] and gestational development at some more convenient and opportune time. Do these involve some danger to the biological integrity of the conceptus? How does this fit in with our responsibility to future generations?

The list of objections is long and growing; and they are as diverse as the backgrounds and concerns as the people who voice them. But there are also considerations on the other side. Obviously—because otherwise the techniques would not be developed and applied in practice.

The most common reason for using these techniques is that they allow people who would otherwise be unable to have children, to have biological offspring of their own. Other reasons include the need for experimentation of fertilized ova to solve problems of embryonic development, to develop techniques of gene therapy, and so on.[32]

We cannot here give a detailed analysis and evaluation of all of the considerations we have mentioned. That would require a treatise in itself. Instead, we shall focus on some of the aspects that strike us as more or less central.

Analysis and Replies[33]

First, is the claim that *in vitro* fertilization and its related technologies violate the sacredness of the family unit. This claim could be criticized from several angles. For instance, it is based on the Western notion of the nuclear family unit as basic to society, and it assumes that this type of family unit is in fact sacred. However, this premise is not shared by a large part of the world.[34] Western society may consider it basic, but there are all sorts of cultural variations. There is no ethical principle which requires that a family unit must have a certain constitution—a female and a male person—or that the adult persons involved in it must be related by a contract (i.e., marriage).

Furthermore, this criticism would be appropriate if and only if there was something inherent in the procedure itself that did violence to the family unit. It is difficult to see how such could be the case. Unless, of course, it was assumed as a matter of principle that using gametes other than those of the spouses should present an ethical problem.

However, in the first place, the underlying premise here is factually mistaken. Not all procedures of artificial insemination or in vitro fertilization use donor gametes. AIH is an accepted procedure; and *in vitro* fertilization does not have to involve donor sperm or donor ova.

In the second place, it is unclear why the use of donor gametes should pose a threat to the family unit. There is no principle which says that the children involved in a family unit must be genetically derived from the adult members of the unit. There may be religious conventions to that effect, or cultural or legal traditions. These may even reflect the commonly held perceptions and ethos of the society in which the family unit is embedded. However, that does not turn these conventional relationships and expectations into ethical principles. Nor do the sociological and psychological data support the contention that genetic relatedness is a requirement for the success of a family relationship. The institution of adoption is predicated on the very opposite.

The claim that *in vitro* fertilization interferes with the bonds of motherhood, is also open to criticism. From a factual perspective, there are no data that support such a contention; therefore the contention lacks factual basis. Furthermore, adoptions would be indicted by the same reasoning. If the bonds of motherhood depended on the mechanics of biological origin, then maternal relations in adoptions would be seriously compromised. That does not appear to be the case.

However, there is an ethical consideration that is much more fundamental than either of these: If we allow the relationship between mother and child to be threatened by the fact that artificial insemination and in vitro fertilization, etc., are not "natural," then what we are really saying than is that the way in which someone comes into the world—the person's origin—is ethically relevant when it comes to dealing with the individual as a person. That is indefensible from a deontological perspective. Persons are persons. As persons, they are all equal. To allow considerations of origin to intrude into the relationships surrounding a person is to deny the principle of autonomy and respect for persons.[35] And to say that a technique should be rejected because it allows people the opportunity to discriminate in this fashion is to legitimate such a perspective. It may be that a particular person has difficulty with the techniques for personal psychological reasons. That, however, does not mean that the technique per se poses a problem. The problem belongs to the person.

We can put the point more generally. Neither the nature nor the ethical status of a person is affected by how that person was generated. Nor is it affected by who did the generating. Facts such as these—i.e., that the origin involved external help, that the genetic origin lies outside of the family unit, or that the genesis involved artificial assistance and was not wholly "natural"—these may be of sociological, legal, scientific or even doctrinal significance. Ethically speaking they are neutral. Even where the child's gestation occurred—whether it grew in one uterus rather than another, or even an artificial uterus—has nothing to do with the ethical status of the child. The child is a person. Where a person comes from or how a person came into being is ethically irrelevant to the ethical status of that person. To argue otherwise is to commit the genetic fallacy. It is to confuse the nature of a being with the nature of its origin.

Of course, this does not mean that someone may not have a specific psychological attitude towards a child because of how that child came into the world. That is perfectly understandable in cases such as incest or rape. However, factors that would play such a role in these cases are absent in cases where a woman voluntarily undergoes a process that involves *in vitro* fertilization. Therefore, if she has a negative attitude towards the child that she bears as a result of that process, it means that the woman needs help, not that the process itself is objectionable. The same thing holds true for fathers or male persons.

The objection that the children produced by such means would be harmed psychologically if they found out the nature of their origin is equally as untenable. First of all, there are no data that support such a claim. Second, even if there were, that would not necessarily make artificial insemination, *in vitro* fertilization, etc.

ethically objectionable. How children see themselves depends on what they are told, how they are told and on what they experience in their environment. Therefore the appropriate thing to do would not be to stop using these techniques but to change the attitudes that would cause this psychological harm. It is the attitude that would give rise to psychological problems that is objectionable, not the techniques themselves.

The suggestion that the nature of a person's origin violates the rights of that new person or constitutes an affront to the person's dignity, is merely a different version of the same mistake. Furthermore, there is no right to be born. Who would be the holder of that right? Consequently, there can be no right to be born in a certain way. The situation would be different if the way in which a person was conceived marked the beginning of a causal chain that became a completed injury when the fetus became a person. However, the only way in which that would follow is if a certain kind of parentage or a certain process of conception belonged to persons as a matter of right. However, that is the very assumption to be proved. Therefore this sort of argument begs the question.

The objection that this sort of technology involves human interference in a natural process is also difficult to sustain. If the underlying principle of this perspective were to be applied consistently, we would be forced to abandon all medicine and all technology. Both interfere with natural processes. That is their very raison d'être. Of course strictly speaking this does not entail that we should therefore permit the use of these reproductive technologies after all. We could equally as consistently draw the conclusion that we should drop medical and technological interventions in all human endeavours. However, this would be a bit extreme.

It would also conflict with the ethics of causality. If we can prevent harm from occurring without undue danger to ourselves and yet we fail to do so, then we become ethically guilty to the extent that we could have prevented that harm.[36] To prevent someone from exercising what is their right is to produce harm. Everyone has a *prima facie* right to have children. If someone wants to exercise that right—that is to say, if someone wants to have children—and it is possible for that person to have children if the available technology were to be employed, then to prevent that person from having access to that technology is to harm that person psychologically and ethically. Of course, the right to have children is conditioned by social circumstances and by the competing rights of others. However, these are not what are here at issue.

In general, parentage, family ties and "naturalness" are legal and culture-bound notions. If our society did not have the ethos of a particular type of legally recognized parentage, AI and surrogate motherhood would be no more of a problem than adoption. And if its traditional ethos did not equate "natural" with "ethically ideal" and "artificial" with "ethically suspect," the difficulties that are presumed to surround in vitro fertilization and artificial placentas would not even arise. Ethos is one thing; ethics is another. If artificial insemination, in vitro fertilization and the other techniques we have mentioned do encounter ethical problems, these problems have to be grounded in some way other than by merely pointing to the fact that ethos and tradition say so.

It is not surprising that these techniques and practices raise legal problems. It would be surprising if it were otherwise. By its very nature, the law is reactive. At least, this is true about the common law. It is a creature of interpretation. It is built over time by judges who interpret statutes and apply socially accepted standards. The law therefore lags behind social changes, and alters its position only after an established tradition no longer holds. Therefore, the fact that something presents legal problems does not necessarily indicate that it is an ethical problem. It may simply reflect the fact that the law is not geared to anticipate problems. It may also reflect the fact that legal considerations are not necessarily ethically motivated. They also include considerations of social policy, which may have a political orientation.

As to the risks inherent in this and similar procedures—we should always try to avoid risks to persons. However, even here we must strike a balance. When the risks are no greater than those encountered under ordinary circumstances, then it is not clear that the mere presence of a risk-factor constitutes an ethically valid objection. As we indicated in our discussion of abortion, there is a high rate of genetic error that occurs in conception and gestation under "normal," "ordinary" circumstances. If the percentage of these errors is not increased by the artificial techniques in question, then it is difficult to see how the fact that their use involves some risk could be a matter of ethical concern. It may be that at the present time the techniques do not have the same risk-factor as "natural" fertilization. If that is true, things are different. But it would still not mean that artificial insemination, *in vitro* fertilization and similar procedures should not be developed.[37] It would merely mean that it was premature to use them at the present time, and that they should be developed further.

There remains the fact that this development would involve the use of human beings as experimental objects. Spare embryos would have to be deliberately produced and discarded—which is to say, they would have to be brought into being first and then be killed or allowed to die.[38] This seems ethically objectionable on several grounds: It would involve treating humans like mere objects—which would contravene the principle of respect for persons. It would coarsen our sensibilities—which would cheapen the moral sensitivity of our society. And it would encourage an instrumentalistic view of persons.

However, these considerations would require us to accept either of two assumption, or both. The first is that an embryo is a person from the moment of conception. The second is that human beings, whether they are persons or not, may never be treated as mere biological organisms. We have already seen that there are good reasons for questioning both of these considerations: in our discussion of abortion and in our discussion of death. Therefore, if our reasoning then was correct, these assumptions fail, and the objection with it.

This does not mean that the treatment of fertilized ova would not be subject to strict guidelines. The very fact that they are *human* fertilized ova would bring all sorts of values and interests into play. The Warnock Commission in Great Britain[39] suggested some guidelines years ago, and the Medical Research Council of Canada[40] and the Law Reform Commission of Canada[41] have recently followed suit. Other countries have also considered the matter from more or less restrictive perspectives.[42] But in all of these cases it is useful to keep in mind that guidelines such as these reflect more than ethical reasoning. They also reflect—and sometimes are motivated by—political, sociological and religious considerations. The standards of ethical experimentation should always be followed, and the value of respect for life should also be honoured. However, this does not rule out research and development; and that is important.

Gene Therapy and Genetic Engineering[43]

We have already dealt with some aspects of this new reproductive technology when we considered genetic and prenatal screening. However, as we said then, advances in reproductive technology have gone far beyond screening. The very developments that have made genetic screening possible have also opened to the door to further developments. The ability to isolate human DNA has gone hand-in-hand with the developments of techniques that allow us to excise segments from the DNA molecule and to replace them with others. Since it is these segments of DNA—these codons—that form the basis of human heredity, it means that with these developments we have acquired the ability to modify the genetic inheritance of humanity itself.[44]

Not that interference with genetic inheritance is something entirely new. Humanity has always interfered with (and to a certain extent, determined) its genetic make-up.[45] However, when it occurred, it was unconscious and non-deliberate. Inchoate social forces were at work. There was no preconceived plan, nor a program of deliberate implementation.

Furthermore, the control and determination that were exercised involved culturally related standards of beauty, physiological characteristics and the like.[46] This resulted in an enhancement and/or retention of some traits that otherwise would not have been retained or that would not have been maintained to that degree. It also resulted in the loss or attenuation of others. The racial variations among contemporary humanity are at least in part ascribable to such factors.[47]

However, whatever channelling of inheritance occurred was holistic in nature. It did not focus on specific human persons; nor was it directed towards the very basis of their characteristics. It involved individuals only as members of a society: so to speak, as tokens of a type. And if one can speak of direction in this context at all, it was directed at the characteristics themselves, not at their genetic base.

Furthermore, an important factor that is distinctive about past human interference in the process of inheritance is that is was essentially self-limiting. Any change or alteration that took place, no matter how it was brought about, had to occur within the limits of survival.

The reason was simple. The utter lack of reproductive technology itself required that the changes that went on should not impair the reproductive success of the adult members of the community, and the relative absence of medical services demanded that the survival rate of children to reproductive age should not be seriously affected. This put a lower limit on the nature and degree of changes that could be tolerated. To some extent this was offset by the development of a cooperative social lifestyle.[48] These limits were extended still further with the discovery and introduction of more and better pharmacological and medical devices, techniques and procedures. The overall situation, however, was not really changed by this in any fundamental way until recent times.

The advent of modern medicine caused the first fundamental change. It expanded the traits that could be selected for and that could be retained or enhanced. Traits whose distribution had previously been self-limiting because they limited the survival or reproductive chances of the individual who carried them—traits like haemophilia, cystic fibrosis, pelvic disproportionment, diabetes and epilepsy[49]—no longer meant severe selective disadvantage, because medicine and health care guaranteed the survival of those who had such traits. And even when they did not guarantee their survival in individual cases, they were successful in raising the survival rate of persons who carried these traits in a statistically significant sense. Previously, these genetic traits would have been lethal or would have seriously disadvantaged their carriers and the carriers' children (if any). Therefore in the long run, their distribution in the human gene pool would have been restricted in a self-limiting sense or eliminated entirely.

However, modern medicine and health care could deal with their effects on individual carriers and their offspring. At least to some degree. Consequently the genetic factors responsible for them could be bred back into the gene pool and begin to spread.[50] As a result some geneticists have begun to feel that the human gene pool is becoming more and more permeated by disadvantageous genes that in many cases, but for the grace of modern medicine itself, would be lethal.[51]

The obvious implication of these considerations is that all members of society should be responsible in their reproductive acts. If they carry deleterious genes, then they should refrain from having children. We discussed the pros and cons of this in the previous chapter.[52]

That solution may be satisfactory from the standpoint of society. However, it is unlikely to satisfy the desires and aspirations of the individual. As we saw in our discussion of the right to have children, there is a strong presumption in our society that people want to have biological offspring of their own. There is also a strong presumption that giving birth to one's own biological children and of having of biological offspring of one's own is a matter of fundamental right.[53] That presumptions finds strong support in the law.

If the considerations that we raised in the preceding chapter are correct, then the unfortunate individuals who carry deleterious genes will be at a disadvantage. Their negative genetic load would seem to impose on them the duty of refraining from having biological offspring of their own. That means that they would be less-than-equal. They would become the unfortunate victims of a capricious nature.

Thesis

The development of new reproductive technologies provides the possibility of changing all this. At least in principle, the direct manipulation of germ plasm would allow us to correct the genetic flaws that exist. Therefore, it would allow people who otherwise would be disadvantaged to avail themselves of the opportunities open to all other members of society. The privilege of having children would be open to them as well. The techniques have already been applied in animal models, so we know it can be done.[54] If society did not follow this path and develop these technologies; and having developed them, if society did not give everyone equitable access to them, it will perpetuate discrimination on the basis of genetic inheritance— not perhaps by law, as it would if it enacted eugenic statutes, but by moral suasion. The effect, however, would be the same.

However, this is not all. The drive to reproduce is one of the most fundamental of all biological drives. It is unrealistic to expect that all who know that they are carriers of deleterious genes will let their reason rule their gonads. Not everyone who should be morally persuaded not to have children because of carrier status in fact will refrain from having them. Therefore, if this technology is not developed, the result will be that children will be continue to be born who suffer from serious genetically caused diseases and conditions. These children have a right to health care. Equality and justice demand they receive it. However, the cost of providing that health care has to be defrayed from the same resource pool that pays for social health care in general. This in turn means that the resources available for providing health care for society in general are diminished in an unnecessary way, and because of this people suffer needlessly. Therefore, unless society develops and applies these technologies, it will carry the blame.

There is also the perspective of the children who will receive the defective genes. They will suffer the effects of these genes, and therefore will be suffering a preventable harm.[55] Gene therapy could prevent such suffering:

> From the viewpoint of the integrity of the person, gene therapy in the early embryonal stage (with unavoidable effects on the germinal line) is no more problematical that treatment shortly before birth or on children after birth at an age when they are incapable of giving consent.[56]

Furthermore, those who are in a position to prevent that suffering would share the blame for the suffering of the future offspring if they did not act in a positive fashion. They would be part of the causal chain that leads up to that suffering. Through inaction, they would have let these children come to harm.[57] These children would therefore be in a position similar to that of the fetuses whose genetic abnormalities have been detected by genetic screening but where neither the parents nor any other appropriate decision-maker took appropriate action.

Of course, abortion is always an option, as are abstinence and contraception. Therefore, it could be argued that the truly responsible decision-maker would seek to prevent such suffering by taking the appropriate steps before the suffering becomes real. However, the fact is that this solution has its own problems. The reproductive drive is strong. Accidents do occur. Furthermore, the values of the individual may not allow for abortion or contraception.[58] Finally, why not use techniques that are being developed in any case? Are animals and plants more worthy of these techniques than humanity?

Antithesis

So much for presenting the initial case in favour of the therapeutic use of genetic engineering. The case does not stand unopposed. One of the objections is already familiar from our discussion of genetic screening. It is based on the fear of discrimination. Leon Kass has argued that to interfere deliberately and actively with the human genetic code is to make a statement about the variety of human genotypes.[59] Those whose genes are singled out for attention and action are in effect characterized as being inferior. With this, however, we should be denying the equality of all humanity.

A similar suggestion is made by Murray. Once we allow such manipulation as a matter of choice, the element of choice soon disappears. A social stigma will become attached not only to being a carrier, but also to being the recipient of genes that have been identified as defective. As a result, the genetically uncorrected and unimproved person will become the second class citizens of tomorrow.[60]

Another objection takes its cue from the fact that developments in germinal line therapy will involve the "destructive use of human embryos."[61] Even though the techniques themselves can be developed on animal models, they must ultimately be tested on human embryos. That means that we would have two classes of human fetuses: those whose life and development was governed by the principle of respect for human life, and those whose development and life are not seen from that perspective but may be treated like experimental animal material.

This would not only be utilitarian in the worst sense of the term, it would also be in contravention of the revised Declaration of Helsinki/Tokyo. Its relevant section reads as follows:

> In experiments on human beings, the interests of science and society should never take precedence over considerations that concern the well-being of the experimental subject.[62]

In another vein, some commentators have argued that it is dangerous even to consider genetic improvement or innovation at the present time.[63] We know far too little about the cross-linkages and polymorphisms of the various genetic traits.[64] We have already misidentified some genetic abnormalities as undesirable when in fact they were quite neutral. The experience with the XYY controversy is a very good example.[65]

Alternatively we might alter what we thought was a defective gene and replace it with what we thought was a beneficial one. However, in the process we might lose an advantage that the original gene conferred. Future generations would then be worse off because of our precipitous action.[66] Or the altered gene might interact with the others in a way that had new and negative consequences of its own. As the Medical Research Council of Canada put it:

> However, if a normal gene is expressed inappropriately as a result of this insertion, the outcome for the patient is unknown and the possibility of a disease such as cancer is a concern.[67]

The old adage, *primum non nocere*, which has served health care for so long, should always be considered guiding. Unless we can be sure that the cure is not going to be worse than the disease, we should leave matters well enough alone.

Moreover, the success of a species depends not only on its adaptation to its present environment but also on its having sufficient genetic variety to include some individuals who could survive in any future environment. Therefore, if cloning were extended to the point of markedly homogenizing the population, it could create an evolutionary danger that might threaten the very survival of the species.[68]

We also cannot discount the possibility of a slippery slope.[69] From small beginnings, large consequences grow. To approach the human genetic code as something to be fixed, to be repaired and manipulated bespeaks a view of humanity that sees human beings like pieces of machinery: to be designed, redesigned and moulded. If that perspective becomes accepted, then the human person in general, and not merely the genetically unimproved or non-regularized individual, will lose all dignity as an autonomous being. With the abandonment of the inviolability of the genetic code in some cases, the door will be opened to further changes. There will be the very real danger that what began as a matter of therapy might slowly devolve in to a diabolical practice that will outstrip even the most fecund imagination.[70]

Furthermore, as C.S. Lewis has pointed out, there is unimaginable power in the application of genetic engineering:

> If any one age really attains, by eugenic means and scientific education, the power to make its descendants what it pleases, all men who live after it are patients of that power. They are weaker, not stronger ... Mans' conquest of Nature, if the dreams of the scientific planners are realized, means the rule of a few hundreds of men over billions upon billions of men.[71]

That power of course exist in all sorts of contexts: in medicine, technology and so on. However, nowhere is it as profound; and nowhere is it as dependent on the private conception of the good held by a few people.[72]

Furthermore, the underlying logic of genetic engineering is a two-edged sword. If it were applied consistently, we would also have to heed it when it comes to saving and/or sustaining individuals who carry deleterious and potentially deadly genetic loads. The laws of genetic distribution entail that if we employ the resources of modern medicine, pharmacology and bio-technology to assist such people to survive and reproduce, then their genes will spread in an almost geometrically progressive fashion throughout the population. That means that the incidence of homogenous expressions of these genes will increase proportionally. That would also be an evolutionary danger. A consistent application of the logic of this argument would therefore require that we should not save or sustain the lives of these people.

Closely associated with this is the danger that genetic engineering will be used to solve what are social problems. Discrimination on the basis of skin colour is one example. Such discrimination is ethically unacceptable, and there are laws explicitly aimed at preventing it. Genetic engineering might foster the tendency to remove discrimination by altering the gene for skin colour instead of solving the problem by attacking its root. The example might strike us as extreme, and the solution as unlikely. However, the fact remains that when a technique becomes easy to use, those who suffer will be tempted to use it. There is the historical precedent of skin-whitening creams that were sold in the 1920s and 30s.

This concern can be generalized. If there is a technique of dealing with the overt manifestations of a problem and that technique is cost-effective and easy to use, then there is a tendency to adopt that technique and to see it as solving the problem without ever asking whether it is ethically appropriate. In the case of discrimination on the basis of colour, the problem is an ethically indefensible attitude towards people as people. In the case of workers exposed to dangerous chemicals, radiation or a generally hostile working environment genetic engineering offers the possibility of altering the genetic make-up of people so that they will not be so susceptible to the negative effects of this working environment. But in doing this, genetic engineering solution would address the effect, not the cause. It would encourage an instrumentalistic view of people, and it would ignore the fundamental ethical issues that are here at stake.[73]

The introduction of genetic engineering as a socially acceptable tool would also have the power to alter the very rationale of social problem-solving from cause-oriented to effect-directed. However, an effect-directed approach to problem-solving is essentially an approach that seeks to solve problems by compensating, not by addressing their root. By that very token it tends to see situations in isolation, independently of the context in which they are embedded. Therefore, it runs the danger of compensating in one area—of "solving" the initial problem—by introducing new variables that do indeed address the initial issue, but which present new problems in another area that have to be addressed in turn. Therefore, this whole approach may well lead to a magnification of the problematic—to a heterodyning, rather than a solving of issues.

Analysis

Like most topics in biomedical ethics, genetic engineering tends to polarize opinions to a remarkable degree. What we have just sketched is but a small sampling of the diversity of positions that exists about genetic engineering as a means of therapy.

The diversity grows even more pronounced when it comes to genetic engineering for non-therapeutic purposes: for instance, to create chimera or human-animal crosses, to imbue humans with special properties or characteristics, and so on. It may be due in part to the fact that biomedical issues generally have that effect, in part to certain ingrained and culturally established beliefs and perspectives of a religious nature.[74]

Furthermore, the manipulation of genes touches the reproductive stability of the species itself. That provokes natural and justified caution: not only in terms of the survival of the species itself, but also in terms of what the underlying attitude which allows for such manipulation says about our view of humanity itself.

However, whatever the reasons for this diversity and opposition, it is easy to lose sight of what is really ethically relevant. Therefore, it may be useful to keep in mind some of the considerations that follow.

Somatic versus Germ Line Therapy

First, we have to distinguish between germ line therapy and somatic therapy.[75] Germ line therapy is the manipulation of human genetic material in fertilized ova or zygotes in the expectation that the genetic changes that are produced will be passed on to all the cells of the developing embryo, including the germ cells. These changes would then be passed on to future generations.[76]

Somatic cell genetic manipulation, as its name says, alters the genetic structure only in somatic cells of a specific population that can be isolated and treated. An example here would be gene therapy aimed at sickle cell anemia. Bone marrow cells could be removed from the affected person, their genetic structure altered and returned to the original person. The marrow cells would continue to reproduce and would produce healthy red blood cells.[77] Since these are not involved in reproduction, any changes that are made here would not be passed on to future generations. In the words of the President's Commission:

> Gene therapy carried out on somatic cells, such as bone marrow cells, would resemble standard medical therapies in that they all involve changes limited to the cells of the person being treated. They differ, however, in that gene therapy involves an inherent and probably permanent change in the body rather than requiring repeated applications of an outside force or substance. An analogy is organ transplantation, which also involves the incorporation into an individual of cells containing DNA of: "foreign" origin.[78]

We can therefore see that if there are objections to germ cell therapy and manipulation, these objections do not automatically apply to somatic cell manipulation; and vice versa. Their relevance would have to be established independently and on other grounds. This means that most of the concerns that have been expressed about the future effects of genetic engineering really have only limited validity. They apply only to germ cell genetic manipulation. Only that sort of intervention has any effect on future generations.[79]

General Considerations

If we now turn to the pros and cons of the discussion itself, there are several points that we should try to keep in mind. The first is procedural. As we pointed out in the discussion of genetic screening, it is irrational (and possibly unethical) to ignore data that are relevant to a particular decision-making process. That applies here as well. To ignore the data on genetic engineering and not even consider their application to the human context is to decide *a priori* that genetic engineering must be bad. To do so is neither rational nor ethical.

Somatic therapy illustrates this well. The people who suffer from a genetically caused defect may wish to try the treatment on an experimental basis. If the strictures that apply to experimentation in general are met here, there is no reason why these people should not be offered the choice. Especially since it may be the only chance of treatment there is. To deny them that choice is to violate the principle of autonomy. It would also violate the principle of equality, for in all other contexts we do allow choice.

Nor does the use of genetic engineering necessarily mean that people are being treated like objects. That is to say, it is sometimes objected that the development and use of genetic engineering techniques will produce two classes of embryos: those that will be considered as worthy of protection, and those that will be treated like mere organic tissue. This objection derives its force from an extreme position on the nature of the human person. It identifies being a human being with being a person. As we suggested in our previous discussion,[80] a fetus does not start as a person. It becomes a person at some stage in its development. Therefore, it is true that the development and application of gene therapy involves the destruction of human fetuses. It is also true that this involves treating these fetuses like pieces of organic matter, and therefore like objects. But this does not mean that it involves treating human persons as pieces of organic matter. Being a human being and being a person are just not the same.

We have to distinguish clearly between the body and the person. The reason for the development of the therapy is not because we have a purely objective and instrumentalistic view of the person. It is because we see the body as something to be used by the person, not as identical with the person itself. In germ line therapy it is the body that is the target of alteration, not the person. It is precisely because we respect the offsprings as persons that we want to change their body and their bodily functions so as to prevent suffering. Germ line therapy, which is intended to change inherited physiological flaws, simply happens to be a most effective means of doing that. Of course there are other ways. We have explored some of them in the preceding chapter. However, most of these entail that some people will not be able to have biological offspring of their own. Germ line therapy has the potential for solving the problem without limiting anyone's *prima facie* right to have children.

It is possible that germ line therapy might be used for the sorts of purposes indicated by Murray and others. If that did happen, then of course its use would be unethical. It would involve the instrumentalistic perspective of humanity that was suggested. However, this use is not something that is inherent in the techniques themselves; nor do we have an instrumentalistic perspective of humanity when we use the techniques to help and to cure.

We use gene therapy precisely because we respect the individuals who suffer here and now as persons and we want to change the genetic cause of their suffering. It is not that we think the people who suffer from genetically caused diseases are inferior. We think they are worthy of help. We would use other means if we could. Unfortunately, so far most other means have proven ineffective. Huntington's chorea and cystic fibrosis are but two of a series of examples where there appear to be no other effective ways of dealing with the diseases and conditions that exist. And in many cases where there are other ways or providing relief, these usually address the symptoms, not the underlying cause itself. The treatment for PKU here comes to mind. In these cases treatment will have to be on a continuing basis. That can be very expensive in the long run, which has ethical implications in terms of allocation of resources. It also subjects the individuals themselves to an inefficient and burdensome method of treatment when a better one is available. It thereby violates their dignity and the principle of best action.

Nor is there anything inherently undignified about being the subject of genetic engineering. The words of the President's Commission here come to mind:

> An analogy is organ transplantation, which also involves the incorporation into an individual of cells containing DNA of "foreign" origin.[81]

The same objection of indignity to the person was originally advanced against transplantation. We have come to see that it was, and is, unjustified. It would be undignified if the dignity of the individual lay in the fact of suffering. That, however, would be to put the cart before the horse. While there may be dignity in the way in which people respond to the suffering that they experience, the suffering itself holds no dignity. Such suffering is a curse. That is why we try to alleviate it. Furthermore, the people who are relieved of their suffering have no less dignity as persons because they no longer need to suffer. If that were true, then all medical intervention and all attempt to alleviate the suffering of humanity would lessen humanity's dignity.

As to the objection that the introduction of these techniques will soon turn something that is a matter of choice into a matter of obligation, here we have to ask ourselves whether there are ever any reason to suppose that the use of these techniques should be a matter of obligation. If we are going to be intellectually honest about it, we cannot simply assume that the answer has to be a No. What we said in the preceding chapters about allocation of resources may be relevant in the case of somatic therapy. Do we have a right to persist in having a condition that requires expensive medical treatment if a cheaper, or more effective method of treatment is available? As to germ line therapy, we might want to hark back to the discussion of genetic and prenatal screening. It is just possible that some of the considerations that deal with preventing harm, and that focus on the notion of an injury becoming complete are relevant here.

There is no question that techniques of genetic engineering, whether directed at germ lines or merely somatic, are liable to abuse. But this is not something unique to genetic engineering. We can say it about all sorts of scientific developments. Medical, pharmacological and biological techniques, for example, can all be misused. What is more, they can be misused in ways that have equally as horrendous consequences as those described for genetic engineering. And when we consider these other areas in retrospect, we could construct all sorts of tutioristic slippery slope arguments against their introduction and use. Something as harmless as antibiotics would even fall into this category. For instance, it could have been argued that antibiotics might be used only selectively, for those who are deemed politically acceptable. Or, it could have been argued that their use would initiate a lowering of our sensibilities towards suffering because we could deal with it so easily. It could even have been argued that their use would lead to a stigmatization of those who required them because they obviously lacked the inherent genetic mechanisms of resistance to infection. These arguments may strike us as fanciful today. However, they bear a close resemblance to some of the arguments that have been raised against genetic engineering.

This is not to dismiss the slippery slope arguments out of hand. They have a valid point to make. However, their point is not logical but heuristic. They sound a warning. Techniques of genetic engineering must be used with care because they carry the potential for disaster. But that holds true of many biological, medical, pharmacological and engineering techniques. In fact, to a greater or lesser degree it holds true of just about everything that humanity has ever developed. The invention of something as simple as the wheel is a case in point. The fact that it has been misused does not mean it should not have been developed and used under appropriate circumstances.

We cannot dismiss out of hand the danger of misidentifying a particular genetic component as deleterious or of developing something that will have serious negative consequences. Such errors have occurred, as for instance in the case of the XYY problem; and they may occur again. But that does not mean that we should refrain from using these techniques. It means that we should try to be extremely careful. It is reliably reported that approximately one in five medications administered by health care professionals in the hospital context are in error. Some of these errors result in severe morbidity and even mortality.[82] It is also estimated that approximately 40 percent of all throat ailment diagnoses are in error—and of course that subsequent treatment modalities are mistaken.[83] However, this does not mean that therefore medications should not be given out, diagnoses made, or treatments initiated. It simply means that we have to take the appropriate steps to reduce the possibility of error.

The same reasoning applies in this case. The fact that mistakes may be made does not militate against the use of bioengineering techniques. It argues for extreme care in their employment. Because here as there, we if do not attempt to employ them, the arsenal of health care will be impoverished, and the health of humanity will suffer needlessly.

The claim that a stigma might come to be attached to those who have been "improved" may be true. We have no way of knowing. Stranger things have happened. However, it is important to remember that a stigma can be attached to all sorts of things. It can be attached to something as reasonable as going to night-school to finish one's education or to having cosmetic surgery to improve a psychologically debilitating nasal profile. The problem lies not in these actions but in the attitude towards them and in the social context that allows them to be stigmatized. And the solution is not to get rid of the stigma by leaving those who might be stigmatized in a disadvantaged position and depriving them of the possibility of relief from what otherwise would be a burdensome lot. The solution is to deal with the root of the problem: to address the social process of stigmatization itself. Stigmatization is a form of discrimination. In it lies the problem; not in the fact that someone is freed from the probability of a lower quality of life.

In general, we would agree with the Medical Research Council of Canada's cautions in accepting somatic gene therapy:

> Any attempt to treat an inherited disease by somatic cell gene transfer should be regarded as a research protocol, and subject to procedures and considerations [outlined by the Council and by] the MRC's *Guidelines on Research Involving Human Subjects* (1987).[84]

However, we would also agree with the President's Commission that somatic gene therapy should be seen as what it really is: a species of medicine. We would extend this to germ line therapy as well. It should be seen as a species of preventive medicine. The following thought-experiment might loosen the hold that preconceived notions may have on us in this regard. Let us suppose that we had an ointment that would cure a particular congenital condition—say, hemophilia. Let us suppose further that use of the ointment would guarantee that hemophilia would no longer be passed on to any offspring. We might have initial qualms about using the ointment. In the end, however, our misgivings would probably give way to our appreciation of its salubrious effects. The fact that from a longitudinal perspective these effects would be severe, irreversible and alter the nature of the offsprings would probably give us pause. But it would probably not stop us from using it.

Of course, this analogy breaks down. Analogies always do. That is why they are analogies. However, it does point to an important fact. A great deal of the objection to genetic engineering appears to be not so much against its effects as against the means by which its effects are brought about. In other words, a great deal of the objection seems to be directed not against what is done, but against how it is done. But this has to be examined in its own right. Unless how it is done can be shown to be unethical in itself, or unless there is something ineluctably unethical in the conditions of its use, it would be premature to say that bioengineering technology has to be rejected for ethical reasons.

We could go further. We could argue that we have to distinguish between technologies that are designed with the express purpose of dehumanizing people or of hurting them and whose use is inherently destructive, and technologies that may be misused. The various genetic engineering techniques, both extant as well as in the offing, do not fall into the first category. They are ethically inherently neutral. Unlike the rack, the thumbscrew or the electric chair, they are not developments whose purpose is inherently to inflict harm or to degrade. They are biochemically sophisticated tools of preventive medicine: contemporary equivalents of vaccination.

The comparison to vaccination is of course only an analogy; and being an analogy, it breaks down. However, it is sufficiently close to make a useful point. The purpose and function of these techniques is to assist in the delivery of health care. They should therefore be viewed from that perspective and according to the same rules that we use in all other cases of health care technology—without any pre-conceived bias. Perhaps they are too dangerous to use at the present time, because we cannot evaluate them sufficiently. That would be a valid objection. Perhaps their development would require too many resources. That would be another. It may even be that their development and use would contravene fundamental ethical principles. That would be the most important reason of all. But none of this can be assumed. It has to be shown.

There remains the complex of questions that centre around decisions-making. What conditions should be targeted for treatment, and who should decide? We can offer no ready answer. All we can do is suggest that this problematic is not unique to bioengineering, but something that faces the development and application of all new health care technologies. Our society has begun to develop some ways of dealing with it. It has begun to institutionalize the notion of Ethics Review Boards for all experimental procedures involving human subjects; it has begun to establish a national mechanism for developing ethical guidelines for experimental and innovative procedures,[85] and so on. All levels of government concerned with the delivery of health care have struck committees; commissions have been set up; and the various professions have started to keep a watchful eye on these developments from their own perspective. All this suggest that in the end it is probably society itself that will make the relevant decisions. However, to make decisions properly, society needs information. Perhaps it is here that we should begin to concentrate our efforts as a society: to make sure that all the relevant information reaches the public. That is probably the best way to ensure that none of the decisions that will undoubtedly be made, will be made without input from those who are intimately and ultimately affected.

Cloning

We will now take a brief look at cloning. Cloning is the production of genetically identical individuals. It can occur naturally—for example with identical twins, triplets, etc.—or artificially, through the use of bioengineering techniques. Is cloning unethical?

We have already given part of an answer to the question. If the objection to cloning is based on the fact that an artificial means of reproduction is used, then the objection fails. The fact that something is artificial does not stamp it as unethical. If the objection is based on the expectation of psychological damage that will be suffered by the children who will be genetically identical, then the objection has to be based on a factual premise. Therefore we need some data that support this factual claim. There are no such data.

The objection may based on the perception that a deliberate duplication of genetic heritage offends the dignity of the individual.[86] Each person is a unique individual, and to deprive someone of that uniqueness is to deprive that person of his or her identity.

If that is the basis of the objection, then it is not as convincing as it may sound at first. The uniqueness of persons as persons is not determined by their genetic heritage. That would be true if persons were the same as their bodies. In that case, however, any material change in the body would alter the identity of the person.[87]

The uniqueness of persons resides in their persona: that is to say, in their mental identity. The body, and therefore the genetic heritage, may provide the material basis for developing such an identity. However, the one cannot be reduced to the other without doing violence to the notion of personhood itself.[88]

Furthermore, identical twins share the same genetic heritage. There is nothing undignified about being an identical twin; nor is their dignity diminished by being natural clones of each other. Of course it could be argued that it is really the deliberateness of the duplication that constitutes the indignity. However, that would follow only if the dignity of the individual depended on material uniqueness and if deliberateness itself were ethically objectionable. As we suggested, this is not the case. If existence as determined by a genetic code is ethically unobjectionable, then so is there being two (or more) people having the same code. Duplication is not identical with ethical risk. Nor is doing something deliberately, that otherwise occurs by chance, necessarily the doing of something unethical. It all depends on what is done; and herewith we are back to the issue of duplication—of there being several individuals who are identical.

There is the pragmatic concern that cloning may lead to an impoverishment of the genetic diversity of the human race and therefore threaten its existence. However, this concern would have force only if in fact cloning was practised on such a large scale that humanity's genetic diversity was threatened. That need not be the case. Furthermore, the consideration derives whatever ethical force it has from the assumption that there would be something unethical about the disappearance of the human race. That assumption would have to be argued on independent grounds.

The last consideration we want to mention takes us back to something we already touched on in other contexts: the attitude that cloning would foster. It is argued that it would promote an instrumentalistic view of humanity, and that it would encourage the perception that humanity has not only the ability but also the right to control its destiny.

There are several ways of responding to this. However, no matter how we respond, we should always keep in mind a very simply but very important fact. Everything humanity does has an impact on the direction of its destiny; whether that be developing new antibiotics, instituting sanitation and housing programs for the poor or developing a new branch of mathematics. So the real issue is not the fact of control: it is its deliberateness and the perspective that underlies it. That perspective need not be instrumentalistic. However, chances are that in the case of cloning it is. It is that fact that would be worrisome, not the fact of control itself.

Surrogate Motherhood

Surrogate motherhood is currently one of the most controversial topics in reproductive ethics.[89] There are several ways in which the notion can be understood. The Law Reform Commission of Ontario gives the following list:[90]

1. a woman is artificially inseminated *in vivo* by sperm of a donor and, upon birth, custody of the child is surrendered to the sperm donor;
2. a woman's extracted ovum is fertilized *in vitro*, the embryo is transplanted into the uterus of another woman who is able to bear a child and, upon birth, the child is surrendered to the ovum donor;
3. a woman is fertilized *in vivo*, the embryo is flushed from her by means of lavage and transplanted into the uterus of another woman who is able to bear a child and, upon birth, the child is surrendered to the ovum donor; and
4. a woman's ovum is fertilized *in vitro*, or *in vivo* followed by recovery through lavage, and transplanted into the uterus of a second woman and, upon birth, the child is surrendered to a third person, such as the sperm donor and his wife.

The Law Reform Commission continues:

> A surrogate motherhood arrangement involves an agreement between the woman who is to bear the child and the persons who are to receive it to raise as their own. While a variety of terms may be agreed upon by the parties, the heart of any arrangement is a promise on the part of the surrogate mother to undergo the medical procedure necessary to achieve a pregnancy and to surrender custody of the child irrevocably upon birth, and a reciprocal promise on part of the other party or parties to accept the child.[91]

Almost all jurisdictions in the world have begun to examine the issue.[92] Canada has recently struck a Royal Commission on New Reproductive Technologies, and surrogate motherhood is on its agenda. Ontario and British Columbia have considered it already, as have several professional organizations. The only thing that we can say about the positions that have been published is that they disagree. For instance, Ontario has recommended acceptance and legal recognition of surrogate motherhood arrangements subject to certain conditions; the Warnock Commission in Great Britain has recommended rejection; the American College of Obstetricians and Gynecologists has expressed "significant reservations about this approach to parenthood," but left its members free to decide whether to participate in such arrangements.[93] The American Medical Association has rejected it,[94] but the Canadian Medical Association has followed the lead of the Society of Obstetricians and Gynaecologists of Canada and allows it, at least in a research context and under strictly monitored guidelines.[95]

The fact that opinion is thus divided is not surprising.[96] Surrogate motherhood presents many social, legal and ethical questions. Implicated are issues of legitimacy of the child,[97] economic coercion of the surrogate,[98] the relationship between genetic parents and their offspring,[99] autonomy of women, children as objects and so on. Given the differences in professional, legal and cultural perspective from which the issue has been approached, it would be surprising if unanimity did exist. Or even general agreement.

We cannot mention, let alone deal with, all of the issues that are raised by the topic. The reason we mention surrogate motherhood at all is that it brings together several fundamental questions that are central to having children. One is of course the question of the right to have children. Does that right extend to all people or only to people who live in certain kinds of socially approved relationships? Equality and justice are implicated here. Then there is the question of genesis. Does the way in which, and the reason for which, a child is engendered and brought into the world constitute an ethical affront to the child? All techniques of reproductive technology, whether artificial or natural, have to address this troublesome question. There is also the question of autonomy: All other things being equal, does a woman have the right to do with her body as she pleases? Equality and autonomy once more into the forefront.[100]

The last question we want to mention takes us back to the child. What should the primary consideration in childbearing be: The welfare of the child, the expectations of society or the feelings of the parents? The thing we always have to remember is that progenitors of the child have a choice in the matter, limited as such a choice may be. The child that results from that choice has none. Yet, nonetheless, it is a person.

The questions that we have just mentioned will not determine how the issue of surrogate motherhood is to be resolved. They will have to be combined with considerations that we raised in the preceding chapters: informed consent and proxy decision-making, the right to have children, equality and autonomy and respect for persons, experimentation, allocation of resources, and so on. However, unless and until the questions we have just raised are answered in a satisfactory fashion, the issue of surrogate motherhood will remain a Gordian knot.

Conclusion

Like everything else in this book, our discussion of reproductive ethics has been from a deontological perspective. With that as a given, we would like to conclude with a few general remarks about the ethics of reproductive technology as a whole.

First, it strikes us that here as anywhere else, the primary and indeed ultimate concern must be for the individual persons who are involved. Their status as persons, their rights and obligations, the way they are embedded in the social context—all these have to be taken into account. These matters cannot be dealt with on the basis of emotions, however deeply they may be felt.[101] Nor can they be resolved on the basis of private beliefs, however sincerely these may be held. Appeals to the law or to tradition are relevant only insofar as the law or tradition define the problem. They do not provide a solution. If the solution is to be ethical, it has to be justifiable in ethical terms. And it cannot be held against the solution that it conflicts with some preconceived stance or intuition.

Second, the fact that techniques of new reproductive technology are artificial, non-natural or whatever, does not itself mean that they are therefore ethically unacceptable. If that were true, then all achievements of civilization would be ethically objectionable as well. Of course that does not mean they aren't. For all we know, they might well be. But that they are must be shown on independent grounds.

Third, if there is a way of ameliorating a problem that is not itself unethical and does not cause problems on its own, then those who have the problem have a *prima facie* right to see whether they can adopt that way. Our discussion of the ethics of causality and responsibility focused on that fact. We see no reason why reproductive ethics should be different. Ethics is not an *ad hoc* affair.

This is important in the context of reproductive technology. The current world situation in general and limitations of resources within our society in particular result in the delivery of less-than-optimal care for those who are already on the scene. It could therefore be argued that the resources that are being spent to develop ways of producing more children would be used ethically more appropriately by meeting the needs of those who currently go without adequate health care, who suffer from inadequate nutrition, education and housing, and so on. Perhaps this is true; perhaps not. In any case, the subject warrants closer scrutiny.

ENDNOTES

[1] British Columbia, Royal Commission on Family and Children's Law, *Ninth Report of the Royal Commission on Family and Children's Law: Artificial Insemination* (Victoria, 1975); Alberta Institute of Law Research and Reform, *Status of Children* (Report No. 20, 1976); Ontario Law Reform Commission, *Report on Human Artificial Reproduction and Related Matters* (Toronto: Ministry of the Attorney General, 1985); Gouvernement du Quebec, Conseil du Statut de la Femme, *General Opinion of the Conseil du Statut de la Femme in*

Regard to New Reproductive Technologies (Quebec City, 1989); Law Reform Commission of Saskatchewan, *Tentative Proposals for a Human Artificial Insemination Act* (1981).

[2] The British Columbia Bar Association, *Report of the Special Task Force Committee on Reproductive Technology of the British Columbia Branch*, The Canadian Bar Association (Vancouver, June, 1989); the Canadian Medical Association, the Society of Obstetricians and Gynaecologists of Canada (1990).

[3] The mandate of the Commission is to consider all aspects of new reproductive technologies, together with problems of infertility, surrogate motherhood and the like. It is to present its report in the Fall of 1992.

[4] See British Columbia Royal Commission on Family and Children's Law, *Ninth Report of the Royal Commission on Family and Children's Law: Artificial Insemination* (Victoria: 1975); Ontario Law Reform Commission, Report on Human Artificial Reproduction and Related Matters (Toronto: Ministry of the Attorney General, 1985); Health and Welfare Canada, *Report of the Advisory Committee on the Storage and Utilization of Human Sperm* (Ottawa: HWC, 1981); Law Reform Commission of Saskatchewan, *Tentative Proposals for a Human Artificial Insemination Act* (1981); South Australia, *Report of the Working Party on In Vitro Fertilization and Artificial Insemination by Donor* (1984); Australia, Victoria Committee to Consider Social, Ethical and Legal Issues Arising from In Vitro Fertilization, *Report on the Disposition of Embryos Produced by In Vitro Fertilization*; Australia, Queensland, *Report of the Special Committee Appointed by the Queensland Government to Enquire into the Laws Relating to Artificial Insemination, In Vitro Fertilization and Other Related Matters* (1984); U.K., Department of Health and Social Security, *Report of the Committee of Inquiry into Human Fertilization and Embryology* (Cmnd. 9314, 1984).

[5] Heather Bryant, *The Infertility Dilemma: Reproductive Technologies and Prevention*, (Calgary: Canadian Advisory Council on the Status of Women, February, 1990) 4.

[6] See *Ethical Considerations*, (ref. note 7 below) Combined Report Section II.

[7] See *Ethical Considerations of the New Reproductive Technologies*, Report of the Ethics Committee of the American Fertility Society, *Fertility and Sterility* 46: 3 (Sept., 1986) Suppl. 1.at v.

[8] Sometimes and not always, because there are occasions when the sperm of the donor is directly inserted into the vagina of the women, or when the sperm of the husband is collected, concentrated or treated, and then inserted directly into the woman's vagina.

[9] See below, at 374.

[10] Geoffrey Chamberlain, "An Artificial Placenta," *American Journal of Obstetrics and Gynecology*, 100: 24 (March 1, 1968). Y. Kuwabara, "Development of Extrauterine Fetal Incubator," *Asian Medical Journal* 32(8), 1989, 419–425. Time of life in artificial womb (fetal incubator) since 1960 has gone up from 19 hrs (Callaghan, *Canadian Journal of Surgery* 8: 2496, 1982) to 55 hours (Zapol, *Science* 166: 617, 1969). Kuwabara initially reported an improvement to 165 hours in 1987, using an extracorporeal membrane oxygenator *(Artificial Organs* 11: 224–227, 1987). In 1989, with this report, Kuwabara indicates an extension for fetal sheep to 236 hrs. (p. 420) The survival rate was 5 out of 9 in their system I. The cause of death was heart failure. The projected use is for premature infants and for fetal therapy for pulmonary hypoplasia due to hydropsis fetalis or diaphragm hernia due to heart deformities.

[11] See also *Ethical Considerations of the New Reproductive Technologies,* A Report of the Combined Ethics Committee of the Canadian Fertility and Andrology Society and the Society of Obstetricians and Gynecologists of Canada (1990).

[12] See *Ethical Considerations*, ref. note 11, 22.

[13] See *Ethical Considerations*, ref. note 11, for a brief discussion. See also M.A. Field, *Surrogate Motherhood* (Cambridge and London: Harvard Univ. Press, 1988) Chapter 3.

[14] See B.M. Ashley and K.D. O'Rourke, *Health Care Ethics: A Theological Analysis* (St. Louis: Catholic Hospital Assoc., 1982).

[15] See Ontario Law Reform Commission Report, ref. note 4, for a rejection of this.

[16] *Ethical Considerations*, ref. note 11, 27. See also Field, ref. note 13 above.

[17] See below, at 356, ref. note 23.

[18] See Field, ref. note 13.

[19] Ashley and O'Rourke, ref. note 14, 322. Most other religions have avoided public statements. See also Theresa Mady, "Surrogate Mothers: The Legal Issues," *American Journal of Law and Medicine*, 9: 1 (Spring 1983), 323f. See also Sacred Congregation, for the Doctrine of Faith, "Instructions," Rome: Vatican, 1987.

[20] For a different view, see T.H. Milby, "The New Biology and the Question of Personhood: Implications for Abortion," *American Journal of Law and Medicine* 9: 1 (Spring 1983), 31–41.

[21] Paul Lauritzen, "What Price Parenthood?" *Hastings Center Report* 20: 2 (March/April 1990) 38–46, 41.

[22] See Mady, ref. note 19, for some discussion of this and related issues.

[23] See Margaret Atwood, *The Handmaiden's Tale* (Toronto: McClelland and Stewart, 1985.) Atwood's story follows a line familiar to science fiction readers for decades.

[24] See Society of Obstetricians and Gynaecologists of Canada, "Statements on In Vitro Fertilization and Embryo Transfer," Bulletin of the SOGC 6: 3 (May/June 1984); American Fertility Society, "Ethical Statement on In Vitro Fertilization," *Fertility and Sterility* 41: 12 (1984).

[25] The use of spare ova and spare embryos is considered by the Warnock Commission in its report to parliament.

[26] See British Columbia Royal Commission, and Ontario Law Reform Commission Report, ref. note 4.

[27] See the Reports of the British Columbia Bar Association, Ontario Law Reform Commission, Society for Andrology and Society of Obstetricians and Gynecologists of Canada, ref. note 2.

[28] The Swedish model allows for children to request knowledge of the identity of their genetic fathers. While this initially resulted in a drop in donation, the trend seems to be reversing again.

[29] See the Ontario Law Reform Commission, ref. note 1. See also E.-H W. Kluge and C. Luckock, *New Reproductive Technologies: A Preliminary Perspective of the Canadian Medical Association*, (Ottawa: CMA, 1991).

[30] Compare Paul Ramsey, *The Ethics of Fetal Research* (New Haven: Yale, 1975) for a dated but classic exposition of some of the issues; J.L. Lenow, "The Fetus as Patient: Emerging Rights as a Person?", *American Journal of Law and Medicine*, 9: 1 (Spring 1983), at 1–29 for a more legal perspective. See also the various reports by the Medical Research Council of Canada and the National Committee for Bioethics in Human Research in the bibliography, below.

[31] For a discussion of some problems from the legal perspective, see David Westfall, "Beyond Abortion: The Potential Reach of a Human Life Amendment," *AJLM*, 8: 2 (Summer 1982), 97–135. The reason for cryo-preservation is to allow testing of donors for diseases like AIDS at an interval of several months.

[32] See American Fertility Society, suppl.1; SOGC, ref. note 24.

[33] Compare *Report on Human Artificial Reproduction*, vol. 2, at 218–272, for an extended and on the whole positive discussion.

[34] See John Caldwell and Pat Caldwell, "High Fertility in Sub-Saharan Africa," *Scientific American* (May, 1990) 118–125.

[35] See *Ethical Considerations*, ref. note 11, 22 and elsewhere.

[36] See Law Reform Commission of Canada, Working Paper 46, ref. note 11, 41 and elsewhere. See also p. 248ff. above.

[37] Unless the increased margin of risk is inherent in the procedure which is here assumed not to be the case. That matter, however, must be decided upon individual inspection.

[38] See the Address of the Bishop of York to the House of Lords (HL, 7 December, 1989). See also the Victoria Report, ref. note 4, at various points.

[39] Great Britain, Dept. of Health Services, *Report of the Committee of Inquiry into Human Sterilization and Embryology*, ed. M. Warnock (London: H.M. Stationery Offices, 1984).

[40] Medical Research Council of Canada, *Research on Gene Therapy in Humans: Background and Guidelines* (Ottawa: MRC, 1990).

[41] Law Reform Commission of Canada, Working Paper 61, *Biomedical Experimentation Involving Human Subjects* (Ottawa: Ministry of Supply and Services, 1989) at 3: iv.

[42] See note 4 above. Germany has one of the most restrictive set of regulations in the world at the present time. It grew out of the *Report of the Commission of Enquiry of the German Bundestag, Prospects and Risks of Genetic Engineering*, Parts I and II (Deutscher Bundestag, 10. Wahlperiode: Bonn 1987; the so-called *Inquiry Commission*). Other countries, like the U.S., have a mixture of voluntary controls and federally imposed regulations.

[43] Compare Medical Research Council of Canada, *Research on Gene Therapy in Humans: Background and Guidelines* (Ottawa: MRC 1990).

[44] Compare Mitchell Golbus, "Advances in Fetal Diagnosis and Therapy," in M.W. Shaw and A.E. Doudera, eds., *Defining Human Life: Medical, Ethical and Legal Implications*, (Ann Arbor, Mich: AUPHA, 1983), 73–83.

[45] President's Commission for the Study of Ethical Problem in Medicine and Biomedical and Behavioral Research, *Splicing Life: a Report on the Social and Ethical Issues of Genetic Engineering with Human Beings* (Washington, D.C.: U.S. Govt. Printing Office, 1982) 8.

[46] Psychological characteristics, if they have a material basis, will also be implicated.

[47] See any standard text in human genetics dealing with phenotype, blood-type prevalence, the ability to metabolize bovine milk proteins, etc.

[48] All human developments in medicine, hygiene, etc. are here implicated.

[49] See Golbus, ref. note 44. See also Leon Rosenberg, "Toward an Even Newer Genetics," in Shaw and Doudera, ref. note 44; and T.M. Powledge, "Genetic Screening and Personal Freedom," in R. Munson, ed., *Intervention and Reflection*, (Belmont, Calif.: Wadsworth, 1979) 371.

[50] See H.T. Mueller, "Human Evolution by Voluntary choice of Germ Plasm," in R. Munson, ed., *Intervention and Reflection*, (Belmont, Calif.: Wadsworth, 1979) 349–358, 349 f.; see also E. Goodman and D. Goodman, "The Overselling of Genetic Anxiety," *Hastings Center Report*, 12: 5 (Oct. 1982), at 21.

[51] Mueller, as above; Goodman and Goodman, as above.

[52] See Powledge, ref. note 49.

[53] See *Re Eve* [1987], 3 D.L.R. (4th) S.C.C., [1987] 2 S.C.R. 388 (S.C.C.) which, while it talks about the "fundamental privilege," definitely gives the impression that it sees this "fundamental privilege" almost as a right.

[54] See V.G. Pursel, C.A. Pinkert, K.F. Miller, D.J. Bolt, R.G. Campbell, R.D. Palmiter, R.L. Brinster and R.E. Hammer, "Genetic Engineering of Livestock," *Science* 244 (16 June, 1989) 1281–1288. The animals successfully involved include chickens, cows, fish, mice, pigs, rabbits and sheep.

[55] For progress in human gene therapy see T. Friedmann, "Progress Towards Human Gene Therapy," *Science* 244 (16 June, 1989) 1275–1281. Friedmann concludes with the observation that gene therapy is a "conceptually new approach [which is] a response to a medical need and is achieving increasing medical, scientific, and ethical acceptance" (1280).

[56] *Report of the Commission of Enquiry of the German Bundestag, Prospects and Risks of Genetic Engineering*, Parts I and II (Deutscher Bundestag, 10. Wahlperiode: Bonn 1987), 188a.

[57] As above.

[58] J. Fletcher, *The Ethics of Genetic Control* (New York: Doubleday, 1974); L.M. Purdy, "Genetic Diseases: Can Having Children Be Immoral?" in J.J. Buckley, ed., *Genetic Now: Ethical Issues in Genetic Research* (Wash., D.C.: Univ. Press of America, 1978) for analogous reasoning.

[59] Compare Leon Kass, "Implications for Prenatal Diagnosis for the Human Right to Life," in T.A. Mappes and J.S. Zembaty, eds., *Biomedical Ethics* (New York and London: McGraw-Hill, 1978) 464–468. For a variant view, see P. Reilly, *Genetics, Law and Social Policy* (Cambridge: Harvard Univ. Press, 1977).

[60] Compare R.H. Murray, "Problems Behind the Promise," *Hastings Center Report*, (April, 1979) 10–12; Kass, ref. note 59, 466f.

[61] Report of the Commission of Inquiry of the German Bundestag, at 188bff. See also Address of the Bishop of York, ref. note 38.

⁶² Declaration of Helsinki. "Recommendation for Doctors Working in Human Biomedical Research." Revised version of the 29th General Assembly of the World Medical Association, Tokyo, 1975.

⁶³ Compare Lawrence E. Karp, "The Prenatal Diagnosis of Genetic Disease," in T.A. Mappes and J.S. Zembaty, eds., *Biomedical Ethics* (New York and London: McGraw-Hill, 1979), 358–364.

⁶⁴ For a discussion of the various issues involved, see Goodman and Goodman, ref. note 50. Compare also European Medical Research Council: *Draft Guidelines for the Application of Gene Therapy to Human Beings*, (Strasbourg: undated); NIH Recombinant DNA Advisory Committee, Human Gene Therapy Subcommittee, *Points to Consider in the Design and Submission of Protocol for the Transfer of Recombinant DNA into Human Subjects*, (Nat. Inst. Health: Bethesda, Va., June 21, 1989); World Council of Churches, Working Group Sub-Unit on Church and Society, " Manipulating Life," *Church and Society*, 1982 (Sept./Oct.).

⁶⁵ See also Loretta Kopelman, "Ethical Controversies in Medical Research: The Case of XYY Screening," *Perspectives in Biology and Medicine* 2 (Winter, 1978), 196–204.

⁶⁶ *Splicing Life*, ref. note 45, 63.

⁶⁷ Medical Research Council, ref. note 43, 21.

⁶⁸ Compare *Splicing Life*, ref. note 45, 62–64.

⁶⁹ See Report of the Commission of Enquiry of the German Bundestag, ref. note 42, 188b–189b.

⁷⁰ See also Lisa Sowle Cahill, "Moral Tradition, Ethical Language, and Reproductive Technologies," *The Journal of Medicine and Philosophy* 14: 5 (October, 1989) 497–522, whose general tone of argument in response to the Report of the Ethics Committee of the American Fertility Society is along these lines.

⁷¹ C.S. Lewis, *The Abolition of Man* (New York: Collier-Macmillan, 1965) 70.

⁷² See Report of the Commission of Enquiry of the German Bundestag, ref. note 42, 187ff. for a discussion of similar considerations.

⁷³ President's Commission for the Study of Ethical Problems in Medicine and Biomedical and Behavioral Research, *Splicing Life: The Social and Ethical Issues of Genetic Engineering with Human Beings*, (Wash., D.C.: U.S. Govt. Printing Office, 1982) 72.

⁷⁴ See the general sentiment expressed in and underlying *Donum vitae*: "Instruction on Respect for Human Life in its Origin and on the Dignity of Procreation—Replies to Certain Questions of the Day," given at Vatican City, Rome, from the Sacred Congregation for the Doctrine of the Faith, approved and ordered for publication by the Supreme Pontiff, John Paul II, February 22, 1987.

⁷⁵ For an example of somatic therapy, see B.J. Culliton, "One Step Closer for Gene Therapy," *Science* 248 (8 June, 1990) 1182, which discussed approval given by the U.S. National Institute of Health for experimental adenine deaminase treatment by inserting the ADA gene into patients who are not doing well on alternative methods of treatment.

⁷⁶ Medical Research Council, ref. note 43, 1.7 and elsewhere; *Splicing Life*, ref. note 45, 45–48; Report of the Commission of Enquiry on "Prospects and Risks of Genetic Engi-

neering," German Bundestag, 10th legislative Period, (January 1987) Sections C: 6, Section D.

[77] Richard Roblin, "Human Genetic Therapy: Outlook and Apprehensions," in G.K. Chacko, ed., *Health Handbook* (New York: Elsevier-North Holland Pub. Co., 1979) 108–112. For a failed early experiment along these lines, see W. French Anderson, "Genetic Therapy," in M.P. Hamilton, ed., *The New Genetics and the Future of Man* (Grand Rapids, Mich.: William B. Eerdmans Pub., 1972) 109, 118.

[78] *Splicing Life*, ref. note 45, 45. For a similar position, but one which was ultimately rejected, see Report of the Commission of Inquiry of the German Bundestag, at 188a.

[79] See *Splicing Life*, ref. note 45.

[80] See above, Chapter 11, "Abortion," pp. 275–301.

[81] See *Splicing Life*, ref. note 45, 45. See also Medical Research Council of Canada, *Discussion Report: Research on Gene Therapy in Humans* (Ottawa: MRC, 1989) 1.6–1.7.

[82] "One in Five Done Wrong," *RNABC News*, Sept./Oct. 1984, 20f.

[83] The implication is not necessarily that this is a matter of incompetence. It may lie in the nature of the situation as a whole, or a whole series of other factors.

[84] Medical Research Council, *Guidelines for Research on Somatic Cell Therapy in Humans*, (Ottawa: Medical Research Council, 1990) 24.

[85] The National Committee for Bioethics in Human Research is a body that was recently established federally to audit in this regard.

[86] See Address of the Bishop of York to the House of Lords, ref. note 38.

[87] This is the core of the classical problem of personal identity.

[88] There is a whole philosophical literature that has grown around the notion of personal identity ever since Plato indirectly raised the issue with his Myth of Er. For more on the subject; see the works of David Hume, Thomas Aquinas, Terence Penelhum, P.F. Strawson, P.T. Geach, Gilbert Ryle, J.J.C. Smart, G.W. Leibniz—to mention but a few of the better-known classic authors.

[89] See M.A. Field, *Surrogate Motherhood* (Cambridge and London: Harvard University Press, 1988) for a good introductory discussion of some of the legal issues from a U.S. perspective.

[90] Law Reform Commission of Ontario, *Report on Human Artificial Reproduction and Related Matters* (Toronto, Ministry of the Attorney General, 1985) 218.

[91] As above, 218–19.

[92] In the U.S., Louisiana (1987), Nebraska (1988) and Michigan (1988) statutes reject surrogacy contracts as unenforceable, while New Jersey, Maryland, New York, Rhode Island and Delaware are currently looking at various bills. In the Kentucky case of *Surrogate Parenting Associates, Inc. vs. Kentucky*, 704 S.W. 2d. 209 (Ky. Supreme Court 1986), the court held that surrogate contracts do not violate the state's statute against bay-selling, but the surrogate mother has an absolute right to change her mind within five days after the baby's birth. In the New Jersey case of *In re Baby M* [*Family Law Reporter* 14 (1988) at 2010] the Supreme Court held that paid surrogacy contracts are illegal and unpaid contracts are unenforceable. The matter was also raised at the federal level with

proposal prohibiting surrogacy arrangements on a commercial basis.

In the U.K., the case of *A. vs. C.* (1985) F.L.R. 445 (Eng. Ct. App. 1978) held that to make surrogate contracts enforceable would be against public policy; a position that was reflected in the Warnock Report. The matter was settled by the *Surrogacy Arrangements Act,* 1985, Ch.49, which bans commercial surrogate arrangements but not private ones. Furthermore, only agencies and go-betweens are criminally liable, not those who use the services.

In France, surrogacy is considered baby-selling and hence is considered illegal, and all parties are liable. In Germany the courts have ruled that surrogacy contracts are unenforceable and that they are against good social morals (*contra bonos mores*). See *Family Reporter* 13 (1987), at 1260.

[93] American College of Obstetricians and Gynecologists, "Ethical Issues in Surrogate Motherhood," (May 1983).

[94] Judicial Council Report I–83 (1983).

[95] SOGC, *Ethical Considerations,* ref. note 11, Ethical Issue No.7, "Surrogacy."

[96] The 1987 survey of the U.S. Office of Technology Assessment reports that only approximately 1% of physicians specializing in artificial insemination and the use of new techniques of reproductive technology reject the use of surrogate motherhood. Of the remainder, 29% believe the price should be state controlled, 42% believe it should be federally controlled and 27% believe that there should be no regulation at all. U.S. Office of Technology Assessment, Washington, DC., 1987, *Artificial Insemination,* 55–56, table 2–60.

[97] See Law Reform Commission of Ontario Report, 260f. For a general discussion of the legal issues of legitimacy, see Law Reform Commission of Canada, Working Paper 6, *Family Law* (1976).

[98] See Amicus Brief (Rutger's Women's Rights Litigation Clinic), 217 N.J. Super. 313, 525 A.2d 1128 (1987); and M.J. Radin, "Market-Inalienability," *Harvard Law Review,* 100 (June 1987), 1930. See also G. Corea, *The Mother Machine: Reproductive Technologies from Artificial Insemination to Artificial Wombs* (New York: Harper and Row, 1986) 214f.

[99] See G.R. Dunstan, "Moral and Social Issues Arising from AID: Law and Ethics of AID and Embryo Transfer," *CIBA Foundation Symposium* 17 (1973).

[100] The recent Canadian cases of *Re Eve, Morgentaler* and *Daigle* give authoritative examples of where the courts have insisted that this right is supreme. This may be a clear reflection of the fact that Canada would allow surrogate motherhood—at least in some sense or other.

[101] As Kant put it in his *Foundations of the Metaphysics of Morals,* ethics "does not rest at all on feelings, impulses and inclination; it rests merely on the relation of rational beings to one another." [434]

SUGGESTED READINGS

- Canadian Fertility Society and Society of Obstetricians and Gynecologists of Canada. *Ethical Considerations of the New Reproductive Technologies* (1990).

  The official position of the two societies who are most intimately connected with the delivery of reproductive technology to Canadian health care consumers. It was the result of over two years of study and discussion within the societies.

- Feldman, David M. "The Ethical Implications of New Reproductive Techniques," in Rabbi Levi Meier, ed., *Jewish Values in Bioethics*. New York: Human Sciences Press, 1986, 174–182.

  A judaic perspective of some of the issues that surround the use of new reproductive technologies. It might profitably be read in conjunction with works by Catholic and Protestant thinkers.

- Law Reform Commission of Ontario. *Report on Artificial Human Reproduction*. Toronto: Ministry of the Attorney General, 1985.

  The classic Canadian study of new techniques of reproductive technology from a judicial perspective. However, it also contains good analyses of some of the major ethical issues like *in vitro* fertilization and surrogate motherhood.

- Medical Research Council of Canada. *Guidelines for Research on Somatic Cell Gene Therapy in Humans*. Ottawa: Medical Research Council, 1990.

  Guidelines for somatic cell gene therapy research by the national Canadian body responsible for setting research guidelines and standards. It includes a brief scientific discussion of gene therapy.

- President's Commission for the Study of Ethical Problems in Medicine and Biomedical and Behavioral Research. *Splicing Life: A Report on the Social and Ethical Issues of Genetic Engineering with Human Beings*. Washington, DC: U.S. Government Printing Office, 1982.

  An introductory study of genetic engineering from a legislative perspective. It contains a brief historical sketch of developments in the field until 1982. Although dated, the study is a good introduction to many of the issues.

- Purdy, L.M. "Genetic Diseases: Can Having Children Be Immoral?" in J.J. Buckley, ed., *Genetics Now: Ethical Issues in Genetic Research*. Washington, D.C.: University Press of America, 1978.

  A thought-provoking article by a well-known writer on the ethics of genetic technology in the human context. The author defends the claim that having children can be immoral under certain genetically determined conditions.

Glossary

a priori: deductive; reasoning based solely on principles; considered independently of existing facts.

absolute value: value that something has whether someone values it or not.

absolutism: the ethical theory that ethical principles, properties and facts do not depend on people.

act-utilitarianism: a kind of utilitarianism that judges the utility of a given act on its own terms and independently of any reference to rules.

active euthanasia: euthanasia that involves an action to bring about the death of the individual.

advance directive: a directive given by a competent person about what kind of medical treatment the person does or does not want when that person is no longer competent and in a position to make medical decision her- or himself. When advance directives are used, they usually focus on cessation-of-treatment orders.

agapistic: an ethical theory that is love oriented; sometimes referred to as the "ethics of brotherly love." This ethical approach usually emphasizes respect for life.

agency or engineering model: a model of the health care professional relationship that portrays the relationship of the professional to the patient as one where the patient gives the orders and the professional follows them without question.

AIDS: Acquired **I**mmune **D**eficiency **S**yndrome.

AIH: Artificial **I**nsemination by **H**usband.

alpha-fetoproteins: proteins which, if they are detected in the blood of a pregnant woman, indicate the likelihood of a neural tube defect in the fetus.

Alzheimer's disease: a progressive neurological disorder of the brain involving diffuse cortical atrophy, increasing dementia, memory loss and general cognitive impairment.

amniocentesis: insertion of a hollow needle into the amniotic sac surrounding the fetus, withdrawing of amniotic fluid and testing of the fluid for abnormalities, especially neural tube defects and serious genetic abnormalities.

anencephaly: a congenital condition resulting from a failure of the neural tube to close during gestation. It involves an open skull and an absence of all brain matter except a brain stem. The condition is incurable and invariably fatal.

spina bifida: a congenital condition characterized by the failure of the spine to close properly during fetal development. The spinal cord in that area is exposed, unprotected and may be defective. It is usually associated with a degree of physical handicap whose precise nature depends on the degree of defect.

applied ethics: ethical theory as applied to problems of every-day life.

artificial insemination: the introduction of semen into the vagina by artificial means.

artificial placenta: a device that allows a fetus to develop outside of a uterus; very much experimental in nature and so far confined only to animal models. Strictly speaking, the phrase is a misnomer. It should be "artificial uterus."

auto-induced needs: needs that are preventable but that the person who has these needs has brought on by her or his own actions.

autonomy, principle of: the principle that all persons have a fundamental right to self-determination that is limited only by unjust infringement on the rights of others. It is central to deontological ethics.

beneficence, principle of: has been characterized as the "duty to help others further their important and legitimate interest" when we can do so with minimal risks to ourselves. We can distinguish two components: a positive duty to bring about the good for others if it lies within our power to do so without harm to ourselves, and a general duty to attempt to bring about a balance of good over harm in situations that allow for various choices.

best action, principle of: the principle that whoever has an obligation also has the ethical duty to discharge it in the best manner possible under the circumstances.

bioethics: ethical theory applied to issues in health care and biology; a species of applied ethics.

carrier: a term used in genetics to indicate that someone carries a particular kind of gene.

CAT scan: derived from the phrase **C**omputerized **A**xial **T**omography. It refers to a computer-assisted technique of taking a series of X-rays of the body and visualizing the inside of the body as a series of stacked planes. It is an exceedingly useful diagnostic tool.

categorical imperative: refers to Kant's statement that we should never treat any person, inclusive of oneself, solely as means to an end but that we should always treat persons as ends in themselves.

chemotherapy: usually treatment of cancer by chemical agents. These tend to be exceedingly toxic, with severe side-effects, and therefore their use has to be monitored and controlled very closely.

chromosome: the genes of human beings are carried in 23 pairs of chromosomes, where one member of each pair is contributed by the mother, the other by the father.

cloning: a technique of growing an exact genetic duplicate of a living thing.

co-operation model: an approach to the professional-patient relationship that sees the professional as engaged in a co-operative enterprise with the patient.

coercion: forcing someone to do something against that person's will.

cognitive significance: meaningfulness on a symbolic level.

collegial model: an approach to the professional-patient relationship that sees the professional and the patient on the model of colleagues engaged in a common enterprise.

collateral risks: a risk associated with a given undertaking.

comatose: being in a persistent coma, or being deeply unconscious for a protracted period of time, usually as the result of some injury.

competence: the ability to understand, reason, and make judgements and decisions on the basis of reasonable values and without serious volitional or emotional compromise.

compliance: giving in to the wishes, desires or directives of others. Excessive compliance may be an indication of volitional incompetence.

conception: fertilization of an ovum or egg.

conceptual framework: the system of concepts that allow us to think and that make our experiences cognitively meaningful.

conceptual competence: the condition of being impaired in one's ability to reason, understand and remember.

confidentiality, duty of: the duty of a professional not to reveal information of which he or she has become aware in the context of the professional-client relationship. The duty may be breached only under rare conditions.

congenital: term used to describe a disease or condition that is present at birth.

congenitally incompetent: the state of being incompetent from birth. All infants are congenitally incompetent. However, normally their competence increases with age, until they become fully competent as older children or young adults.

consequentialistic: goal- or end-oriented.

contraceptive: something that prevents conception.

contractual model: an approach to the professional-patient relationship that characterizes this relationship on the model of a contract.

coronary bypass surgery: surgery that by-passes defective heart arteries by replacing them with suitable veins taken from some other part of the body.

cost/benefit: an evaluation of possible courses of action that compares the relative cost of competing undertakings against their expected benefits.

cost/effectiveness: an evaluation of possible courses of action that compares their relative costs measured against their degree of effectiveness in bringing about a certain state of affairs.

cross-linked: characteristics whose genetic basis is contained in more than one gene.

cross-over: a method of controlling bias in drug experiments. It involves switching the group of subjects that were on the drug to a placebo, and vice versa.

cryo-preservation: preservation or storage at extremely low temperatures.

cystic fibrosis: an inherited disease in which the pancreas fails to produce enzymes necessary to break down foods, and in which the glands lining the bronchial tubes of the lungs produce a thick, sticky mucus that tends to remain. It is associated with respiratory infections and early death.

de-identified: having identifying marks or names removed.

debriefing: telling the subjects of an experiment what occurred in the experiment.

decerebrate: without a functioning cerebrum or higher brain centres.

deontological pluralism: an ethical theory which says that there is more than one basic deontological principle.

deontological: rule or law-centred; an approach to ethics which says that the nature of what is right and what is wrong does not depend on outcome but on certain principles or fundamental and objective rules.

depatterning: a psychiatric technique to change the basic personality structure or pattern of an individual.

disciplinary hearings: a hearing called by the disciplinary body of a professional association to decide on whether an accused professional is guilty of not having followed the guidelines set by the profession.

disclosure: the disclosure of information to a patient. It may be either full, professional, subjective or objective.

DNA: deoxyribonucleic acid; the double helix molecule that carries genetic information characteristic of an organism.

double-blind experimental studies: experimental studies where neither the subject nor the experimenter know whether the subject is receiving the drug to be tested or a placebo.

durable power of attorney: power of attorney that endures even when the person who has given it has become incompetent.

effective: a right is effective when the conditions under which the right comes into force in fact obtain.

electroconvulsive shock treatments: therapy that involves the conduction of electric current through the brain of an individual. It has been used for a variety of conditions, including severe depression.

embryo: the generic word for a young organism in early stages of development; in human beings, the product of conception from the moment of conception to the eighth week after fertilization;

emergent: something is emergent if it cannot be reduced to an additive sum of its parts.

emergent qualities: qualities that cannot be analyzed in additive terms.

emotional incompetence: incompetence centering in extreme emotions that interfere with the ability to make appropriate decisions.

emotivism: an approach to ethics that reduces all ethical statements to expressions of emotions.

epidemiological: dealing with incidence patterns of diseases or health conditions.

equality and justice, principle of: the principle that a right is effective to the degree that it preserves or promotes equity and justice.

ethos: the system of standards and beliefs that a particular group of people professes.

estrogen: one of the main hormones responsible for female sex characteristics.

ethical voluntarism: the theory that what is ethically right or wrong depends on what someone decides it should be.

ethical justification: the justification of something solely in terms of ethical relationships or characteristics.

ethical: having to do with ethics.

ethics review boards: also called ERB's. Board whose function it is to assess the ethical acceptability of a project, action or undertaking.

etiquette: rules of how to behave appropriately; manners.

eudaemonistic: happiness-oriented.

eugenics: the theory that the genetic characteristics of a species ought to be improved by deliberate interference. It may be either positive or negative.

euthanatize: to kill a person in order to prevent suffering; to give an easy death.

experimental therapies: therapies that are not standard, that involve a great deal of uncertainty and whose use involves among other things the desire to gather more data.

expertise, fallacy of: the fallacious belief that expertise in one area translates into expertise in another unrelated area.

extra-ordinary means: means that transcend what the ordinary person would find acceptable or too burdensome under the circumstances. The notion is context-dependent.

extra-billing: the practice of charging patients more than is provided for by a provincial fee schedule.

fee schedule: the set fee schedule that a provincial ministry of health considers appropriate for health care services.

fetoscopy: technique that involves inserting a light-conducting tube through the woman's abdominal wall into the womb.

fetus: in human beings, the developing human being in the uterus from the ninth to the fortieth week of development;

fibrillations: extremely rapid contractions of the heart muscles.

fiduciary: based on trust.

Friedreich's ataxia: an inherited disease that involves increasing loss of coordination, especially in walking, standing, speaking and use of arms; no known treatment.

friendship model: an approach to the professional-client relationship that sees the professional and the client acting in a relationship of friendship.

gene therapy: manipulation of genetic material in order to cure a genetically caused defect.

genetic engineering: manipulation of the genetic code.

genetics: the study of the genetic code of organisms.

genome: a complete set of hereditary factors.

germ line therapy: gene therapy that involves a change in the genetic material of ova or sperm, and that will therefore be passed on to future generations.

gestation: the development of a fertilized ovum in the uterus until birth of the organism.

gestational motherhood: the practice whereby a woman agrees to gestate a child for another woman, where that child has no genetic relationship to the gestational mother.

haemophilia: a bleeding disorder that is genetically sex-linked involving the deficiency or absence of a plasma coagulant, therefore preventing the blood from clotting appropriately.

health potential: the level of health that an organism can potentially reach.

hedonistic: having to do with pleasure.

hepatitis: a highly infectious viral disease of the liver.

hetero-induced needs: needs that are not within the control of the individual who has them.

heterozygous: having two members of one or more genes dissimilar.

homeostatic balance: the ability to respond to the challenges of the environment while at the same time maintaining functional integrity. We refer to such a state as a state of homeostatic balance.

homo sapiens: human beings.

Huntington's chorea: or Huntington's disease; an inherited progressive disease of the central nervous system characterized by progressive spastic involuntary and convulsive movements, dementia and disturbed speech. It is incurable, and its usual onset is in adult life.

hysterectomy: partial or total removal of the uterus

ideal utilitarian: a version of utilitarianism that involves a series of rules centering around ideal values such as generosity, justice, etc.

impossibility, principle of: the principle that a right that cannot be fulfilled under the circumstances is ineffective as a right, and that an obligation that cannot be met under the circumstances ceases to be effective as an obligation.

impure placebos: pharmacologically active substances which are not known to be specific or even appropriate for the condition in question.

***in vitro* fertilization:** fertilization outside of the body of a woman, usually in a petri dish.

***in vivo*:** in a living body

incommensurable value: a value that cannot be expressed in arithmetic or calculable terms.

indirect euthanasia: euthanasia that takes place with the aid of intervening causal agents or steps.

induced abortions: an abortion that is brought about deliberately, or induced.

infanticide: legally, the killing of a new-born by its mother within the first year of the neonate's life; in general, the killing of a neonate.

infertility: the inability to procreate when physiologically the individual should be capable of doing so.

informed consent: the process of giving voluntary and competent consent to an undertaking after having received and understood all relevant and appropriate information.

innovative procedures: procedures or modalities which are already known from another area but which are adapted to a new context without there being as much certainty as there is in the standard uses.

institutionalization: being placed into the formally structured context of an institution. This need not involve residence or presence in a certain building.

institutionalized context: the context of an institutional setting.

intrinsic value: the value that something has independently of being valued by anyone; the value inherent in it as such.

involuntary sterilization: sterilization against one's will.

isolation, fallacy of: the mistake of trying to evaluate the ethical nature of a decision or course of action independently of the context in which that decision or action takes place.

IUD: intra-uterine device. A device that prevents implantation of a fertilized ovum into the uterine wall.

living wills: an advance directive in anticipation of possible incompetence and inability to make health care decisions for oneself. It outlines under what conditions a person wants to be allowed to die.

locum: temporary replacement for a physician absent from practice.

macro-allocation: allocation of resources between competing areas of health care or between different groups of health care consumers.

maxim: the generalized rule or principle of a particular act.

meningitis: an inflammation of the meninges or membranes of the brain or spinal cord.

meso-allocation: allocation involving competition between a specific individual and a group of individuals.

meta-ethics: theories dealing with the nature of ethics and of ethical theories.

micro-allocation: allocation involving competition between individuals.

minimal harm: harm that is no greater than that encountered in the ordinary everyday context of life.

mixed utilitarianism: utilitarianism that combines hedonistic and ideal elements.

monistic: having only one basic principle or basis.

MRI: Magnetic **R**esonance **I**maging; a computer-assisted technique for visualizing cellular structures in the body by exposing them to alternating magnetic fields.

multiple sclerosis: a progressive disease of the nervous system that involves loss of the insulating covering of the neurons and the formation of plaques.

nationality, fallacy of: the fallacy that what is ethically right or wrong depends on nationality and therefore differs from nation to nation.

neural tube defect: a defect of the developing neural tube of an embryo.

neurosis: one of the two major categories of emotional maladjustment; usually involving anxiety.

non-cognitivistic: having no cognitive meaning or significance.

non compos mentis: not of sound mind; incompetent;

non-malfeasance, principle of: may be expressed in the following two statements: "Do not intentionally or knowingly injure the patient" and "Do not intentionally or knowingly expose the patient to unjustified risk."

non-voluntary: without voluntary permission or agreement.

non-therapeutic experimentation: experimentation where the primary concern is the advancement of knowledge.

non-validated: therapy that has not been systematically tested and approved for therapeutic use.

nuclear family: the traditional Western notion of a family as composed of two parents and children.

objectivism: the theory that ethics is not relativistic but has an objective basis independent of subjective attitudes.

obligation of ubiquity: the obligation to make health services reasonably available independently of location.

obligation: duty

oncology: the study of neoplastic growth or cancer.

ontologically basic: something that cannot be analyzed into more basic components.

ordinary means: means that are usually accepted by the majority of the population and that are considered standard treatment for a particular disease or condition.

ova: female gamete.

palliative: providing only comfort care.

parens patriae: the powers of the judiciary to make decisions on behalf of members of society; usually exercised only on behalf of congenitally incompetent persons.

particularize: to make specific to a particular context or set of circumstances.

passive euthanasia: allowing death to occur even though it could be prevented or staved off at that point in time.

paternalistic: overriding the wishes of someone motivated solely by the desire to do good for that other person.

personhood: the state of being a person; having the present capacity for sapient cognitive awareness.

PET scan: **P**ositron **E**mission **T**omography scan; a nuclear diagnostic tool.

pharmaco-kinetic: having to do with the kinetic action of a drug in the body.

physician/patient relationship: a fiduciary relationship that comes into being between physician and patient as soon as the physician interacts with a person in a professional capacity as physician.

physiologically: opposed to psychologically; having to do with the body.

PKU: acronym for phenylketonuria: an inheritable recessive metabolic disorder that results in the presence of increased amounts of phenylalanine and phenylpyruvic acid in the urine; if untreated, it leads to retardation, eczema, and occasionally seizures.

placebo effect: the effect of an otherwise ineffective drug, procedure or undertaking that cannot be accounted for in terms of its pharmacological or other effectiveness; the psychosomatic effect of a placebo.

placebos: any therapy or component of therapy that is deliberately used for its non-specific, psychological or psychophysiological effect, or that is used for its presumed specific effect but is without specific activity for the condition being treated (see also impure placebos, and pure placebos).

podiatry: diagnosis and treatment of disorders of the feet.

poliomyelitis: a viral disease that involves upper respiratory and gastrointestinal symptoms, but which may progress to nerve involvement and lead to paralysis.

pre-natal screening: screening of a fetus or an embryo for anomalous conditions.

premature birth: birth of a human infant prior to the 37th or 38th week of gestation.

priestly model: an approach to the professional-patient relationship that sees the professional as the ultimate decision-maker whose task it is to decide for the good of the patient; also called the paternalistic model.

prima facie: at first sight; on first impression; without taken relevant differences into account.

primary macro-allocation: the general level of macro-allocation that is based on the average health status of members of society.

primum non nocere: above all, do not harm; a classic expression of the principle of non-malfeasance.

priority, principle of: the principle that rights can be ranked according to logical, natural, and voluntary priority

pro-life: an attitude that values life itself more than quality of life.

prognosis: forecast, based on diagnosis, of what is likely to happen in a particular context.

proxy decision-making: decision-making by someone who takes over the decision-making role for someone who is making a decision on her or his own behalf.

psychic driving: an experimental psychiatric technique similar to brain-washing, used by Dr. Cameron in his CIA sponsored experiments.

psycho-social: psychological factors in their collective or social context.

psychoses: an impairment of mental functioning so extensive that it interferes greatly with a person's ability to function; included are paranoias, affective disorders and schizophrenias.

psychotropic drugs: drugs that have a special affinity for or effect on the mind.

pure placebos: pharmacologically inert substances used as placebos.

QALY's: **Q**uality **A**djusted **L**ife **Y**ears; an economic measure used to compare the cost of a given intervention with the improvement in the quality of life that results over the number of years involved.

quadriplegic: paralysed in all four limbs.

quality control: an attempt to monitor and control the quality of a given undertaking.

quality-enhancing: something that enhances the quality of life of a person.

quasi-legal document: a document that has no legal binding power but is regulatory in nature and that may influence the direction of a legal decision on the subject at issue.

recombinant DNA technology: technology that involves the decomposition of the DNA molecule into its component parts and recombing it either in a different form or with different segments of DNA inserted into the old molecule.

reductio ad absurdum: a method or reasoning that shows that following a given assumption leads to a contradiction.

relativism: the theory that ethics is not universally valid but relative to a society or a given perspective.

relevant difference, principle of: the principle that a right is effective to the degree that nothing in the relevant circumstances contravenes the conditions under which it arose.

research: investigation or experimentation; in the medical context, it may be either therapeutic or non-therapeutic experimentation.

review ethics boards: ethics review boards.

rights: claims that someone has on others, where others have corresponding duties.

rule utilitarianism: a version of utilitarianism that believes that specific actions should not be evaluated for their utility but that instead what has to be established is the utility of rules of action.

screening: checking for anomalies.

secondary macro-allocation: allocation that looks at the justification for providing additional resources for disadvantaged groups of individuals.

self-determination: deciding for oneself.

service monopoly: monopoly on providing a particular kind of service.

sex-determination: the determination of the sex of an embryo or fetus before it is born.

sickle cell anemia: an inheritable disease of the red blood cells in which hypoxia causes red blood cells to assume a sickle shape.

social preference utilitarianism: a version of utilitarianism that attempts to identify what constitutes the good to be aimed at by reference to what society prefers.

socialization: the process of acquiring social values and norms, and of fitting into society.

somatic cell therapy: therapy that affects only the somatic cells of the body and gametes.

speciesm: the charge that a particular position favours a particular species in a discriminatory fashion.

sperm: male gamete

spina bifida: a congenital defect in the spinal cord, which has failed to close; usually associated with protrusion of the covering and sometimes of the nerve tissue of the spinal cord itself; often associated with more or less severe disabilities.

steatopygia: an inherited disposition to accumulate large amounts of adipose tissue in the buttocks; characteristic of certain African indigenous peoples.

sterilization: the process or procedure of rendering someone incapable of procreation.

substituted judgement: an approach to proxy decision making for congenitally incompetent persons that asks the proxy decision-maker to place him- or herself into the place of the congenitally incompetent person and make the decision from that perspective.

sui generis: unlike any other kind of thing; unique in nature.

super-ovulation: the production of more than one ripe ovum at a time.

surrogate motherhood: the practice whereby a woman agrees to bear a child for some other woman and then to relinquish to that woman any rights of a mother that she might otherwise have.

Tay-Sachs: a heritable fatal neurological disorder; also known as infantile amaurotic familial idiocy.

teleological: a goal directed approach to ethics; the end or outcome is more important than the means used for attaining that outcome.

thalidomide: a medication that was once prescribed for morning sickness; it has unfortunate side-effects that involve, among other things, severe interference with the development of fetal limbs.

therapeutic privilege, doctrine of: the doctrine that a physician has the privilege to withhold information if the disclosure of that information will harm the patient.

therapeutic experimentation: takes place when the primary aim of the protocol is to benefit the patient.

transfer payments: funds transferred by the federal government to the various provinces.

trisomy: the presence of three of a given chromosome rather than the normal two.

tubal ligation: binding off the tubes that carry ova from the follicles to the uterus; a popular method of female sterilization.

tutioristic: a line of reasoning that suggests that we should err on the side of safety.

typhoid fever: a highly infectious and dangerous acute systemic infection.

uniqueness, fallacy of: the fallacy of assuming that something of special interest should be treated as though it were ethically unique.

uraemia: accumulation of various metabolic byproducts as a result of kidney failure.

utilitarian: a teleological ethical theory.

validated procedure: a procedure that has gone through standard methods of testing and that has been approved for medical practice by the relevant bodies or agencies.

valuational competence: competence with respect to the values that someone holds.

value-free definition: a definition that does not depend on and does not include any reference to values.

values: action potentials; beliefs that motivate someone to act.

vasectomy: cutting of the vas deferens; a popular method of male contraception.

vitalism: the position or belief that life has absolute value and should be protected if at all possible.

volitional competence: the uncompromised ability to make decisions and to put them into practice.

whole-brain criterion: a criterion for the determination of death; it requires that the whole brain, inclusive of the brain stem, be permanently dysfunctional.

wrongful life: a legal action brought by a child on the grounds that it should not have been borne because the quality of its life is unacceptably low.

Bibliography

"Active and Passive Euthanasia," Editorial, *New England Journal of Medicine* 292: 2 (Jan. 9, 1975): 78–80.

"Embryos Again," Editorial, *Ethics and Medicine* 5: 2(1989):17.

"The XYY Man: Do Criminals Really Have Abnormal Genes?", *Science Digest* 79 (Jan. 1976): 33–38.

Alberta Institute of Law Research and Reform. *Report for Discussion No.6,* "Sterilization Decisions: Minors and Mentally Incompetent Adults," (Edmonton, 1988).

Alberta Institute of Law Research and Reform. *Report No.52,* "Competence and Human Reproduction" (Edmonton, 1989).

Alberta Institute of Law Research and Reform. *Report No.20,* "Status of Children" (Edmonton, 1976).

American College of Physicians. "Cognitively Impaired Subjects, " *Annals of Internal Medicine* 111:10 (Nov. 15, 1989): 843–848.

American Fertility Society. "Ethical Considerations of the New Reproductive Technologies," *Fertility and Sterility* 46:3 (Sept., 1986) Supplement.

American Fertility Society. "Ethical Statement on In Vitro Fertilization," *Fertility and Sterility* 41:12 (1984).

American College of Obstetricians and Gynecologists. "Ethical Issues in Surrogate Motherhood," (May 1983). *Ethical Considerations, Ethical Issue No.7,* "Surrogacy." SOGC.

American Medical Association. "Persistent Vegetative State and the Decision to Withdraw or Withhold Life Support." *Report of the Council on Ethical and Judicial Affairs, No.19,* June 1989.

Anderson, French W. "Genetic Therapy," in *The New Genetics and the Future of Man.* Ed. Hamilton, M.P. Grand Rapids, Mich.: William B. Eerdmans Pub., 1972.: 109-118.

Anglican Church of Canada. *On Dying Well.* Anglican Church Information Office (1972).

Annals of the Royal College of Physicians and Surgeons of Canada. "Informed Consent: Ethical Considerations for Physicians and Surgeons," 21:1 1988 (approved, Sept.) 1987.

Annas, George J. "The Emerging Stowaway—Patients' Rights in the 1980s." *Law, Medicine and Health Care* (1982): 32–35.

Annas, George J. "Righting the Wrong of 'Wrongful Life.'" *Hastings Center Report* 11:1 (Feb. 1981).

Annas, George J. "A French Homonculus in a Tennessee Court." *Hastings Center Report* 19:6 (Nov. Dec. 1989): 20–22.

Annas, G.J., L.H. Glantz, and B.F. Katz. *Informed Consent to Human Experimentation: The Subject's Dilemma.* Cambridge, Mass.: Ballinger Publication Co., 1977.

Anscombe, Elizabeth. "Who Is Wronged?" *The Oxford Review* 5 (1967): 16–17.

Ashley, B.M. and K.D. O'Rourke. *Health Care Ethics: A Theological Analysis.* St. Louis: Catholic Health Association, 1982.

Australia."Victoria Committee to Consider Social, Ethical and Legal Issues Arising from In Vitro Fertilization," *Report on the Disposition of Embryos Produced by In Vitro Fertilization.*

Ayer, A.J. *Language, Truth and Logic.* London: Gollanz, 1948.

Babikian, H.N. "Abortion," in *Comprehensive Handbook of Psychiatry*, 2nd ed. Eds. Kaplan, H.I. and A.M. Freedman. Baltimore: Williams and Wilkins, 1975: 1496–1500.

Bacon, F. *The New Atlantis.*

Barnes, H.E. *The Repression of Crime: Studies in Historical Penology.* Montclair, N.J.: Patterson Smith, 1969; reprint of the 1918 edition.

Bartholome, W.G. "Parents, Children, and the Moral Benefits of Research," in *Medical Research with Children: Ethics, Law and Practice.* Ed. R.H. Nicholson, Oxford: Oxford University Press, 1986: 146–151.

Bayles, Michael. *Professional Ethics.* Englewood Cliffs, N.J.: Prentice Hall, 1985.

Bayles, Michael. "Harm to the Unconceived," *Philosophy and Public Affairs* 5:3 (1976).

Bayles, Michael. *Reproductive Ethics.* Englewood Cliffs, N.J.: Prentice-Hall, 1984.

Beauchamp, T.L. and J.F. Childress. *Principles of Biomedical Ethics.* New York and Oxford: Oxford University Press, 1979.

Beauchamp, T.L. and L.B. McCullough. *Medical Ethics: The Moral Responsibility of Physicians.* Englewood Cliffs, N.J.: Prentice-Hall, 1984.

Becker, M., and L. Maiman. "Strategies for Enhancing Patient Compliance," *Journal of Community Health*, (1980): 113–132.

Beckwith, Jon. "Social and Political Uses of Genetics in the United States: Past and Present," in Munson, ed., *Intervention and Reflection.* Belmont, Calif.: Wadsworth, 1979: 384–392.

Beecher, H.K. *Experimentation in Man.* Springfield, Ill.: Charles C. Thomas, 1959.

Beecher, H.K. "Ethics in Clinical Research," *New England Journal of Medicine* 274 (1966): 1350–60.

Beecher, H.K. "The Powerful Placebo," *JAMA* 159 (1955): 1602–1606.

Bennett, Kathryn and David Feeny. "Clinical and Economic Evaluation of Therapeutic Technologies: The Case of neonatal Intensive Care Programs" in *Health Care Technology: Effectiveness, Efficiency and Public Policy.* Eds. Feeney, D., G.Guyatt, and P.Tugwell. Montreal: Institute for Research on Public Policy, (1986): 199–223.

Bennett, Jonathan, "Whatever the Consequences," *Analysis* 26:3 (1966): 83–97.

Bentham, J. *The Principles of Morals and Legislation.* London, 1789.

Bergsma, D., ed. *Ethical, Social and Legal Dimensions of Screening for Human Genetic Disease*, Birth Defect Series, vol. 10. New York: Stratton-Intercontinental.

Bishop of York, Address to the House of Lords (H.L. 7 December, 1989).

Bok, S. *Lying.* New York: Random House, 1978.

Boorse, C. "Health as a Theoretical Concept," *Philosophy of Science* 44 (1977): 542–573.

Brandt, R.B. *Ethical Theory.* Englewood Cliffs, N.J.: Prentice Hall, 1959.

Brandt, R.B. *A Theory of the Good and the Right.* Oxford: Clarendon Press, 1979.

British Columbia, Royal Commission on Family and Children's Law. *Ninth Report of the Royal Commission on Family and Children's Law: Artificial Insemination,* (Victoria, 1975).

British Columbia Bar Association. *Report of the Special Task Force Committee on Reproductive Technology of the British Columbia Branch, Canadian Bar Association.* Vancouver: June, 1989.

Brody, Howard. "The Lie That Heals: The Ethics of Giving Placebos." *Annals of Internal Medicine* 97:1 (1982): 112–118.

Brown, Barry F. "Proxy Consent for Research on Incompetent Elderly" in *Ethics and Aging: The Right to Live, the Right to Die.* Eds. Thornton, J.E. and E.R. Winkler. Vancouver: The University of British Columbia Press, 1988: 183–193.

Brown, W. Miller. "On Defining 'Disease,'" *Journal of Medicine and Philosophy* 10:4 (1985): 311–328.

Bryant, Heather. *The Infertility Dilemma: Reproductive Technologies and Prevention.* Calgary: Canadian Advisory Council on the Status of Women,(February, 1990).

Buchanan, Allen. "Medical Paternalism," *Philosophy and Public Affairs* 7 (1978): 370–390.

Buchanan, Allen. "The Right to a Decent Minimum of Health Care," in the President's Commission for the Study of Ethical Problems in Medicine and Biomedical Behavioral Research, *Securing Access to Health Care: The Ethical Implications of Diferences in the Availability of Health Services,* 43 vols.(U.S. Govt. Printing Office: Washington D.C., 1983.) Volume 2, 207-238.

Buchanan, Allen and Dan W.B.Brock. *Deciding for Others: The Ethics of Surrogate Decision Making.* Cambridge and New York: Cambridge University Press, 1989.

Buchanan, A. "Philosophical Foundations of Beneficence" in *Beneficence and Health Care.* Ed. Shelp, E., Dordrecht and Boston: Reidel, 1982. 33–62.

Burns, Chester R. "The Nonnaturals: A Paradox in the Western Concept of Health," *The Journal of Medicine and Philosophy* 1:3 (1976): 202–211.

Cahill, Lisa S. "Moral Tradition, Ethical Language, and Reproductive Technologies," *The Journal of Medicine and Philosophy* 14:5 (October, 1989): 497–522.

Caldwell, J. and P. Caldwell. "High Fertility in Sub-Saharan Africa," *Scientific American* (May, 1990): 118–125.

Callahan, Joan C."Paternalism and Voluntariness," *Canadian Journal of Philosophy* 16:2 (1986): 199–220.

Callahan, Daniel. "The WHO Definition of Health," *Hastings Center Studies,* 1:3 (1973): 77–87.

Canadian Fertility Society and Society of Obstetricians and Gynecologists of Canada. "Ethical Considerations of the New Reproductive Technologies," (1990).

Canadian Medical Association. "The Ethical Status of the Human Fetus: A Discussion Paper." Ottawa: C.M.A., 1989.

Canadian Medical Association, The. *Canadian Medical Association Code of Ethics.* Ottawa: C.M.A., 1987 and 1990.

Canadian Medical Association, The Guide for the Treatment of Terminally Ill Patients. Ottawa: C.M.A., 1987.

Canadian Nurses Association, The. *Code of Ethics.* Ottawa: C.N.A., 1987.

Cassileth, B.R., E.J. Lusk, D.S. Miller et al. "Psychological Correlates of Survival in Advanced Malignant Disease," *New England Journal of Medicine*, 312 (1985): 1551–1555.

Cass, Leon. "Coronary Artery Surgery Study: A Randomized Trial of Coronary Bypass Surgery," *Circulation* 68 (1983): 939–950.

Cassell, Eric. "Autonomy and Ethics in Action," *New England Journal of Medicine* 297 (1977): 33–34.

Chamberlain, Geoffrey. "An Artificial Placenta," *American Journal of Obstetrics and Gynecology*, 100:24 (March 1, 1968).

Chambers, D. "The Right to the Least Restrictive Alternative," in *The Mentally Retarded Citizen and the Law*. Eds. Kindred, M., et al. New York: Free Press, 1976.

Childress, James I. and Mark Siegler "Metaphors and Models of Doctor-Patient Relationships: Their Implication for Autonomy," *Theoretical Medicine* 5 (1984): 17–30.

Chinen, A. "Modes of Understanding and Mindfulness of Clinical Medicine," *Theoretical Medicine* 9:1 (Feb. 1988): 45–72.

Chisholm, R. *Realism and the Background of Phenomenology*. New York: Glencoe, 1969.

Clark, J.T.R. "Screening for Carriers of Tay-Sachs Disease: Two Approaches," *Canadian Medical Association Journal*, 119 (1978): 450.

CMA Policy Summary on Induced Abortion, CMAJ 1176A (1988).

CMA Position, "Resuscitation of the Terminally Ill," CMAJ vol.136 (Feb.15, 1987).

Cohen, C. "Medical Experimentation on Prisoners," *Perspectives in Biology and Medicine*, Vol. 21, No. 3 (Spring 1978): 357–372.

Combined Ethics Committee of the Canadian Fertility and Andrology Society and the Society of Obstetricians and Gynecologists of Canada. *Ethical Considerations of the New Reproductive Technologies*. Toronto: SOGC, 1990.

Conference on Transcultural Dimensions (Washington: Fidia Research Group, 1990).

Connery J.R. "The Moral Dilemma of the Quinlan Case," *Hospital Progress* 56:17 (Dec. 1975): 18–19.

Corea, G. *The Mother Machine: Reproductive Technologies from Artificial Insemination to Artificial Wombs*. New York: Harper and Row, 1986: 214f.

Council on Scientific Affairs of the American Medical Association, "Societal Effects and Other Factors Affecting Health Care for the Elderly," *Archives of Internal Medicine*. 150:6 (June 1990): 1184–1189.

Crane, Diana. *The Sanctity of Social Life: Physicians' Treatment of Critically Ill Patients*. New York: Russell Sage Foundation, 1975.

Culliton, B.J. "One Step Closer for Gene Therapy," *Science* 248 (8 June, 1990): 1182.

Daniels, Norman. *Just Health Care*, Cambridge and London: Cambridge University Press, 1985.

Daniels, Norman. "Equity of Access to Health Care: Some Conceptual and Ethical Issues," *Milbank Memorial Fund Quarterly*, 60: 1 (1982), reprinted in *Securing Access to Health Care* vol. 2, especially 41–47.

Dennett, D.C. *Content and Consciousness*. London: Routledge and Kegan Paul, 1969.

Denton, F.T. and B.G. Spence. "Population Aging and the Economy: Some Issues in Resource Allocation," in *Ethics and Aging: The Right to Live and the Right to Die*. Eds. Thornton, J.E, and E.R. Winkler. Vancouver: UBC Press, 1988: 98–123.

Dickens, B. "The Role of the Family in Surrogate Medical Consent," *Health and Law in Canada* 1: 3 (1980): 49–52.

Dickens, B. "Comparative Legal Abortion Policies and Attitudes Towards Abortion," in *Defining Human Life: Medical, Legal and Ethical Implications.* Eds. Shaw, M. and A. Doudera. Ann Arbor: AUPHA Press, 1983.

Dickens, B. "What Is a Medical Experiment? " *Canadian Medical Association Journal,* 113 (Oct. 4, 1975): 635–639.

Doane, B.K. and B.G. Quigley. "Psychiatric Aspects of Therapeutic Abortions," *Canadian Medical Association Journal,* 125 (1981): 427–432.

Doerflinger, Richard "Assisted Suicide: Pro-Choice or Anti-Life? " *Hastings Center Report* 9:1 (Jan/Feb 1989) suppl.: 16–19.

Donagan, Alan. "Informed Consent in Therapy and Experimentation," *The Journal of Medicine and Philosophy* 2:4 (Dec. 1977): 319–318.

Donceel, J.F. and S.J. Donceel "Abortion: Mediate and Immediate Animation," *Continuum* 5 (1967): 167–71.

Dorland's Medical Dictionary, 27 ed. Philadelphia: W.B.Saunders Co., 1988.

Drower, S. and E. Nash. "Therapeutic Abortion on Psychiatric Grounds," *South African Medical Journal* (1980) 54: 604–608 and 55: 643–647.

Drummond, M.F. *Principles of Economic Appraisal in Health Care.* Oxford: Oxford Medical Publications, 1980.

Drummond, Michael. "Guidelines for Health Technology Assessment: Economic Evaluation," in *Health Care Technology: Effectiveness, Efficiency and Public Policy.* Eds. Feeny, D., G. Guyatt, and P. Tugwell. Montreal: Institute for Research on Public Policy, 1986.

Dubos, Rene. "Health as Ability to Function" in *Contemporary Issues in Bioethics.* Eds. Beauchamp, T.C., and L. Walters. Belmont, Calif.: Dickenson Publishing Co., 1978.: 96–99.

Dunstan, G.R. "Moral and Social Issues Arising from AID: Law and Ethics of AID and Embryo Transfer," *CIBA Foundation Symposium* 17 (1973).

Dworkin, Ronald. *Taking Rights Seriously.* Cambridge: Harvard University Press, 1977.

Dworkin, Gerald. "Paternalism," *The Monist* 56 (Jan. 1972).

Edelstein, L. "The Professional Ethics of the Greek Physicians," Bulletin of the History of Medicine 1956, Vol. 30 reprinted in *Ancient Medicine.* Ed. Edelstein, L. Baltimore: Johns Hopkins U. Press, 1967.

Emson, H.E. *The Doctor and the Law: A Practical Guide for the Canadian Physician.* Toronto and Vancouver: Butterworths, 1989.

Engelhardt, Jr., H.T. *The Foundations of Bioethics.* Oxford and New York: Oxford University Press, 1986.

Engelhardt, Jr., H. T. "Human Well-Being and Medicine: Some Basic Value-Judgements in the Biomedical Sciences," reprinted in *Biomedical Ethics.* Eds. Mappes, T.A., and J.S. Zembaty. New York and London: McGraw-Hill, 1981.

Entralgo, P.L. *Doctor and Patient.* (trans. F. Partridge). N.Y.:World University Library, 1969.

Ethics Committee of the American Fertility Society, "Ethical Considerations of the New Reproductive Technologies," *Fertility and Sterility* 46:3 (Sept.1986) Supplement 1.

Faden, R.R. and T.L. Beauchamp. *A History and Theory of Informed Consent*. New York and Oxford: Oxford University Press, 1986.

Federation of Medical Women of Canada *Newsletter*, Vol.1 (October, 1989): 1.

Feeny, D., G. Guyatt, and P. Tugwell. *Health Care Technology: Effectiveness, Efficiency and Public Policy*. Montreal: Canadian Medical Association & The Institute for Research on Public Policy, 1986.

Feinberg, Joel. "Disease and Values," in *Doing and Deserving: Essays in the Theory of Responsibility*. Ed. Feinberg. J. Princeton:Princeton Univ. Press, 1974.: 253–55.

Feinberg, Joel. *Social Philosophy*. Engelwood Cliffs, N.J.:Prentice-Hall, 1973.: 52.

Feldman, David M. "The Ethical Implications of New Reproductive Techniques," in *Jewish Values in Bioethics*. Ed. Meier, Rabbi Levi. New York: Human Sciences Press, 1986.: 174–182.

Field, M.A. *Surrogate Motherhood*. Cambridge and London: Harvard Univ. Press, 1988.

Fitzgerald, P.J. "Acting and Refraining," *Analysis* 27:4 (1973): 133–139).

Flaherty, J. and L. Curtin. *Nursing Ethics*. Bowen, Maryland: Bradey, 1982.

Fletcher, Joseph. *The Ethics of Genetic Control*. New York: Doubleday, 1974.

Foot, Philippa. "The Problem of Abortion and the Principle of Double Effect," *Oxford Review* 5 (1967).

Foot, Philippa. "Euthanasia," *Philosophy and Public Affairs* 6:2 (Winter 1977).

Fowler, Gregory, Eric T. Juengst, and Burke K. Zimmerman, "Germ-Line Gene Therapy and the Clinical Ethos of Medical Genetics," *Theoretical Medicine* 10: 2 (June 1989) 151–165.

Frankena, W.K. "The Ethics of Respect for Life," in *Respect for Life in Medicine, Philosophy, and the Law*. Ed. Barker, Stephan F. Baltimore: Johns Hopkins Univ. Press, 1977.: 24–62.

Frankena, W.K. *Ethics*, 2nd ed. Englewood Cliffs, N.J.: Prentice-Hall, 1973.

Freedman, Benjamin and the McGill/Boston Research Group, "Nonvalidated Therapies and HIV Disease," *Hastings Center Report* 19:3 (June 1989): 14–20.

Frenkel, D.A. "Human Experimentation: Codes of Ethic," *Legal Medical Quarterly* 1:1 (1977): 7–14.

Fried, Charles. "The Lawyer as Friend," *The Yale Law Review* 85 (1976): 1060–1089.

Fried, Charles. *Medical Experimentation: Personal Integrity and Social Policy*. N.Y.: American Elsevier, 1974.

Friedman, R.C., J.T. Bigger, and D.S. Kornfeld. "The Intern and Sleep Loss," *New England Journal of Medicine*. 285:4 (July 22, 1971).

Friedmann, T. "Progress Towards Human Gene Therapy," *Science* 244 (16 June, 1989): 1275–1281.

Garbesi, G.C. "The Law of Assisted Suicide," *Issues in Law and Medicine* 1987, 3(2): 93–111.

Garrett, T.M., H.W. Baillie and R.M. Garrett. *Health Care Ethics: Principles and Problems* Englewood Cliffs, N.J.: Prentice- Hall, 1988.

Gauthier, David. "Unequal Need: A Problem of Equity in Access to Health Care," in the President's Commission for the Study of Ethical Problems in Medicine and Biomedical Research: *Securing Access to Health Care: the Ethical Implications of Differences in* the *Availability of Health Services*. U.S. Govt. Printing Office: Washington D.C., 1983. Volume 2, 179-206.: 179–105.

Gaylin, W. and R. Macklin, eds. *Who Speaks for the Child? The Problems of Proxy Consent*. New York and London: Plenum Press, 1982.

Gert, Bernard and Charles M. Culver, "Paternalistic Behaviour," *Philosophy and Public Affairs* 6 (1976): 45–47.

Goodman, E. and D. Goodman, "The Overselling of Genetic Anxiety," *Hastings Center Report*, 12:5 (Oct. 1982): 21.

Goosens, W. "Values in Health and Medicine," *Philosophy of Science* 47 (1980): 100–115.

Gordon, Robert M. *The Structure of Emotions: Investigations in Cognitive Philosophy*. New York: Cambridge Univ. Press, 1987.

Gordon, Harry H. "The Doctor-Patient Relationship: A Judaic Perspective," *The Journal of Medicine and Philosophy* vol. 8 (1983): 243–255.

Goslin, D.A., ed. *Handbook of Socialization Theory and Research*. Chicago: Rand McNally, 1969.

Gouvernement du Quebec, Conseil du Statut de la Femme, *General Opinion of the Conseil du Statu de la Femme in Regard to New Reproductive Technologies*. (Quebec City, 1989).

Gowdy, C.W. "A Guide to the Pharmacology of Placebos," *Canadian Medical Association Journal* 128 (1983): 921–5.

Graber, Glenn C. "On Paternalism in Health Care," in *Contemporary Issues in Biomedical Ethics*. Eds. Davis, John W., Barry Hoffmaster and Sarah Shorten. Clifton, N.J.: Humana Press, 1981.

Great Britain, Dept. of Health and Social Services, *Report of the Committee of Enquiry into Human Sterilization and Embryology*. Ed., Warnock, M. London, Her Majesty's Stationer's Office, 1984: "The Warnock Report".

Grobstein, C.L. "A Biological Perspective on the Origin of Human Life and Personhood," in *Defining Human Life: Medical, Legal, and Ethical Implications*. Eds. Shaw, M.W., and A.E. Doudera. Ann Arbor, Mich: AUPHA Press, 1983: 3-11.

Grubb, Andrew and David Pearl. "Sterilisation and the Courts," *Cambridge Law Journal* 1987 46(3): 439–464.

Guillemin, J.H. and L.L. Holmstrom. *Mixed Blessings: Intensive Care For Newborns*. N.Y. and Oxford: Oxford Univ. Press, 1986.

Hall, A. Emmett. *Report of the Royal Commission on Health Services*. Ottawa: Queen's Printer, 1964.

Hammerman, J. "Health Services: Their Success and Failure in Reaching the Aged Older Adult," in *Dominant Issues in Medical Sociology*. Eds. Schwartz, H.D. and R. Kart. Don Mills: Addison-Wesley, 1978: 407.

Handbook of Living Wills. New York: Society for the Right to Die, 1987.

Hare, R.M. *The Language of Morals*. Oxford: Oxford Univ. Press, 1952.

Harrover, M.R. "Social Status and the Moral Development of the Child," *British Journal of Educational Psychology* 4 (1934): 75–95.

Health Protection Branch and Pharmaceutical Manufacturers' Association of Canada. *Guidelines for the Conduct of Clinical Investigation*. Ottawa: Health Protection Branch, Health and Welfare Canada, 1985.

Health and Welfare Canada. *Report of the Advisory Committee on the Storage and Utilization of Human Sperm.* Ottawa: HWC, 1981.

Hinton, J.M. *Experiences.* Oxford: Clarendon Press, 1979.

Hobbes, Thomas. *Leviathan.* Harmondsworth: Pelican, 1968.

Hoffman, M.L. "Moral Development," in *Carmichael's Manual of Psychology*, 3rd. Ed. Mussner, P.H. New York: John Wiley and Sons, 1970, vol.2: 276–281.

Hofling, C.K., E. Brotzman, S. Dalrymple, N. Graves, and C.M. Pierce, "An Experimental Study in Nurse-Physician Relationships," *Journal of Nervous and Mental Disease* 143 (August 1966): 171–80.

Hume, David. *Treatise on Human Nature*, 2nd. edition. Ed. Selby-Bigge, L.A., Oxford: Clarendon Press, 1967.

Idler, Ellen. "Definition of Mental Health and Illness and Medical Sociology," *Society, Science and Medicine* 3A: 723–31.

Ingarden, Roman. *Man and Value.* (trans. A. Szylewicz) Dordrecht: Philosophia, 1984.

Ingelfinger, Franz. "Arrogance," *New England Journal of Medicine* 303 (1980): 1509.

Ingelfinger, Franz J. "Informed (But Uneducated) Consent," *The New England Journal of Medicine* 287 (August 31, 1972): 465–466.

Jackson, David L., and Stewart Youngner, "Patient Autonomy and 'Death With Dignity,'" *New England Journal of Medicine* 301 (1979): 404–408.

Jameton, A. *Nursing Practice: The Ethical Issues.* Toronto: Prentice Hall, 1984.

Jonas, Hans. "Philosophical Reflections on Experimenting with Human Subjects," in *Experimentation with Human Subjects.* Ed. Freund, P.A. New York: American Academy of Arts and Sciences, 1970.

Jones, J.H. *Bad Blood.* New York: Free Press, 1981.

Jospe, M. *The Placebo Effect in Healing.* Lexington, Mass.: Heath, 1978.

Kamisar, Yale. "Some Non-Religious Objections Against Proposed Mercy-Killing Legislation," *Minnesota Law Review* 42 (May 1958): 969–1042.

Kane, F.J., M. Feldman, J. Susheila, M.A. Lipton, "Emotional Reactions in Abortion Services Personnel," *Archives of General Psychiatry* 28 (1973): 409–414.

Kant, Immanuel. *Foundations of the Metaphysics of Morals.* New York: Bobbs-Merrill, 1959.

Kant, Immanuel. *Critique of Pure Reason.*

Karp, Lawrence E. "The Prenatal Diagnosis of Genetic Disease," in *Biomedical Ethics.* Eds. Mappes T.A. and J.S. Zembaty. New York and London: McGraw-Hill, 1978.: 458–64.

Kass, Leon. "Implications of Prenatal Diagnosis for the Human Right to Life," in *Biomedical Ethics.* Eds. Mappes T.A. and J.S. Zembaty. New York and London: McGraw-Hill, 1978.: 465.

Kass, Leon. "Regarding the End of Medicine and the Pursuit of Health," in *Contemporary Issues in Bioethics.* Eds. Beauchamp, T.L. and L. Walters. Belmont, Calif.: Wadsworth, 1981.:99-108. (Reprinted from *The Public Interest* 40 (Summer 1925).

Katz, Jay. *The Silent World of Doctor and Patient.* Free Press: New York, 1984.

Katz, Jay., and A.M. Capron. *Catastrophic Diseases: Who Decides What.* New York: Russell Sage, 1975.

Katz, Jay. *Experimenting With Human Beings.* New York: Russell Sage, 1972.

Katz, M.M., and G.Benil. "Blood Sugar Lowering Effects of Chlorpropamide and Tolbutamide: A Double Blind Study," *Diabetes* 14 (1965): 650–657.

Kenen, R.H., and R.M. Schmidt. "Stigmatization of Carrier Status: Social Implications of Heterozygote Genetic Screening Programs," *American Journal of Public Health*, 68 (1978): 116–120.

Ketchum, S., and C. Pierce. "Rights and Responsibilities," *Journal of Medicine and Philosophy* (1981): 271–279.

Keyserlingk, Edward W. *The Unborn Child's Right to Prenatal Care: A Comparative Law Perspective.* Montreal: McGill Legal Studies No.5, 1984.

Keyserlingk, Edward W. "Fetal Surgery: Establishing the Boundaries of the Unborn Child's Right to Prenatal Care," in *Biomedical Ethics and Fetal Therapy*. Eds. Nimrod, Carl, and Glenn Griener. Waterloo, Ont.: Wilfrid Laurier Press, 1988: 81–105.

Keyserlingk, Edward W. *Sanctity of Life or Quality of Life in the Context of Ethics, Medicine, and the Law.* Study Paper for the Law Reform Commission of Canada, Ottawa: Law Reform Commission, 1979.

Kirchheimer, Otto. "Criminal Omissions," *Harvard Law Review* 55 (1942).

Klarman, H.E., J.D. Francis, G.D. Rosenthal. "Cost-Effectiveness and Analysis Applied to the Treatment of Chronic Renal Disease," *Medical Care* 6 (1968): 48–54.

Klerman, Gerald L. "Mental Illness, the Medical Model, and Psychiatry," *The Journal of Medicine and Philosophy* 2:3 (1977): 222–243.

Klopfer, B. "Psychological Variables in Human Cancer," *Journal of Project Techniques* 21 (1957): 331–340.

Kluge, E.H.W. The Calculus of Discrimination: Discriminatory Resource Allocation for An Aging Population," in *Ethics and Aging: The Right to Live, the Right to Die.* Eds. Thornton, J.E. and E.R. Winkler. Vancouver: Univ. of B.C. Press, 1988: 84–97.

Kluge, E.H.W. "The Profession of Nursing and the Right to Strike," *Westminster Institute Review* 2:1 (1982): 3–6.

Kluge, E.H.W. "St. Thomas, Abortion and Euthanasia," *Philosophical Research Archives*, 1981/82.

Kluge, E.H.W. *The Ethics of Deliberate Death.* Port Washington: National University Publications, 1980.

Kluge, E.H.W. "Experimenting on Embryos," in *Ethical Problems in Reproductive Medicine*. Eds. Bromham, D., E. Forsyth, and M. Dalton. London: British Journal of Family Planning, 1988, Suppl.

Kluge, E.H.W. *The Practice of Death*. New Haven: Yale Univ. Press, 1975.

Kluge, E.H.W. "Placebos: Some Ethical Considerations," *CMAJ* 142: 4 (Feb.15, 1990): 293–295.

Kluge, E.H.W. "When Cesarian-Section Operations Imposed by Court Order Are Justified," *Journal of Medical Ethics* 14:4 (Dec. 1988): 206–211.

Kluge, E.H.W. "The Euthanasia of Radically Defective Neonates: Some Statutory Considerations," *Dalhousie Law Journal* 6:2 (Nov. 1980): 229–257.

Kluge, E.H.W., "Cerebral Death," *Theoretical Medicine* 5 (1984): 209–231.

Kluge, E.H.W., "Infanticide as the Murder of Persons," in *Infanticide and the Value of Life*. Ed. Kohl, M. Buffalo: N.Y.: Prometheus, 1978.

Kluge, E.H.W. "Medical Informatics and Education: The Profession as Gatekeeper," *Methods of Information in Medicine*. 28 (1989): 196–201.

Kluge, E.H.W. "Behaviour Alteration, the Law Reform Commission and the Courts: An Ethical Perspective," *Dalhousie Law Journal* 11:33 (October 1988): 864–884.

Kluge, E.H.W. "Designated Organ Donation: Private Choice in Social Context," *Hastings Center Report* (Sept./Oct. 1989): 10–16.

Kluge, E.H.W. "After 'Eve': Whither Proxy Decision-Making? ", *Canadian Medical Association Journal* 137 (October 15, 1987): 715–720.

Kluge, E.H.W. "In the Matter of Stephen Dawson: Right vs. Duty of Health Care," *Canadian Medical Association Journal* 129 (October 15, 1983): 815–818.

Kohl, Marvin, ed. *The Morality of Killing: Sanctity-of-Life, Abortion and Euthanasia*. London: Peter Owen, 1974.

Kohlberg, F.L. "Development of Children's Orientation towards A Moral Order: First Sequences in the Development of Moral Thought," *Vita Humana* 6 (1963).

Kopelman, Loretta. "Ethical Controversies in Medical Research: The Case of XYY Screening," *Perspectives in Biology and Medicine* 2 (Winter, 1978): 196–204.

Kuhse, Helga. *The Sanctity-of-Life Doctrine in Medicine: A Critique*. Oxford: Clarendon Press, 1987.

Kuwabara Y. "Development of Extrauterine Fetal Incubator," *Asian Medical Journal* 32 (8),(1989): 419–425.

Lalonde, M. *A New Perspective on the Health of Canadians*. Ottawa: Minster of Supply and Services, 1974.

Lappe, Marc. "The Limits of Genetic Inquiry," *Hastings Center Report* 17:4 (1987): 5–10.

Lauersen, N.H., and Wilson, K.H. "The role of long-acting vaginal suppositories of 15-ME–PGF 2x in first and second trimester abortion," *Journal of Advanced Prostaglandin Thromboxane Research* 8 (1980): 141–143.

Lauritzen, Paul. "What Price Parenthood? " *Hastings Center Report* 20:2 (March/April 1990): 38–46.

Law Reform Commission of Ontario. *Report on Artificial Human Reproduction*. Toronto: Ministry of the Attorney General, 1985.

Law Reform Commission of Canada, (Working Paper 26). *Medical Treatment and the Criminal Law*. Ottawa: Minister of Supply and Services, 1980.

Law Reform Commission of Canada, (Working Paper 33). *Homicide*. Ottawa: Minister of Supply and Services, 1984.

Law Reform Commission of Canada, (Working Paper 6). *Family Law*. Ottawa: Minister of Supply and Services, 1976.

Law Reform Commission of Canada, (Working Paper 61). *Biomedical Experimentation Involving Human Subjects*. Ottawa: Minister of Supply and Services, 1989.

Law Reform Commission of Canada, (Report 20). *Euthanasia, Suicide and Cessation of Treatment*. Ottawa: Minister of Supply and Services, 1983.

Law Reform Commission of Canada, (Working Paper 58). *Crimes Against the Foetus*. Ottawa: Minister of Supply and Services, 1989.

Law Reform Commission of Canada, (Working Paper 24). *Sterilization: Implications for Mentally Retarded and Mentally Ill Persons*. Ottawa: Minister of Supply and Services, 1978.

Law Reform Commission of Canada, (Working Paper 46). *Omission, Negligence and Endangering*. Ottawa: Minister of Supply and Services, 1985.

Law Reform Commission of Ontario. *Report on Artificial Human Reproduction and Related Matters*, 2 vols. Toronto: Ministry of the Attorney General, 1985.

Law Reform Commission of Canada, (Working Paper 28). *Euthanasia, Aiding Suicide and Cessation of Treatment*. Minister of Supply and Services: Ottawa, 1982.

Law Reform Commission of Saskatchewan, *Tentative Proposals for a Human Artificial Insemination Act*. Saskatoon: LRCS, 1987.

Lenow, J.L. "The Fetus as Patient: Emerging Rights as a Person?," *American Journal of Law and Medicine*, 9:1 (Spring 1983): 1–29.

Lewis, C.S. *The Abolition of Man*. New York: Collier-Macmillan, 1965.

Light, D.W. "Corporate Medicine for Profit," *Scientific American* 155:6 (Dec. 1986).

Linden, A. *Canadian Tort Law*, third ed. Toronto: Butterworths, 1982.

Lipkin, M. "Suggestion and Healing," *Perspectives in Biology and Medicine*. 20 (1984): 121–126.

Macklin, R. *Mortal Choices*. N.Y.:Pantheon Books, 1987.

Mady, Theresa. "Surrogate Mothers: The Legal Issues," *American Journal of Law and Medicine* 9:1 (Spring 1983).

Maguire, Daniel. *Death by Choice*. N.Y.: Doubleday, 1974.

Mahowald, Mary B. "Is There Life After Roe v. Wade?" *Hastings Center Report* 19:4 (July/August, 1989): 22–29.

Makdur, I. "Sterilization and Abortion from the Point of View of Islam" in *Islam and Family Planning*, vol. 2 (271).

Mallary, S.D., B. Gert and C.M. Culver. "Family Coercion and Valid Consent," *Theoretical Medicine* 7:2 (June, 1986): 123–126.

Mangan, J.T., (Jesuit), "A Historical Analysis of the Principle of Double Effect," *Theological Studies*, 10 (1949): 40–61.

Martin, D.C., J.D. Arnold, T.F. Zimmermann, R.H. Richart. "Human Subjects in Clinical Research—A Report of Three Studies," *New England Journal of Medicine*, 279 (1968).

Masters, Roger. "Is Contract and Adequate Basis for Medical Ethics?" *Hastings Center Report* 5 (Dec. 1975): 24–28.

May, R. "Code and Covenant or Philanthropy and Contract?" in *Ethics in Medicine: Historical Perspectives and Contemporary Concerns*. Eds. Reiser, S.J., A.J. Dyck, and W.J. Curran. Cambridge, Mass.: MIT Press, 1977: 65–76.

McCormick, R.A. "Proxy Consent in Experimentation Situation," *Perspectives in Biology and Medicine* 18:1 (1974): 3–20.

McCormick, R.A. *Health and Medicine in the Catholic Tradition*. New York: Crossroad, 1984.

McLaren, Angus. "The Creation of a Haven for 'Human Thoroughbreds': the Sterilization of the Feebleminded and the Mentally Ill in British Columbia," *Canadian Historical Review*, 67 (2) (1986): 127–50.

Medical Research Council of Canada. *Guidelines on Research Involving Human Subjects*. Ottawa: Medical Research Council, 1987.

Medical Research Council of Canada Discussion Paper. *Guidelines for Research on Somatic Cell Therapy in Humans*. Ottawa: Medical Research Council, 1990.

Mehler, Barry. "Eliminating the Inferior: American and Nazi Sterilization Programs," *Science for the People* 19:6 (1987): 14–18.

Melzack, R. *The Puzzle of Pain.* New York: Basic Books, 1973.

Milby, T.H. "The New Biology and the Question of Personhood: Implications for Abortion," *American Journal of Law and Medicine* 9:1 (Spring 1983): 31–41.

Millis, J.S. "Wisdom? Health? Can Society Guarantee Them?", *New England Journal of Medicine,* 283 (July 30, 1970): 260–61.

Milner, E. *Human Neural and Behavioural Development.* Springfield: Thomas, 1967.

Milunsky, A. and G.J.Annas. eds. *Genetics and the Law.* New York: Plenum Press, 1976.

Moore, G.E. *Principia Ethica.* Oxford: Oxford Univ. Press, 1928.

Moore, G.E. *Ethics.* London: Cambridge Univ. Press, 1912.

Morreim, Haavi. "The Concepts of Patient Competence," *Theoretical Medicine* 4:3 (October 1983): 231–51.

Moskop, John C. "The Nature and Limits of the Physician's Authority," in *Doctors, Patients and Society: Power and Authority in Medical Care.* Eds. Staum, Martin S. and Donald E. Larson. Waterloo: Wilfred Laurier Univ.Press, 1981: 29–44.

Mueller, H.J. "Genetic Progress by Voluntary Conducted Germinal Choice," in *Fabricated Man: The Ethics of Genetic Control.* Ramsey, Paul. New Haven and London: Yale University Press, 1970.

Mueller, H.J. "Human Evolution by Voluntary Choice of Germ Plasm," reprinted in *Interpretation and Reflection: Basic Issues in Medical Ethics.* Ed. Munson, Donald. Belmont, Calif.: Wadsworth, 1979.: 349-358.

Murray, R.F. "Problems Behind the Promise: Ethical Issues in Mass Genetic Screening," *Hastings Center Report* 2 (April 1979): 46–7.

Murray, T.H.E. "Gifts of the Body and the Needs of Strangers," *Hastings Center Report* 17:2 (1987): 30–38.

Muyskens, J. *Moral Problems in Nursing: A Philosophical Investigation.* Lanham, M.D.: Rowman & Littlefield, 1982.

National Commission for the Protection of Human Subjects of Biomedical and Behavioral Research. *The Belmont Report: Ethical Principles for the Protection of Human Subjects of Research.* (Washington, D.C: U.S. Government Printing Office, 1978) pub. no. 78–0012, App. 1–0013, App. 2–004.

National Commission for the Protection of Human Subjects of Biomedical and Behavioral Research, Report and Recommendation. *Research Involving Children.* (Washington, D.C. DHEW 1977).

National Commission for the Protection of Human Subjects of Biomedical and Behavioral Research. *Appendix: Research on the Fetus* (1975) DHEW No. (05): 76–128.

Ney, P.G. and A.R. Wickett. "Mental Health and Abortion: Review and Analysis," *Psychiatric Journal of the University of Ottawa* 14:4 (Nov., 1989): 506–516.

Nicholson, R.H. *Medical Research with Children: Ethics, Law and Practice.* Oxford: Oxford University Press 1986.

Nirje, B. "The Normalization Principle and its Human Management Implications," in *Changing Patterns in Residential Services for the Mentally Retarded.* Eds. Kugel, R.B. and W. Wolfensburger. Resident's Committee on Mental Retardation: Waskington, D.C.: Govt. Printing Office, 1969.

Nordenfelt, Lennart. *On the Nature of Health.* Dordrecht and Boston: D.Reidel Pub.Co.: 1987.

Nuremberg Code, in *Trials of War Criminals before the Nuremberg Military Tribunal*. Washington D.C.: U.S. Government Printing Office, 1948.

O'Hair, Dan. "Patient Preference for Persuasion," *Theoretical Medicine* 7 (1986): 147–164.

Omran, A. R. "Abortion in the Natality Transition in Moslem Countries," in *Islam and Family Planning* 2 (271).

Outka, Gene. "Social Justice and Equal Access to Health Care," reprinted in *Biomedical Ethics*. Eds. Mappes T.A. and J.S. Zembaty. New York and St. Louis: McGraw-Hill, 1981: 523–531.

Overall, Christine. *Ethics and Human Reproduction: A Feminist Analysis*. Boston: Allen and Unwin, 1987.

Parks, L.C. et al. "Effects of Informed Consent in Research Patients and Study Results," *Journal of Nervous and Mental Diseases* 195 (1976): 349–357.

Parsons, Talcott. *Essays in Sociological Theory*. Glencoe, Ill.: The Free Press, 1954.

Parsons, F.M. "Selection of Patients for Haemodialysis," *British Medical Journal*. (March 11, 1967): 622–624).

Patenaude, Andrea Farkas, Joel M. Rappeport, and Brian R. Smith. "Physician's Influence on Informed Consent for Bone Marrow Transplantation," *Theoretical Medicine* 7 (1986): 165–179.

Paton, A.J. *The Categorical Imperative*. London: Hutchinson 1947.

Paulson, R. "Fatigue in Medical Personnel," *Journal of the American Medical Association* 246:2 (July 10, 1982).

Percival, Thomas. *Medical Ethics: or a Code of Institutes and Precepts, Adapted to the Professional Conduct of Physicians and Surgeons*. London: Russell and Bickerstaff, 1803.

Perry, Clifton. "Wrongful Life and Comparison of Harms," *Westminster Institute Review* 1:4 (1982): 7–9.

Perry, R.B. *Realms of Value*. Cambridge, Mass.: Harvard Univ. Press, 1954.

Piaget, J. *The Moral Judgement of the Child*. (trans.) London: Routhledge and Kegan Paul, London, 1932.

Picard, E. *Legal Liability of Doctors and Hospitals in Canada*. Toronto: Carswell 1984.

Picard, Ellen. "The Doctor-Patient Relationship and the Law," in *Doctors, Patients and Society: Power and Authority in Medical Care*. Eds. Staum, M.S., and D.E. Larsen. Waterloo, Ont.: Wilfrid Laurier University Press, 1981: 45–57.

Pilpel, H. "Personhood, Abortion and the Right to Privacy" in *Defining Human Life*. Eds. Shaw M.W., and A.E. Doudera. Ann Arbor: AUPHA Press, 1983: 154.

Plato, *Republic*.

Pope Paul VI, Encyclical Letter "Humanae Vitae," *Acta Apostolicae Sedis* LX: 9 (1968).

Pope Pius XII, "Prolongation of Life: Allocution to an International Congress of Anesthesiologists," Nov. 24, 1957. *Osservatore Romano* 4 (1957).

Pope John Paul II, *Donum vitae*: "Instruction on Respect for Human Life in its Origin and on the Dignity of Procreation—Replies to Certain Questions of the Day," given at Vatican City, Rome, from the Sacred Congregation for the Doctrine of the Faith, approved and ordered for publication by the Supreme Pontiff, John Paul II, February 22, 1987.

Powledge, T.M. "Genetic Screening and Personal Freedom," in *Intervention and Reflection.* Ed. Munson, Donald. Belmont, Calif.:Wadsworth, 1979.: 371-375.

Powledge, T.M., and Joseph Fletcher. "Guidelines for the Ethical, Social, and Legal Issues in Prenatal Diagnosis," *New England Journal of Medicine* 300:4 (1979): 168–172.

President's Commission for the Study of Ethical Problems in Medicine and Biomedical and Behavioral Research. *Securing Access to Health Care,* (3 vols.) Washington D.C.: U.S. Govt. Printing Office, 1983.

President's Commission for the Study of Ethical Problem in Medicine and Biomedical and Behavioral Research. *Splicing Life: a Report on the Social and Ethical Issues of Genetic Engineering with Human Beings.* Washington, D.C.: U.S. Govt. Printing Office, 1982.

President's Commission of the Study of Ethical Problems in Medicine and Biomedical and Behavioral Research. *Deciding to Forego Life-Sustaining Treatment: A Report on the Ethical, Medical and Legal Issues in Treatment Decisions.* Washington D.C.: U.S. Govt. Printing Office, 1983.

Prosser, W.L. *Handbook of the Law of Torts.* 4th ed. Minnesota: West Publishing Co., 1971.

Purdy, L.M. "Genetic Diseases: Can Having Children be Immoral? " in *Genetics Now: Ethical Issues in Genetic Research.* Ed. Buckley, J.J. Washington, D.C.: Univ. Press of America, 1978.

Pursel, V.G. et al. "Genetic Engineering of Livestock," *Science* 244 (16 June, 1989): 1281–1288.

Queensland, *Report of the Special Committee Appointed by the Queensland Government to Enquire into the Laws Relating to Artificial Insemination, In Vitro Fertilization and Other Related Matters* (1984)

Rachels, James. L.C. Parks and L. Covi. "Non-blind Placebo Trials," *Archives of General Psychiatry* 124 (1965): 334–345.

Rachels, James F. "Euthanasia," in *Matters of Life and Death: New Introductory Essays in Moral Philosophy.* Reagan, Tom. New York: Random House, 1980.: 28–38.

Rachels, James F. "Who Shall Live When Not All Can Live? " *Soundings: An Interdisciplinary Journal* 53 (Winter, 1970): 339–355.

Radin, M.J. "Market-Inalienability," *Harvard Law Review,* 100 (June 1987): 1930.

Ramsey, P. *The Patient as a Person.* New Haven: Yale, 1970.

Ramsey, P. *The Ethics of Fetal Research.* New Haven: Yale, 1975.

Rawls, John. *A Theory of Justice.* Cambridge: Harvard Univ. Press, 1971.

Reilly, P. *Genetics, Law and Social Policy.* Cambridge: Harvard Univ. Press, 1977.

Report of the Commission of Enquiry of the German Bundestag, Prospects and Risks of Genetic Engineering, Parts I and II (Deutscher Bundestag, 10. Wahlperiode: Bonn 1987).

Report of the Consultative Group on Ethics, The Canada Council. *Ethics.* Ottawa: Minister of Supply and Services, 1977.

Rescher, Nicholas. "The Allocation of Exotic Medical Lifesaving Therapy," *Ethics* 79 (1969): 173–180.

Roblin, Richard. "Human Genetic Therapy: Outlook and Apprehensions," in *Health Handbook.* Ed. Chacko, G.K. New York: Elsevier-North Holland Pub. Co., 1979.: 108–112.

Rosenberg, Leon. "Towards Newer Genetics," in *Defining Human Life*. Eds. Shaw, M.W., and A.E. Doudera. Ann Arbor: AUPHA Press, 1983.

Rosner, F. *Modern Medicine and Jewish Law*. New York: Yeshiva University. 1972.

Ross, W.R. *The Right and the Good.* Oxford: Clarendon Press, 1938.

Rozovsky, L.E. *Canadian Hospital Law: A Practical Guide*. Ottawa: Canadian Hospital Association, 1979.

Rozovsky, L.E. and F.A. "Suicide and the Law," *Canadian Critical Care Nursing Journal* 5:3 (Sept/Oct., 1988): 24–25.

Sacred Congregation for the Doctrine of the Faith. *Declaration on Procured Abortion*. Rome: Vatican, 1985.

Sade R.M, and A.B.Redfern. "Euthanasia," *New England Journal of Medicine*. 292:16 (April 17, 1975).

Sade, R.M. "The Patient's Right to Choose," IATROFON 10:1 (1990).

Sade, R. M. "Medical Care as a Right: A Refutation," *New England Journal of Medicine* 285:23 (Dec.2, 1971): 1288–92.

Savage, H. S., and Carla McKague. "Competency and Proxy Decision-Making," in *Mental Health Law in Canada*. Savage, H. S., and Carla McKague. Toronto and Vancouver: Butterworths, 1987: 114–124.

Savage, H. S. and Carla McKague. *Mental Health Law in Canada*. Toronto and Vancouver: Butterworths, 1987.

Schelling, Thomas. "The Life You Save May Be Your Own," in *Problems in Public Expenditure Analysis*. Ed. Chase, Jr., S.B. Washington, D.C.: The Brookings Institute, 1966.: 127–166.

Schmeiser, Douglas A. "Living Wills and Medical Treatment of the Terminally Ill," *Health Management Forum* 2:3 (Fall 1989): 32–37.

Schweitzer, Albert. *Civilization and Ethics*, 3rd ed. London: Black, 1949.

Sedgewick, Peter. "What is Illness? " *The Hastings Center Studies* 1:3 (1973).

Shaw, J. "Dilemmas of 'Informed Consent' in Children," *New England Journal of Medicine*. (1973): 805A.

Shaw, Margery. "Preconception and Prenatal Tests," in *Genetics and the Law II*. Eds. Milunsky, A. and G. Annas. New York: Plenum Press, 1980.

Sider, R.C. and C.D. Clements, "Patients' Ethical Obligation for their Health," *Journal of Medical Ethics* 1984; 10: 142.

Sidgewick, Henry. *The Methods of Ethics*. London, 1847.

Siegler, Mark. "A Right to Health Care: Ambiguity, Professional Responsibility and Patient Liberties," *Journal of Medicine and Philosophy* 4:2 (1979): 148–57.

Silvestre, L., C. Dubois, M. Renault, Y. Rezvani, E. Baulieu, and A. Ulmann. "Voluntary Interruption of Pregnancy with Miferistone (RU–486) and a Prostaglandin Analogue: A Large-scale French Experience," *New England Journal of Medicine* 322:10 (March 8, 1990): 645–648.

Sim, M. and R. Neisser. "Postabortive Psychosis: A Report from Two Centers," in *The Psychological Aspects of Abortion*. Eds. Mall, D. and F. Watts. Washington: Univ. Publications of America, 1979.: 1–13.

Simmons, Beth. "Problems in Deceptive Medical Procedures: An Ethical and Legal Analysis of the Administration of Placebos," *Journal of Medical Ethics* 4 (1978): 172–181.

Simon, Nathan M. "Psychological and Emotional Indications for Therapeutic Abortion," in *Abortion*. Ed. Sloane, R.B. New York: Grune and Stratton, 1971.

Singer, Peter. *Animal Liberation*. New York: Avon Books, 1975.

Singer, Peter. "A Review of Public Policies to Procure and Distribute Kidneys for Transplantation," *Archives of Internal Medicine* 150:3 (March 1990): 523–527.

Slevin, M.L., L.H. Stubbs, J. Plant, P. Wilson, W.M. Gregory, P.J. Armes, and S.M. Dower, "Attitudes to Chemotherapy: Comparing Views of Patients with Cancer with those of Doctors, Nurses, and the General Public," *British Medical Journal* 300 (June 2, 1990): 1458–1460.

Sloate, M. "The Morality of Wealth," in *World Hunger and Moral Obligation*. Eds. Atkins, H.D., and H. La Follette. Englewood Cliffs, New Jersey: Prentice-Hall 1977.

Smith, O.H., H.A. Twig, and I.L. Croft, "Prostaglandins in Gel: A Method to Minimize Nursing Involvement," *British Medical Journal* 282: 2012, (1981).

Smith, David H., and Lloyd S. Pettegrew, "Mutual Persuasion as a Model for Doctor-Patient Communication," *Theoretical Medicine* 7 (1986): 127–146.

Society of Obstetricians and Gynaecologists of Canada, "Statements on In-Vitro Fertilization and Embryo Transfer," *Bulletin of the SOGC* 6:3 (May/June 1984).

Somerville, M. "Structuring the Issues in Informed Consent," *McGill Law Journal* 26 (1981).

Somerville, M. *Consent to Medical Care*. Study Paper for the Law Reform Commission of Canada (Ottawa, 1980).

Somerville, M. "Birth Technology, Parenting and 'Deviance'," *International Journal of Law and Psychiatry* 5 (1982): 123.

South Australia, *Report of the Working Party on In Vitro Fertilization and Artificial Insemination by Donor* (1984).

Spiro, H.K. "The Placebo Response," in *Modern Perspectives in World Psychiatry*, 2nd ed. Ed. Howells, J.G. Edinburgh: Oliver and Boyd, 1971.

Spiro, H.K. and E. Spiro. "Patient-Provider Relationship and the Placebo Effect," in *Behavioral Health: A Handbook of Health Enhancement and Disease Prevention*. Malarazzo, J.D., S.M. Weiss, J.A. Hurd, and N.E. Miller. New York: John Wiley and Sons, 1984.: 372.

Spiro, H.K. *Doctors, Patients and Placebos*. New Haven: Yale Univ. Press, 1986.

Stanton, J.R. and R.L. Maker. "The Suicide Sell," *Senior Patient* (Nov./Dec. 1989): 51–54.

Steinbacher, Roberta. "Futuristic Implications of Sex Preselection," in *The Custom-Made Child? Women-Centered Perspectives*. Eds. Holmes, H.B., B.B. Hoskins and M. Cross. Clifton, N.Y.: Human Press, 1981.

Stevenson, C.L. *Ethics and Language*. New Haven: Yale Univ. Press, 1944.

Storch, Janet. *Patients' Rights, Ethical and Legal Issues in Health Care and Nursing*. Toronto: McGraw-Hill, 1984.

Sugden, R. and A. Williams. *The Principles of Practical Cost-Benefit Analysis*. Oxford: Oxford University Press, 1978.

Sumner, L.W. "Toward a Credible View of Abortion," *Canadian Journal of Philosophy* 4 (Sept., 1974): 163–181.

Swartz, N., ed. *Perceiving, Sensing, Knowing*. New York: Doubleday, 1964.

Swint, J.H., V.L. Carson, L.W. Reynolds, G.H. Thomas, and H.H. Kazazian, "The Economic Returns to a Community and Hospital Screening Program for a Genetic Screening," *Preventive Medicine*, 8 (1979): 465–470.

Szaz, T.S. and Marc H. Hollender, "A Contribution to the Philosophy of Medicine: The Basic Models of the Doctor-Patient Relationship," *Archives of Internal Medicine* 97 (1956): 585–592.

Szaz, T.S. *Ideology and Insanity*. New York: Doubleday, 1970.

Szaz, T.S. *The Myth of Mental Illness: Foundations of a Theory of Personal Conduct*. New York: Hoeber-Harper, 1961.

Templin, M.S. et al., "Placebos: How Much Do You Know About Them?" *Nursing Life* 4 (Nov./Dec. 1984): 52–53.

Thielicke, H.T. *Theologische Ethik*. Tubingen, 1964.

Thielicke, H. T. "The Doctor as Judge of Who Shall Live and Who Shall Die," in *Who Shall Live? Medicine, Technology, Ethics*. Ed. Vaux, K. Philadelphia: Fortress Press, 1970.

Thomasma, D.C. "Beyond Medical Paternalism and Patient Autonomy: A Model of Physician Conscience for the Physician-Patient Relationship," *Annals of Internal Medicine* 98:3 (Feb.1983): 243–247.

Thornton, J., and E. Winkler. *Ethics and Aging*. Vancouver: U.B.C. Press, 1988.

Tomlinson, Thomas. "The Physician's Influence on Patients' Choices," *Theoretical Medicine* 7:2 (June, 1986): 109–121.

Tooley, Michael. *An Analysis of Abortion and Infanticide*. Oxford: Clarendon Press, 1983.

Tooley, Michael. "Abortion and Infanticide," *Philosophy and Public Affairs* 2:2 (1972): 137–165.

Tormey, J.F. "Ethical Considerations for Prenatal Genetic Diagnosis," *Clinical Obstetrics and Gynecology* 19 (Dec. 1976): 957–963.

Trubo, Richard. *An Act of Mercy*. Los Angeles: Nash, 1973.

U.S. Office of Technology Assessment. *Artificial Insemination*. (Washington, D.C. 1987)

U.K., Department of Health and Social Security. *Report of the Committee of Inquiry into Human Fertilization and Embryology* (Cmnd. 9314, 1984).

Urmson, J.O. "Saints and Heroes," reprinted in *Moral Concepts*. Ed. Feinberg, Joel. Oxford: Oxford Univ. Press, 1979.

Veatch, Robert M. "Just Social Institutions and the Right to Health Care," *Journal of Medicine and Philosophy*, 4: 2 (1979).

Veatch, Robert M. *Death, Dying and the Biological Revolution: Our Last Quest for Responsibility*. New Haven: Yale Univ. Press, 1976.: 18–19.

Veatch, Robert M. "Generalization of Expertise," *Hastings Center Studies* 1:2 (1973): 29–40.

Veatch, Robert M. "Who Should Pay for Smokers' Medical Care?", *Hastings Center Report* 4 (Nov.1974): 8–9.

Veatch, Robert M. "Editorial," *Medical Ethics Advisor* 6:1 (1990).

Veatch, Robert M. *A Theory of Medical Ethics*. New York: Basic Books, 1981.

Veatch, Robert M., "Models for Ethical Practice in a Revolutionary Age," *Hastings Center Report* 2:3 (1972): 5–7).

Veatch, Robert M. "Medical Ethics: Professional or Universal?" *Harvard Theological Review* 65 (1972): 531–559.

Vines, Gail. "Bangladeshis Coerced into Sterilization," *New Scientist*, 19 Sept. 1985, 107(1474): 21–22.

Wanzer, S.H., Federman, D.D., Adelstein, F.S.J., et al., Letter in the *New England Journal of Medicine*, 1989; 320: 844–849.

Wasserstrom, R., "Ethical Issues Involved in Experimentation on the Non-viable Human Fetus," in U.S. National Commission for the Protection of Human Subjects, *Research on the Fetus*. Dept. of Health, Education, and Welfare: Washington, D.C., 1975.: 9-1--9-10.

Weithorn, L.A. and S.B. Campbell. "The Competency of Children and Adolescents to Make Informed Treatment Decisions," *Child Development* 53 (1987): 1589–98.

Wertz, D.C. and J.C. Fletcher. "Moral Reasoning Among Medical Geneticists in Eighteen Nations," *Theoretical Medicine* 10:2 (June 1989): 123–138.

Westermarck, E. *The Evolution and Development of the Moral Ideal*. New York: MacMillan, 1906.

Westermarck, E. *Ethical Relativity*. New York: Harcourt Brace, 1932.

Westfall, David. "Beyond Abortion: The Potential Reach of a Human Life Amendment," *AJLM* 8:2 (Summer 1982): 97–135.

Wikler, D. "Philosophical Perspectives on Access to Health Care: An Introduction," in President's Commission for the Study of Ethical Problems in Medicine and Biomedical and Behavioral Research, *Securing Access to Health Care: The Ethical Implications of Differences in the Availabilty of Health Services*. U.S. Govt. Printing Office: Washington, D.C., 1983.: 3 vols. Volume 2: 109-152.

Wikler, D. "Paternalism and the Mildly Retarded," *Philosophy and Public Affairs* 8 (1979): 337–392.

Williamson, N.E. "Boys or Girls? Parents' Preferences and Sex Control," *Population Bulletin* 33:1 (Jan. 1978): 3–35.

Wilson, R.W. and G.J. Shoichet, eds. *Moral Development and Politics*. New York: Praeger, 1980.

Wilson, R.W. "Voluntary Sterilization: Legal and Ethical Aspects," *Legal Medical Quarterly* 3 (1979): 13–23.

Winslow, Gerald. "Anencephalic Infants as Organ Sources: Should the Law be Changed? A Reply," *The Journal of Paediatrics* 115:5 (Part 1, November 1989): 829–832.

Witkin, A.A. et al., "Criminality in XYY and XXY Men," *Science* 1983 (Aug. 13, 1976): 547–55.

Wittgenstein, Ludwig. *Philosophical Investigations*. Oxford: Blackwells, 1954.

World Health Organization. "The Concept of Health," *The First Ten Years of the World Health Organization* Geneva: WHO, 1958.

World Medical Association, The. "The Declaration of Helsinki," 1964. Reprinted in *The World Medical Association Handbook of Declarations*. Farnborough: WMA, 1985.

World Medical Association, The. "An International Code of Medical Ethics," *World Medical Association Bulletin* 1: 3 (1949).

Young, Robert. "Some Criteria for Making Decisions Concerning the Distribution of Scarce Medical Resources," *Theory and Decision* 6 (1975): 439–455.

Appendix 1
Guide To The Ethical Behaviour Of Physicians

The Canadian Medical Association, April 1990

RESPONSIBILITIES TO THE PATIENT

An Ethical Physician

Standard of care
1. will practise the art and science of medicine to the best of his/her ability;
2. will continue self education to improve his/her standards of medical care;

Respect for patient
3. will practise in a fashion that is above reproach and will take neither physical, emotional nor financial advantage of the patient;

Patient's rights
4. will recognize his/her professional limitations and, when indicated, recommend to the patient that additional opinions and services be obtained;
5. will recognize that a patient has the right to accept or reject any physician and any medical care recommended. The patient having chosen a physician has the right to request of that physician opinions from other physicians of the patient's choice;
6. will keep in confidence information derived from a patient or from a colleague regarding a patient, and divulge it only with the permission of the patient except when otherwise required by law;
7. when acting on behalf of a third party will ensure that the patient understands the physician's legal responsibility to the third party before proceeding with the examination;
8. will recommend only diagnostic procedures that are believed necessary to assist in the care of the patient, and therapy that is believed necessary for the well-being of the patient. The physician will recognize a responsibility in advising the patient of the findings and recommendations and will exchange such information with the patient as it is necessary for the patient to reach a decision;
9. will, upon a patient's request, supply the information that is required to enable the patient to receive any benefits to which the patient may be entitled;

10. will be considerate of the anxiety of the patient's next-of-kin and cooperate with them in the patient's interest;

Choice of patient

11. will recognize the responsibility of a physician to render medical service to any person regardless of colour, religion or political belief;
12. shall, except in an emergency, have the right to refuse to accept a patient;
13. will render all possible assistance to any patient, where and urgent need for medical care exists;
14. will, when the patient is unable to give consent and an agent of the patient is unavailable to give consent, render such therapy as the physician believes to be in the patient's interest;

Continuity of care

15. will, if absent, ensure the availability of medical care to his/her patients if possible; will, once having accepted professional responsibility for an acutely ill patient, continue to provide services until they are no longer required, or until arrangements have been made for the services of another suitable physician; may, in other situation, withdraw from the responsibility for the care of any patient provided that the patient is given adequate notice of that intention;

Personal morality

16. will inform the patient when personal morality or religious conscience prevent the recommendation of some form of therapy;

Clinical research

17. will ensure that, before initiating clinical research involving humans, such research is appraised scientifically and ethically and approved by a responsible committee and is sufficiently planned and supervised that the individuals are unlikely to suffer any harm. The physician will ascertain that previous research and the purpose of the experiment justify this additional method of investigation. Before proceeding, the physician will obtain the consent of all involved persons or their agents, and will proceed only after explaining the purpose of the clinical investigation and any possible health hazard that can be reasonably foreseen;

The dying patient

18. will allow death to occur with dignity and comfort when death of the body appears to be inevitable;
19. may support the body when clinical death of the brain has occurred, but need not prolong life by unusual or heroic means;

Transplantation

20. may, when death of the brain has occurred, support cellular life in the body when some parts of the body might be used to prolong life or improve the health of others;
21. will recognize a responsibility to a donor of organs to be transplanted and will give to the donor or the donor's relatives full disclosure of the intent and purpose of the procedure; in the case of a living donor, the physician will also explain the risks of the procedure;
22. will refrain from determining the time of death of the donor patient if there is a possibility of being involved as a participant in the transplant procedure, or when

his/her association with the proposed recipient might improperly influence professional judgement;

23. may treat the transplant recipient subsequent to the transplant procedure in spite of having determined the time of death of the donor;

Fees to patients

24. will consider, in determining professional fees, both the nature of the service provided and the ability of the patient to pay, and will be prepared to discuss the fee with the patient.

RESPONSIBILITIES TO THE PROFESSION

An Ethical Physician

Personal conduct

25. will recognize that the profession demands integrity from each physician and dedication to its search for truth and to its service to mankind;
26. will recognize that self discipline of the profession is a privilege and that each physician has a continuing responsibility to merit the retention of this privilege;
27. will behave in a way beyond reproach and will report to the appropriate professional body any conduct by a colleague which might be generally considered as being unbecoming to the profession;
28. will behave in such a manner as to merit the respect of the public members of the medical profession;
29. will avoid impugning the reputation of any colleague;

Contracts

30. will, when aligned in practice with other physicians, insist that the standards enunciated in this Code of Ethics and the Guide to the Ethical Behaviour of Physicians be maintained;
31. will only enter into a contract regarding professional services which allows fees derived from physicians' services to bo controlled by the physician rendering the services;
32. will enter into a contract with an organization only if it will allow maintenance of professional integrity;
33. will only offer to a colleague a contract which has terms and conditions equitable to both parties;

Reporting medical research

34. will first communicate to colleagues, through recognized scientific channels, the results of any medical research, in order that those colleagues may establish an opinion of its merits before they are presented to the public;

Addressing the public

35. will recognize a responsibility to give the generally held opinions of the profession when interpreting scientific knowledge to the public; when presenting an opinion which is contrary to the general held opinion of the profession, the physician will so indicate and will avoid any attempt to enhance his/her own personal professional reputation;

Advertising

36. will build a professional reputation based on ability and integrity, and will only advertise professional services of make professional announcements as regulated by legislation or as permitted by the provincial medical licensing authority;
37. will avoid advocacy of any product when identified as a member of the medical profession;
38. will avoid the use of secret remedies;

Consultation

39. will request the opinion of an appropriate colleague acceptable to the patient when diagnosis or treatment is difficult or obscure, or when the patient requests it. Having requested the opinion of a colleague, the physician will make available all relevant information and indicate clearly whether the consultant is to assume the continuing care of the patient during this illness;
40. will, when consulted by a colleague, report in detail all the pertinent findings and recommendations to the attending physician and may outline an opinion to the patient. The consultant will continue with the care of the patient only at the specific request of the attending physician and with the consent of the patient;

Patient care

41. will cooperate with those individuals who, in the opinion of the physician, may assist in the care of the patient;
42. will make available to another physician, upon the request of the patient, a report of pertinent findings and treatment of the patient;
43. will provide medical services to a colleague and dependant family without fee, unless specifically requested to render an account;
44. will limit self-treatment or treatment of family members to minor or emergency services only; such treatments should be without fee;

Financial arrangements

45. will avoid any personal profit motive in ordering drugs, appliances or diagnostic procedures from any facility in which the physician has a financial interest;
46. will refuse to accept amy commission or payment, direct or indirect, for any service rendered to a patient by other persons excepting direct employees and professional colleagues with whom there is a formal partnership or similar agreement.

RESPONSIBILITIES TO SOCIETY

Physicians who act under the principles of this Guide to the Ethical Behaviour for Physicians will find that they have fulfilled many of their responsibilities to society.

An Ethical Physician

47. will strive to improve the standards of medical services in the community; will accept a share of the profession's responsibility to society in matters relating to the health and safety of the public, health education, and legislation affecting the health or well-being of the community;
48. will recognize the responsibility as a witness to assist the court in arriving at a just decision;

49. will, in the interest of providing good and adequate medical care, support the opportunity of other physicians to obtain hospital privileges according to individual personal and professional qualifications.

"The complete physician is not a man apart and cannot content himself with the practice of medicine alone, but should make his contribution, as does any other good citizen, towards the well-being and betterment of the community in which he lives."

Reprinted with the permission of the Canadian Medical Association.

Appendix 2
Code of Ethics: Canadian Nurses Association

~ PREAMBLE ~

Nursing practice can be defined generally as a "dynamic, caring, helping relationship in which the nurse assists the client to achieve and maintain optimal health."[*] Nurse educators, administrators and researchers, although not necessarily assisting the client directly, have too as their ultimate goal, the maintenance and improvement of nursing practice. "Nurses direct their energies toward the promotion, maintenance and restoration of health, the prevention of illness, the alleviation of suffering and the ensuring of peaceful death when life can no longer be sustained."[**]

The nurse, by entering and maintaining a commitment to the profession, is committed to its professional ethics. As persons and as citizens nurses continue to be bound by the moral and legal norms shared by all other participants in society. In addition, nurses assume a professional commitment to health and the well-being of clients. Nursing as such encompasses moral activities.

The adoption of this Code represents a conscious undertaking on the part of the Canadian Nurses Association and its members to be responsible for upholding the following statements (values, standards, and limitations. This Code expresses and seeks to clarify those ethical principles that are definitive of ethical nursing activity. For those entering the profession, this Code identifies the basic moral commitments of nursing and may serve as a source for education and reflection. For those within the profession, the Code also serves as a basis for self-evaluation and for peer review. For those outside the profession, this Code may serve to establish expectations regarding the ethical conduct of nurses.

ETHICAL PROBLEMS AND DILEMMAS

Ethical **problems** fall into two distinct categories:
   a. Ethical **violations** involve the neglect of moral obligation; for example, a nurse who neglects to provide competent care to a client because of personal inconvenience has ethically failed the client.
   b. Ethical **dilemmas**, however, arise when ethical reasons both for and against a particular action are present. For example, a nurse whose client is likely to refuse

---
[*] Canadian Nurses Association, *A Definition of Nursing Practice, Standards for Nursing Practice*, Ottawa, Canadian Nurses Association, 1980, p. vi.

[**] As above, p. v.

some appropriate form of health care presents the nurse with an ethical dilemma. In this case, substantial moral reasons may be offered on behalf of several opposed options.

This Code provides clear direction with respect to the avoidance of ethical violations. When a course of action is mandated by the Code, and there exists no opposing ethical principle, ethical conduct requires that course of action.

This Code cannot serve the same function for all ethical dilemmas. There is room within the profession of nursing for conscientious disagreement among nurses. The resolution of a dilemma often depends upon the special factual circumstances of the case in question. Resolution may also depend upon the relative weight of the opposing principles, a matter about which reasonable people may disagree.

For dilemmas, no particular resolution may be definitive of good nursing practice. However, the Code constitutes an attempt to provide **guidance** for those nurses who face ethical dilemmas. A proper consideration of the Code may rule out some suggested resolutions of ethical dilemmas. For example, a nurse whose client is likely to refuse some form of appropriate health care, as was noted, presents the nurse with an ethical dilemma. Even so, it would be wrong for the nurse to engineer consent by deceiving the client about the nature of the care to be provided. (For example, see Value II, Standard 4.)

ELEMENTS OF THE CODE

This Code contains different elements designed to help the nurse in its interpretation. The values and standards are presented by topic and not in order of importance. There is variation in the normative (the nurse **should** or **ought to** or is **obliged to**) terminology used in the Code. These terms have been used interchangeably and no difference in moral force of the statements is intended. A number of distinctions between ethics and morals may be found in the literature. Since no distinction has been uniformly adopted by writers on ethics, these terms are used interchangeably in this Code as well.

— **Values** express broad ideals of nursing. They establish the correct directions for nursing. In the absence of a conflict of ethics, the fact that a particular action promotes a **value** of nursing may be decisive in some specific instances. Nursing behavior can always be appraised in terms of values: how closely did it approach the value, how widely did it deviate from it. Because they are so broad however, values may not give specific guidance in difficult instances.

— **Standards** are moral obligations that have their basis in nursing values. Standards provide more specific direction for conduct than do values, however; they spell out what a value requires under particular circumstances.

— **Limitations** describe exceptional circumstances in which a value or standard cannot receive its usual application. Limitations have been included separately to emphasize that, in the ordinary run of events, the values and standards will be decisive.

It is also important to emphasize that even when a value or standard must be limited, it nonetheless carries moral weight. For example, a nurse who is compelled to testify in a court of law regarding confidential matters is still subject to the values and standards of confidentiality. While the requirement to testify is a justified limitation upon confidentiality, in other respects confidentiality must be observed. The nurse must only reveal that confidential information which is pertinent to the case at hand and such revelation must take place within the appropriate context. The general obligation to preserve the client's confidences remains despite particular limiting circumstances.

RIGHTS AND OBLIGATIONS

Clients possess **rights**, both legal and moral. In general, the statements in this Code are cast in the form of the moral obligations of nurses rather than in terms of the rights of clients. Those legal and moral rights exist with or without professional acceptance. The obligations of nurses **exceed** that which would be required by the legal rights of clients and this Code tries to reflect that fact. (For example, see Value II, Standard 3.) In many instances it is beyond the power of nurses to **secure** the right of a client. A client's right to be treated in a dignified fashion must be reflected in the nurse's own behavior towards the client and in attempts to influence the actions of other members of the health care team. The task of this Code is to state clearly the moral obligations that are incumbent upon nurses.

Nurses too possess legal and moral rights, as persons and as nurses. It is beyond the scope of this Code to address the personal rights of nurses. To the extent that conditions of employment are essential to the establishment of ethical nursing, however, this Code must deal with that issue.

The satisfaction of some ethical responsibilities requires action taken by the nursing profession as a whole. The fourth section of the Code contains values and standards concerned with those collective responsibilities of nursing and are particularly addressed to professional associations. Ethical reflection must be an ongoing affair, and its facilitation is a continuing responsibility of the Canadian Nurses Association.

The body of the code is divided into sections that correspond to the sources of nursing obligations:

— **Clients**

— **Health Team**

— **The Social Context of Nursing**

— **Responsibilities of the Profession**

~ CLIENTS ~

I

A nurse is obliged to treat clients with respect for their individual needs and values.

Standards

1. Factors such as the client's race, religion, ethnic origin, social status, sex, age or health status may not be permitted to compromise the nurse's commitment to that client's care.

2. The expectations and normal life patterns of clients are acknowledged. Individualized programs of nursing care are designed to accommodate the psychological, social, cultural and spiritual needs of clients, as well as their biological needs.

3. The nurse does more than respond to the requests of clients, by accepting an affirmative obligation to aid clients in their expression of needs and values within the context of health care.

4. Recognizing the client's membership in a family and a community, the nurse, with the client's consent, attempts to facilitate the participation of significant others in the care of the client.

II

Based upon respect for clients and regard for their right to control their own care, nursing care should reflect respect for the the right of choice held by clients.

Standards

1. The competent client's consent is an essential precondition to the provision of health care. Nurses bear the primary responsibility to inform clients about the nursing care that is available to them.

2. Consent may be signified in many different ways. Verbal permission or knowledgeable cooperation are the usual forms in which clients consent to nursing care. In each case, however, a valid consent represents the free choice of the competent client to undergo that care which is to be provided.

3. Consent properly understood is the process by which a client becomes an active participant in care. All clients should be aided in becoming active participants in their care to the maximum extent that circumstances permit. Professional ethics may require of the nurse actions that exceed the legal requirements of consent. For example, although a child may be legally incompetent to consent, nurses should nevertheless attempt to inform and involve the child in treatment.

4. Force, coercion and manipulative tactics must not be employed in the obtaining of consent.

5. Illness or other factors may compromise the client's capacity for self direction. Nurses have a continuing obligation to value autonomy in such clients, for example, by creatively providing them with opportunities for choices, within their capabilities, thereby aiding them to maintain of regain come degree of autonomy.

6. Whenever information is provided to a client, this must be done on a truthful, understandable and sensitive way. It must proceed with an awareness of the individual client's needs, interests and values.

7. Nurses should respond freely to their client's requests for information and explanation when in possession of the knowledge required to respond accurately. When the questions of the client require information beyond that of the nurse, the client should be informed of that fact and referred to a more appropriate health care practitioner for a response.

III

The nurse is obliged to hold confidential all information regarding a client learned in the health care setting.

Standards

1. The rights of persons to control the amount of personal information that will be revealed applies with special force in the health care setting. It is, broadly speaking, up to clients to determine who shall be told of their condition, and in what detail.

2. In describing professional confidentiality to a client, its boundaries should be revealed:

a) Competent care requires that other members of a team of health personnel have access to be provided with the relevant details of a clients condition.

b) In addition, discussions of the client's care may be required for the purpose of teaching, research or quality assurance. In this case, special care must be taken to protect the client's anonymity.

Whenever possible, the client should be informed of these necessities at the onset of care.

3. An affirmative duty exists to institute and maintain practices that protect client confidentiality, for example, by limiting access to records.

Limitations

The nurse is not morally obligated to maintain confidentiality when the failure to disclose information will place the client or third parties in danger. Generally, legal requirements to disclose are morally justified by these same criteria. In facing such a situation, the first concern of the nurse must be the safety of the client or the third party.

Even when the nurse is confronted with the necessity to disclose, confidentiality should be preserved to the maximum possible extent. Both the amount of information disclosed and the number of people to whom disclosure is made should be restricted to the minimum necessary to prevent the feared harm.

IV

The nurse has an obligation to be guided by consideration for the dignity of clients.

Standards

1. Nursing care should be carried out with consideration for the personal modesty of clients.
2. A nurse's conduct at all times should acknowledge the client as a person. For example, discussion of care in the presence of the client should actively involve or include that client.
3. As ways of dealing with death and the dying process change, nursing is challenged to find new ways to preserve human values, autonomy and dignity. In assisting the dying client, measures must be taken to afford as much comfort, dignity and freedom from anxiety and pain as possible. Special consideration is given to the need of the client's family to cope with their loss.

V

The nurse is obligated to provide competent care to clients.

Standards

1. Nurses should engage in continuing education and in the upgrading of skills relevant to the practice setting.
2. In seeking or accepting employment, nurses should accurately state their areas of competence as well as limitations.
3. Nurses who are assigned to work outside of an area of present competence should seek to do that which, under the circumstances, is in the best interests of their clients. Supervisors or others should be informed of the situation at the earliest possible moment so that protective measures can be instituted. As a temporary measure, the safety and welfare of clients may be better served by the best efforts of the nurse under the circumstances than by no nursing care at all.
4. When called upon outside of an employment setting to provide emergency care, nurses fulfill their obligations by providing the best care that circumstances, experience and education permit.

Limitations

A nurse is not ethically obliged to provide requested care when compliance would involve a violation of her or his moral beliefs. When that request falls within recognized forms of health care, however, the client should be referred to a more appropriate health care practitioner. Nurses who have or are likely to encounter such situations are morally obligated to seek to arrange conditions of employment so that the care of clients is not jeopardized.

VI

The nurse is obliged to represent the ethics of nursing before colleagues and others.

Standards

    1. Nurses serving on committees concerned with health care or research should see their role as including the vigorous representation of nursing's professional ethics.
    2. Many public issues include health as a major component. Involvement in civic activities may afford the nurse the opportunity to further the objectives of nursing as well as to fulfill the duties of a citizen.

VII

The nurse is obliged to advocate the client's interest.

Standards

    1. Advocating the interests of the client includes assistance in achieving access to quality health care. For example, by providing information to clients privately or publicly, the nurse enables them to satisfy their rights to health care.
    2. When speaking to public issues or in court as a nurse, the public is owed the same duties of accurate and relevant information as are clients within the employment setting.

VIII

In all professional settings, including education, research and administration, the nurse retains a commitment to the welfare of clients. The nurse bears an obligation to act in such a fashion as will maintain trust in nurses and nursing.

Standards

    1. Nurses accepting professional employment must ascertain that conditions will permit provision of care consistent with the values and standards of the Code. Prospective employers should be informed of the provisions of the Code so that realistic and ethical expectations may be established at the beginning of the nurse-employer relationship.
    2. Accurate performance appraisal is required by a concern for present and future clients and is essential to the growth of nurses. Nurse administrators and educators are morally obligated to provide timely and accurate feedback to nurses, and their supervisors, student nurses and their teachers.
    3. Administrators bear special ethical responsibilities that flow from a concern for present and future clients. The nurse administrator seeks to ensure that the competencies of personnel are used efficiently. Working within available resources, the administrator seeks to ensure the welfare of clients. When competent care is threatened due to inadequate resources or for some other reason, the administrator acts to minimize the present danger and to prevent future harm.

4. An essential element of nursing education is the student client encounter. This encounter must be conducted in accordance with ethical nursing practices, with special attention to the dignity of the client. The nurse educator is obligated to ensure that nursing students are acquainted with and comply with the provisions of the Code.

5. Research is necessary to the development of the profession of nursing. Nurses should be acquainted with advances in research, so that established results may be incorporated into practice. The individual nurse's competencies and circumstances may also be used to engage in, or to assist and encourage research designed to enhance the health and welfare of clients.

The conduct of research must conform to ethical nursing practice. The self-direction of clients takes on added importance in this context. Further direction is provided in the Canadian Nurses Association publication entitled, *Ethical Guidelines for Nursing Research Involving Human Subjects*.

~ HEALTH TEAM ~

IX

Client care should represent a cooperative effort, drawing upon the expertise of nursing and other health professions. Acknowledging personal or professional limitations, the nurse recognizes the perspective and expertise of colleagues from other disciplines.

Standards

1. The nurse participates in the assessment, planning, implementation and evaluation of comprehensive programs of care for clients. The scope of a nurse's responsibility should be based upon education and experience, as well as legal considerations of licensure or registration.

2. The nurse accepts a responsibility to work with others through professional nurses' associations to secure quality care for clients.

X

The nurse, as a member of the health care team, is obliged to take steps to ensure that the client receives competent and ethical care.

Standards

1. The first consideration of the nurse who suspects incompetence or unethical conduct should be the welfare of present clients or potential harm to future clients. Subject to that principle, the following should be considered:

   a. The nurse is obligated to ascertain the facts of the situation in deciding upon the appropriate course of action.

   b. Institutional mechanisms for reporting incidents or risks of incompetent or unethical care should be followed.

   c. It is unethical for a nurse to participate in efforts to deceive of mislead clients regarding the cause of their injury.

d. Relationship in the health care team should not be disrupted unnecessarily. If a situation can be resolved without peril to present or future clients by direct discussion with the colleague suspected of providing incompetent or unethical care, that should be done.

2. The nurse who attempts to protect clients threatened by incompetent or unethical conduct may be placed in a difficult position. Colleagues and professional associations are morally obliged to support nurses who fulfill their ethical obligations under the Code.

3. Guidance concerning those activities that may be delegated by nurses to assistants and other heath care workers is found in legislation and policy statements. When functions are delegated, the nurse should be satisfied regarding the competence of those who will be fulfilling these functions. The nurse has a duty to provide continuing supervision in such a case.

~ THE SOCIAL CONTEXT OF NURSING ~

XI

Conditions of employment should contribute to client care and to the professional satisfaction of nurses. Nurses are obliged to work towards securing and maintaining conditions of employment that satisfy these connected goals.

Standards

1. In the final analysis, the improvement of conditions of nursing employment is often to the advantage of clients. Over the short term however, there is a danger that action directed towards this goal will work to the detriment of clients. Nurses bear an ethical responsibility to present as well as future clients and so the following principles should be noted:

a. The safety of clients should be the first concern in planning and implementing any job action.

b. Individuals and groups of nurses participating in job actions share this ethical commitment to the safety of clients. However, their responsibilities may lead them to express this commitment in different, but equally appropriate ways.

c. Clients whose safety requires ongoing of emergency nursing care are entitled to have those needs satisfied throughout the duration of any job action. Members of the public are entitled to know of the steps that have been taken to ensure the safety of clients.

d. Individuals and groups of nurses participating in job actions have a duty of coordination and communication to take steps reasonably designed to ensure the safety of clients.

~ RESPONSIBILITIES OF THE PROFESSION ~

XII

Professional nurses' organizations recognize responsibility to clarify, secure and sustain ethical nursing conduct. The fulfillment of these tasks requires that professional organizations remain responsive to the rights, needs and legitimate interests of clients and nurses.

Standards

1. Sustained communication and cooperation between the Canadian Nurses Association, provincial associations and other organizations of nurses, is an essential step towards securing ethical nursing conduct.

2. Professional nurses' associations must at all times accept responsibility for assuring quality care for clients.

3. Professional nurses' associations have a role in representing nursing interests and perspectives before non-nursing bodies, including legislatures, employers, the professional organizations of other health disciplines and the public media of communication.

4. Professional nurses' associations should provide and encourage organizational structures that facilitate ethical nursing conduct.

   a. Changing circumstances may call for reconsideration and adaptation of this Code. Supplementation of the code may be necessary in order to address special situations. Professional associations should consider the ethics of nursing on a regular and continuing basis and be prepared to provide assistance to those concerned with its implementation.

   b. Education in the ethical aspects on nursing should be available to nurses throughout their careers. Nurses' associations should actively support or develop structures designed towards this end.

~

Reprinted, with permission, from the *Code of Ethics for Nursing*, Canadian Nurses Association, March, 1991.

Index

____ v. *Child and Family Services*, 326, 309
abortion, 3, 6, 9, 18, 19, 22, 24, 29, 30, 100, 125, 202, 211, 239, 241, 242, 245, 262, 275-301, 308, 317, 337, 340ff., 344ff., 353, 360, 364
absolutistic, 21
abstinence, 364
act, 50, 97, 238, 244, 246f., 251, 255, 318, 321, 344
act, duty to, 59, 101, 113, 130, 267
act, failure to, 249, 252
act, supererogatory, 114
agapistic, 16, 17ff., 30ff., 41, 43
allocation, 33ff., 42, 72f., 83, 112f., 178, 205-230, 265, 369, 375
allocation committee, 276, 300
allocation, macro-, 205-213, 217, 227
allocation, meso-, 205, 217-221
allocation, micro-, 105, 220-223, 225f., 229
allocation, primary macro-, 214ff., 229
allocation, secondary macro-, 215f., 229f
allowing harm to occur, 100, 341, 347
allowing nature to take its course, 240
allowing to die, 3, 237, 239f., 242, 246, 247, 258, 262f., 273
amniocentesis, 207, 334, 337, 349
anencephalics, 283
anencephaly, 341
arbitration, binding, 70, 75
assent, 97, 108, 148, 156
assent and consent, 97
assent by children, 97
autonomous decision-making, 98. *See also* autonomy.
autonomy, 13, 24, 27, 32, 54-57, 65, 67ff., 82, 89, 95f., 102, 104, 117, 135, 171, 197, 211, 242, 255, 287, 292, 314f., 338ff., 350, 375. *See also* principle of autonomy, self-determination.
autonomy, level of, 156
autonomy, limitations on, 175, 339
autonomy of patient, 77, 81ff., 88, 93, 103, 105, 116f., 135f., 212
autonomy of physician, 67, 69, 82f., 212
autonomy of professional, 83
balance, 17, 22, 24, 81, 155, 162, 171, 214, 330, 340, 354, 360
balance, homeostatic, 191f., 200, 284. *See also* health.
balance of concerns, 65
balance of demands, 208
balance of good over harm, 87
balance of interests, 243. *See also* health care.

balance of quality, 147, 155
balance of rights, 18, 41, 196, 220, 265, 281, 287f., 292
balance of risks, 118, 162, 322
balance of values, 34
belief, fundamental, 19
belief, moral, 82
belief, private, 376
belief, religious, 29f., 162, 367
beliefs, 4, 9, 13, 30, 48, 69, 133, 148, 150, 337
beneficence, 13, 20, 27, 89, 106, 129, 195f. *See also* principle of beneficence.
Borowski v. Canada (Attorney General), 277, 297
brain dead, 265
brain death, 282
Bravery v. Bravery, 327
Canada Health Act, 75, 185, 212, 220, 231
Canadian Human Rights Act, 297, 328
Canadian Nurses Association, 2, 3, 6, 46, 76, 82, 259, 273
Canterbury v. Spence, 117, 137
categorical imperative, 25f., 42
Charter of Rights and Freedoms, 29f., 32, 41, 124, 187, 241, 248, 277, 304, 309
chorionic villi sampling, 335, 349
Christian Scientists, 13, 88, 148
code of ethics, 2, 3, 22, 25, 44, 45-54, 62, 63, 69, 71, 82, 88, 103, 104, 112, 182, 238ff., 245, 258, 262
coerced, 82, 325
coercion, 50, 94, 112, 126, 140, 172f., 333, 375
coercive, 124, 126, 315
competence, 63, 72, 73, 75, 85, 92-99, 107f., 115, 120, 124, 135, 159, 242, 319
competence, diminished, 91
competence, conceptual, 92-93
competence, cognitive, 91, 99, 122
competence, criteria of, 50f., 143f
competence, duration of, 97f
competence, emotional, 91, 94-96, 99
competence, inferential, 92
competence, mnemonic, 92
competence, standards of 65. *See also* competence, criteria of.
competence, valuational, 96f., 99, 108
competence, volitional, 91, 93f., 99, 122
competent patient, 25, 35, 59, 77, 88, 101f., 112f., 128, 131, 136, 140, 146, 157, 198
competent person, request of, 240-244, 260, 264, 267, 293, 319

INDEX

competent physician, *64f., 138*
competent, rights of, *198ff., 263, 266, 268, 293, 321ff*
compliance, *82, 94, 105*
comprehension, *97, 119*
comprehension, standards of, *111, 119.* See also understanding.
confidentiality, *55-63, 168*
confidentiality, duty of, *56f., 64f*
congenital abnormality, *293*
congenital condition, *331, 341, 371*
congenital defect, *202, 290, 342*
congenital disease, *356*
congenital malformation, *285*
congenitally defective, *262*
consent, *67, 88, 92, 97, 108, 111-149, 156, 304, 318, 363.* See also assent.
consent, competent, *55, 120, 161, 290*
consent, entailed, *135f*
consent, implied, *313*
consent in experiments, *160-165, 167f., 170f., 181, 183*
consent, informed, *42, 55ff., 73, 82, 88, 101, 102, 104, 105, 106, 111-149, 157, 160-161, 165, 167, 171, 174, 177, 179, 180, 239, 258, 262, 290, 319, 338, 375*
consent, obtain, *120-123*
consent, process, *122f*
consent, proxy, *108, 156, 158, 159, 173, 181, 313*
consent, surrogate, *159, 173.* See also proxy.
consent to death, *238, 244, 319*
consent to sterilization, *304, 314.* See also proxy)
contraception, *13, 308, 315, 317, 353, 364*
convention, *12, 35f., 85, 145, 267, 357.* See also rules.
cost, *22, 24, 59, 74, 155, 206f., 209f., 212f., 217, 228, 265, 293, 330ff., 335f., 363*
cost/benefit, *21, 31, 212, 223, 231*
cost/effectiveness, *21, 31, 212, 220, 223, 228, 232, 366*
Criminal Code of Canada, *238, 239, 241, 248, 268, 273, 276f., 290, 293*
death, *281ff., 285.* See also person, personhood.
death, deliberate, *237-244, 247, 249, 252f., 258ff., 264, 291, 319, 344*
death, fear of, *25*
death, painless, *246, 262*
death wish, *239, 247, 258, 263f*
deception, *134f., 163, 169ff., 244*
decisive, *133f., 163, 170f., 181*
Declaration of Human Rights, 302, 304
Declaration on Euthanasia, 270
Declaration on Procured Abortion, 301, 350
defective, *311, 332, 334f., 337, 342, 344, 348, 356*
defective genes, *332, 363ff*
defective newborn, *3, 241, 262, 342f*
deontological, *41, 89, 106, 158*
deontological approach to ethics, *16-19, 25ff., 31f., 34, 39, 41*
deontological argument, *29*
deontological ethics, *57, 59, 237, 262*
deontological framework, *263, 291, 293*
deontological perspective, *25, 32, 34f., 40, 53, 58, 88, 102, 214, 340, 358, 376*
deontological pluralism, *26*
deontological principle, *26, 32*
deontological theory, *25, 27, 29, 44*
determination, causal, *250-253, 263*
determination of death, *283*

dignity, *170, 262f., 356, 359, 365, 369, 373*
disciplinary committee, *62, 74, 75*
disclosure, *40, 57, 82, 86, 90, 138, 140, 142, 162f., 182, 351*
disclosure, duty of, *119, 128-131*
disclosure, full, *115*
disclosure, guidelines for, *167*
disclosure, objective reasonable person standard, *119*
disclosure, professional standard of, *115*
disclosure, standards of, *111, 115-119, 128-131*
disclosure, subjective standard of, *117*
discrimination, *5, 8, 143, 205, 212, 216, 222, 224, 227, 230, 235, 241, 279, 321, 323, 335, 344, 346, 363f., 366, 371*
disease, *13, 184, 186f., 190, 192*
disease, genetic, *331, 338ff., 344ff., 356, 369, 371*
donation, organ, *146, 232, 378*
double effect, principle of, *272, 298, 300*
double-blind placebo study, *164*
duty, *13, 27, 35, 55, 61, 87, 113, 115, 196-200, 246, 258, 303, 307*
duty of disclosure, *114, 116, 119, 130f*
duty of nurse, *334, 362*
duty of physicians, *62ff., 66, 70, 74, 79, 81, 85, 99, 101f., 114, 129f., 137, 147, 158, 162, 178, 241*
duty to patients, *21, 56, 58f., 70f., 258, 263f., 277, 294, 314*
duty to prevent harm, *342.* See also good Samaritan.
duty, to treat, *5, 194f., 264f*
Eberhardy, Matter of, 153
egoism, ethical, *20ff*
egoistic, *39f*
embryo, *293, 300, 327, 330, 345, 354, 360, 364, 368, 374*
embryo, spare, *360*
emergency, *69, 105, 114, 170*
emergency, argument from, *100ff*
emergency context, *56, 59, 64, 67f., 69, 74, 85, 101, 121, 140, 144, 179*
emergency, doctrine of, *101, 105, 136, 145*
emergency funds, *210*
emergency health care, *29*
emergency, nature of, *101f*
emergency powers, *109*
emotions, *1f., 5, 14, 94f., 99, 192, 340, 376*
enticement, *161, 172, 174ff* See also reward.
ethical absolutism, *1*
ethics committee, *74, 168, 180, 260, 266, 288*
ethical emotivism, *1, 3-6, 14f*
ethical principles, *1-4, 8f., 12f., 15, 17, 20ff., 25, 29, 31, 35, 37, 38, 47, 52, 53, 62, 68, 86, 118, 255, 286, 316, 357*
ethical relativism, *1, 3, 4, 6, 7-9*
ethics review board, *161, 168, 176, 178, 372*
ethos, *44, 45, 47, 48-50, 71, 213, 357, 359f*
euthanasia, *237-274, 348*
euthanasia, active, *237f., 240f., 246-249*
euthanasia, arguments against, *259-262*
euthanasia, arguments for, *262ff*
euthanasia, direct vs. indirect, *253-255*
euthanasia, meaning of, *243f*
euthanasia, passive, *237, 246-249, 266*
euthanasia, voluntary vs. non-voluntary, *267f*
experiment, *279, 364.* See also experimentation.
experimental, *108, 134, 360*
experimental context, *183*
experiment, double-blind, *244*

experimental failure, *356*
experimental protocol, *356*
experimental technique, *339*
experimental therapy, *230. See also* innovative procedure.
experimentation, *60, 104, 108, 119, 140, 159, 183, 219, 286, 297, 347, 355, 357, 361, 368, 379*
experimenting with human subjects, *160-183, 356*
experiments, guidelines for, *159. See also* experimentation; Medical Research Council of Canada.
expertise, *51ff., 56, 79, 83, 85, 99, 109*
expertise, fallacy of, *47, 56, 83, 116, 144*
expertise, implications of, *59*
expertise in ethics, *56, 182*
expertise of nurses, *121*
expertise of physicians, *83, 116f*
expertise, role of, *1, 51*
expertise, technical, *47, 52, 78-81, 100, 144*
family, *31, 140, 145, 148, 150, 156, 244, 260, 263, 302, 307, 322, 355-359*
Federation of Medical Women of Canada, *280*
fetal, *288f., 294*
fiduciary model of physician/patient relationship, *81ff., 85, 100, 103, 121, 135f*
fiduciary nature of medicine, *89, 114, 137*
fiduciary relationship, *30, 34, 78, 81ff., 102, 105, 122, 147*
fiduciary role of physician, *101, 146*
gatekeeper, physician as, *263f., 278*
genetic code, *191, 331, 353, 364ff., 373*
genetic defect, *335f., 340, 356. See also* defective genes.
Geneva, Declaration of, *46*
good, aimed at, *340*
good effect, *259*
good, maximize the, *20*
good of others, *87*
good of patient, *20f., 129*
good of professional, *20f*
good of society, *170*
good, promote the, *27*
good, the, *21f., 40, 42, 365*
greatest happiness principle, *42*
Hall Report, *185, 212, 235*
Halushka v. The University of Saskatchewan, *162, 179, 183*
harm, *26, 32, 86f., 90, 100, 116, 129ff., 138, 155, 167, 169f., 173, 199, 248, 281, 318, 320, 324, 342, 347, 359*
health, *54f., 184-194*
health care, access to, *60f., 66*
health care, right to, *70, 78, 143ff., 184f., 194-200, 205-208, 211, 214, 228, 235f., 265, 310, 343, 363*
health potential, *54*
hedonistic, *20, 22, 24, 39f., 108*
Helsinki, Declaration of, *76, 182, 364, 381*
Hippocratic Oath, *238, 258*
Hopp v. Lepp, *32, 140*
humility, value of, *355*
In the Matter of Stephen Dawson, *152, 158*
incompetence, *62, 64, 95, 143, 155*
incompetent and experimentation, *160, 172f*
incompetent child, *146, 151*
incompetent, cognitively, *92, 99, 172*
incompetent, congenitally, *109, 144, 151ff., 155, 199, 242, 267, 313, 334*
incompetence, degree of, *97, 156f*

incompetent, emotionally, *94f., 97, 99*
incompetent, ethically, *14*
incompetent, inferentially, *93*
incompetent, mnemonically, *93*
incompetent patient, *56f., 65, 91, 98ff., 109, 114, 136, 141ff., 147, 151, 157, 172, 266*
incompetent person, *65, 98, 143f., 146, 149-153, 155ff., 160, 172f., 198-200, 241f., 267, 293, 302, 313, 321f., 323, 329*
incompetent, rights of, *149, 156, 158, 198ff., 241, 268, 293, 321-*
incompetent, valuationally, *94-97, 99*
324
incompetent, volitionally, *94.See also* compliance.
institution, *66, 68f., 73, 108, 124f., 168, 171, 211, 289, 303, 322*
institutional framework, *94*
institutionalization, *125*
institutionalized association, *51*
institutionalized conditions, *69*
institutionalized context, *58, 90f., 93, 121, 171*
institutionalized person, *161*
institutionalized setting, *58, 120, 124, 166*
Jehovah's Witnesses, *13, 18, 88, 97, 101, 140, 142*
Kelly v. Hazlett, *115, 137*
killing, *2, 8, 248f, 276, 344*
killing, deliberate, *18, 360*
killing patients, *2f., 238, 247, 254*
Lalonde Report, *185, 212, 235*
Law Reform Commission of Canada, *246, 248, 273, 280, 315, 319, 323, 328, 361*
Law Reform Commission of Ontario, *328, 352, 374, 377, 384*
Law Reform Commission of Saskatchewan, *377*
living will, *108, 141, 144, 147ff., 260, 265-267*
Malette v. Shulman, *32, 73, 101, 106, 109, 137, 140, 158, 179, 240*
malfeasance, *62*
Manitoba Human Rights Code, *304*
Matter of C.P. Little, *101, 109*
maxim, *20, 25f., 33, 51, 63, 318*
means, end justifies the, *31, 71*
means, extraordinary, *237, 243, 246*
means, heroic, *18*
means, ordinary, *237, 243, 246*
means to an end, *17, 25f., 256, 258f., 264, 278, 308*
Medical Research Council of Canada, *119, 156, 165, 168f., 175, 361, 365, 371*
mercy-killing, *238, 240, 243, 272. See also* euthanasia.
merit, *27, 217, 337*
meta-ethics, *1f., 6*
Milgram experiment, *181*
monopoly, medicine as, *45, 59-62, 64f., 69f., 74, 114, 264, 292*
Montreal brainwashing experiment, *177f*
Morgentaler v. The Queen, *32, 241, 269, 276ff., 290, 300*
Mulloy v. HopSang, *32, 42, 87f., 105, 106, 137, 162, 240, 244, 250f., 269*
NCBHR, *382*
needs, *3, 58, 61, 80, 196, 213-218, 220, 224, 226, 310, 376*
needs, auto-induced, *225f*
needs, hetero-induced, *225*
negligence, *116, 342f*
non-maleficence, principle of, *27, 89, 177. See also* principle of non-malfeasance.